I0066563

Advanced Dental Biomaterials

Advanced Dental Biomaterials

Edited by Gerard Keith

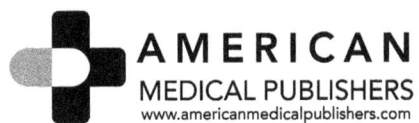

AMERICAN
MEDICAL PUBLISHERS
www.americanmedicalpublishers.com

American Medical Publishers,
41 Flatbush Avenue,
1st Floor, New York,
NY 11217, USA

Visit us on the World Wide Web at:
www.americanmedicalpublishers.com

© American Medical Publishers, 2022

This book contains information obtained from authentic and highly regarded sources. Copyright for all individual chapters remain with the respective authors as indicated. All chapters are published with permission under the Creative Commons Attribution License or equivalent. A wide variety of references are listed. Permission and sources are indicated; for detailed attributions, please refer to the permissions page and list of contributors. Reasonable efforts have been made to publish reliable data and information, but the authors, editors and publisher cannot assume any responsibility for the validity of all materials or the consequences of their use.

ISBN: 978-1-63927-049-1

Trademark Notice: Registered trademark of products or corporate names are used only for explanation and identification without intent to infringe.

Cataloging-in-Publication Data

Advanced dental biomaterials / edited by Gerard Keith.
p. cm.
Includes bibliographical references and index.
ISBN 978-1-63927-049-1
1. Dental materials. 2. Biomedical materials. 3. Dental clinics--Guidebooks. I. Keith, Gerard.
RK652.5 .D46 2022
617.695--dc23

Table of Contents

Preface

This book has been a concerted effort by a group of academicians, researchers and scientists, who have contributed their research works for the realization of the book. This book has materialized in the wake of emerging advancements and innovations in this field. Therefore, the need of the hour was to compile all the required researches and disseminate the knowledge to a broad spectrum of people comprising of students, researchers and specialists of the field.

A substance that is created to interact with biological systems for a medical purpose is known as biomaterials. It can be used for therapeutic or a diagnostic medical purpose. Biomaterials are derived from nature and are even synthesized in the laboratory with the help of various chemical methods such as utilizing metallic components, ceramics, composite material and polymers. Since biomaterials are used for medical applications, they comprise a whole or a part of a living structure which performs, augments and replaces a natural function. Dental biomaterials are specially invented materials, invented for the use in dentistry. They are majorly used in dental implants. There are many different types of dental materials, such as temporary dressings, dental restorations, endodontic materials, impression materials, prosthetic materials, etc. The characteristics of these materials differ according to their planned purposes. This book covers in detail some existent theories and innovative concepts revolving around dental biomaterials. It presents researches and studies performed by experts across the globe. This book will prove to be immensely beneficial to students and researchers in this field.

At the end of the preface, I would like to thank the authors for their brilliant chapters and the publisher for guiding us all-through the making of the book till its final stage. Also, I would like to thank my family for providing the support and encouragement throughout my academic career and research projects.

Editor

Impacted Mandibular Third Molar, Associated Pathoses, and their Relation to Angulation and Impaction Depth: A Cone Beam CT Study

Movahhedian N[a]; Shahidi Sh[b*]; Jozari S[c]; Mosharaf A[d]; Naderi A[e]

[a]Assistant Professor, Department of Oral and Maxillofacial Radiology, Faculty of Dentistry, Shiraz University of Medial Science, Shiraz, Iran
[b]Professor, Department of Oral and Maxillofacial Radiology, Biomaterials Research Center, School of Dentistry, Shiraz University of Medical Sciences, Shiraz, Iran
[c]Undergraduate Student, Student Research Committee, School of Dentistry, Shiraz University of Medical Sciences, Shiraz, Iran
[d]postgraduate student of oral and maxillofacial Surgery, Department of Oral and Maxillofacial Surgery, school of dentistry, Shiraz University of Medical Sciences, Shiraz, Iran
[e]postgraduate student of oral and maxillofacial radiology, Department of Oral and Maxillofacial Radiology, school of dentistry, Shiraz University of Medical Sciences, Shiraz, Iran

ARTICLE INFO

Key words:
Impacted mandibular third molar
Cone beam computed tomography (CBCT)
External root resorption
Caries
Follicular space

Corresponding Author:
Shoaleh Shahidi
Professor, Department of Oral and Maxillofacial Radiology, Biomaterials Research Center, School of Dentistry, Shiraz University of Medical Sciences, Shiraz, Iran
Email: shoalehshahidi@yahoo.com

Abstract

Statement of problem: prophylactic removal of the impacted lower third molar (ILTM) is controversial and accompanying pathologic conditions play an important role.

Objectives: The aim of the present study is to evaluate the prevalence of commonly found pathoses associated with ILTM in relation to angulation and impaction depth in cone beam computed tomography (CBCT).

Materials and Methods: We evaluated CBCT of 500 ILTMs from 235 females (57%) and 177 males (43%) for the presence of caries on the second and third molars, external root resorption (ERR) of the second molar, and follicular spaces (FS) >5 mm in diameter in relation to angulation and impaction depth according to Pell and Gregory and Winter's classifications, respectively.

Results: We observed that 55.6% of ILTM had at least one detectible lesion. ERR was the most frequent pathologic condition (31.2%), followed by caries on the second (26%) and third (13.4%) molars, and FS >5 mm (2.4%). ERR was the only pathology influenced by angulation. There was significantly more ERR in mesioangular ILTMs (40.5%, P<0.001). Most ERR occurred in direct contact with the third molar. Class C showed a lower risk for second and third molar caries (P<0.001), but higher risk for ERR (P=0.008) and FS >5 mm (P=0.035). There were more caries on the second molar (P=0.013) and FS >5 mm (P<0.001) in class III.

Conclusions: Prophylactic removal of ILTMs (especially in mesioangular or horizontal impactions) could be suggested considering the potential for pathologic changes in ILTMs and the propensity for these teeth to cause ERR in second molars.

Introduction

Tooth impaction is defined as the condition in which a tooth fails to erupt into its normal position after root completion due to pathological or developmental factors such as jaw size, eruption pattern, and any barrier to the eruption path [1]. In a survey, researchers have reported that 28.3% of the population had at least one impacted tooth, 82.5% of which was the mandibular third molar [2].The decision regarding prophylactic removal or retention of the impacted third molar has been a challenging and controversial subject for dental professionals [3-6] and accompanying pathologic conditions play an important role in this decision. While some of these impacted lower third molars (ILTMs) may remain with no pathologic or clinical complications, others may develop pathologic conditions that include infection, external root resorption (ERR) or caries of the adjacent teeth, and cystic/tumoral transformation of the follicle [3,7,8]. Radiographs are necessary to evaluate impacted teeth. Compared to conventional techniques, three-dimensional imaging modalities such as computed tomography (CT) and cone beam CT (CBCT) provide more information to analyze impacted teeth, which would not be available otherwise. Additionally, because of less effective radiation dosage, the relatively lower cost, and fewer artifacts, CBCT has proven to be the technique of choice for evaluation of impacted teeth and related pathologic conditions [9-11]. Most data that pertain to the pathos of ILTM is available through panoramic studies [3,7,12-14]. This modality has a number of shortcomings that include lack of detail, distortion, superimposition, and projection errors, which in turn reduces its validity [12].

The objective of this study is to assess the prevalence of the most common pathoses associated with ILTMs that include caries on the second and third molars, ERR of the second molar, and follicular spaces (FS) >5 mm in diameter in relation to their impaction depth and angulation by means of CBCT images. The results of this study may help dental professionals with the risk assessment of removal or retention of an ILTM.

Materials and Methods

In this retrospective cross-sectional study, we analyzed 500 ILTMs from 412 patients. These patients had preoperative radiologic examinations of their third molars over a two-year time frame (February 2014 to February 2016) in a private oral and maxillofacial radiology clinic in Shiraz, Iran. The Ethics and Research Committee of Shiraz University of Medical Sciences approved the study protocol (# 03-9504). All CBCT images were obtained with a NewTom VGi (Quantitative Radiology, Verona, Italy) CBCT unit that operated at 90 kVp and 6 mA with an exposure time of 10 seconds, and voxel size set for 0.3 mm in a 15×15 field of view. The images were evaluated with NNT viewer software (version 4.6, NewTom, Verona, Italy) in all three orthogonal planes (axial, coronal, and sagittal) by two oral and maxillofacial radiologists with consensus. In instances where it was difficult for the two radiologists to reach an agreement, a third expert reviewed the images. The parameters evaluated in the present study were caries on the distal surface of the mandibular second molar, caries of the mandibular third molar, FS of more than 5 mm in diameter around the third molar, and ERR of the second molar (Figure 1). Different degrees of resorption from a mild blunting of the root curvature to resorption that invaded the pulpal structure were considered as the stages of root resorption.The lower third molar impaction depths in relation to the ramus and occlusal plane have been determined according to the Pell and Gregory classification [15], as follows. Class I: the third molar is completely anterior to the anterior border of the ramus; class II: up to half of the third molar crown is covered by the ramus; class III: more than half of the third molar crown is covered by the ramus. Moreover, Class A: the third molar occlusal plane is at the same level or above the second molar occlusal plane; class B: the third molar occlusal plane is between the cervical line and occlusal plane of the second molar; and class C: the third molar is below the cervical line of the second molar.We used the Winter classification [16] to determine the ILTM inclination according to which the angle between the longitudinal axis of the ILTM to the occlusal plane defined the inclination, as follows: 0-30: horizontal; 31-60: mesioangular; 61-90: vertical; and >90: distoangular.This study excluded subjects

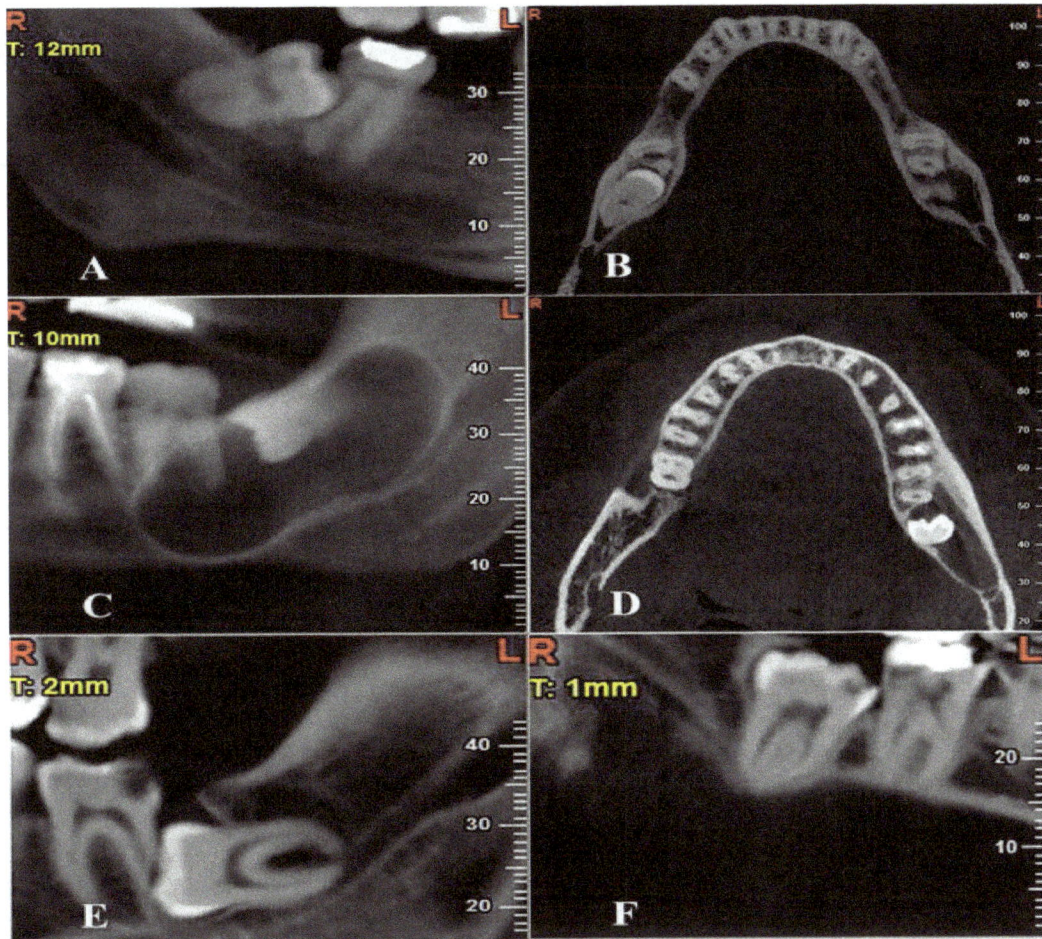

Figure 1: (A, B) External root resorption (ERR) in the sagittal and axial planes. (C, D) Enlarged follicular space (FS) in the sagittal and axial planes. (E) Caries on the second molar. (F) Caries on the third molar

with gross carious lesions, extensive restoration in the second molar, third molars simultaneously in classes I and A, or root development of less than two thirds.

Statistical analysis

We used the chi-square test to assess the relationship between variables. SPSS version 18.0 (SPSS Inc., Chicago, IL, USA) was applied for statistical analysis. $P<0.05$ was considered statistically significant.

Results

The sample for this study consisted of 500 ILTMs from 412 CBCT images of which there were 235 (57%) females and 177 (43%) males. Most cases (51.4%, 257 teeth) were in a mesioangular position, followed by vertical (27.2%, 136 teeth), horizontal (18.4%, 92 teeth), and distoangular (3%, 15 teeth)

positions. Class A comprised 6.4% of the ILTMs, followed by 56.0% for class B, and 37.6% for class C. The impaction depth in the images of the samples were 23.6% (class I), 54.4% (class II), and 22% (class III). Among the evaluated pathologic conditions, ERR of the second molar was the most frequent with a prevalence of 31.2%, followed by caries on the second (26%) and third (13.4%) molars, and FS >5 mm in diameter (2.4%). By taking into consideration the results, we concluded that 222 (44.4%) cases did not have any of the evaluated pathologies and 278 (55.6%) had at least one detectible lesion. Table 1 shows the distribution of evaluated pathologies according to angulation. The only pathologic factor influenced by the angulation of the teeth was ERR ($P<0.001$), which was significantly more prevalent in mesioangular ILTMs (40.5%). The occurrence of caries and FS were not significantly related to ILTM angulation (Table 1). Only one out of 12 enlarged FS was

Table 1: Frequency of pathologic findings in terms of the angulation of the third molar

Type	ILTM(n)	Caries on second molar	Caries on third molar	ERR	FS >5 mm
Mesioangular	257	75(29.2%)	39(15.2%)	104(40.5%)	3(1.2%)
Vertical	136	31(22.8%)	17(12.5%)	17(12.5%)	4(3.0%)
Distoangular	15	3(20%)	1(6.7%)	1(6.7%)	0(0.0%)
Horizontal	92	21(22.8%)	10(10.9%)	34(37.0%)	5(5.4%)
P-value*		0.417	0.602	<0.001	0.115

*Chi-square test (base on Monte-Carlo method)
ILTM = Impacted mandibular third molar, ERR = external root resorption, FS= Follicular space

associated with a horizontally impacted third molar and caused ERR on the second molar. Analysis of the relationship between pathologic conditions and impaction status showed that class C had a lower risk for caries on the second and third molars (both P<0.001). However, as Table 2 shows, we observed an increasing risk for ERR (P=0.008) and FS >5 mm (P=0.035) gradually from class A to class C. Table 2 also shows that class III had significantly more caries on the second molar (P=0.013) and FS

Table 2: Frequencies of pathologic findings in terms of impaction status

Type	ILTM(n)	Caries on second molar	Caries on third molar	ERR	FS >5 mm
Class A	32(6.4%)	11(34.4%)	7(21.9%)	3(9.3%)	0(0.0%)
Class B	280(56.0%)	105(37.5%)	55(19.6%)	84(30.0%)	2(0.7%)
Class C	188(37.6%)	14(7.4%)	3(1.6%)	68(36.2%)	8(4.2%)
P-value*		<0.001	<0.001	0.008	0.035
Class I	118(23.6%)	38(32.2%)	18(15.2%)	32(27.1%)	1(0.8%)
Class II	272(54.4%)	74(27.2%)	41(15.1%)	86(31.6%)	1(0.3%)
Class III	110(22.0%)	17(15.4%)	7(6.3%)	38(34.5%)	8(7.2%)
P-value*		0.013	0.054	0.474	<0.001

*Chi-square test (base on Monte-Carlo method)
ILTM= Impacted mandibular third molar, ERR = external root resorption, FS=Follicular space

>5 mm (P<0.001).

Discussion

The decision to prophylactically remove or retain an ILTM is a matter of great debate with divergent opinions among professionals [3-6]. The complications following extraction of the impacted third molar have tremendous influence on this debate [3]. Oral surgeons should weight the benefits of removing a third molar against the risks. While there is no documented evidence for prophylactic surgery of an asymptomatic third molar, some researches have rejected this idea. However, there is strong indication for removal of the third molar in cases with accompanied pathologic changes [12,17]. In support, the American Association of Oral and Maxillofacial Surgeons (AAOMS) have provided a guideline for the extraction of third molars according to associated lesions [18]. AAOMS has also advocated new studies that concern the evaluation of pathologic conditions accompanied with third molars [12]. Two-dimensional characteristics, as well as the lack of sufficient details, distortion, and potential errors make it difficult for panoramic radiography to detect lesions as precisely as CBCT [8,12,17,19,20]. CBCT allows for the examination of a subject free from overlapping structures in all three orthogonal planes with higher spatial resolution [21]. Studies that examined the ability of panoramic and CBCT radiography to diagnose ERR [22,23] and proximal and occlusal caries [24,25] have confirmed the favorable position of CBCT over panoramic radiography. Oenning et al. [8] reported an agreement of only 4.3% between CBCT and panoramic radiography in ERR detection. They recommended CBCT for its evaluation. Another study by Alqerban et al. [23] had similar results in the ERR of incisor teeth. The higher prevalence of ERR in the present study (31.2%) compared to panoramic studies supported this fact. Similar studies reported incidents for ERR that ranged from 0.3% [7] to 1.4% [13]. Although the overall prevalence of ERR in this study was 31.2%, there were significantly higher incidents of third molars that had mesioangular (40.5%) and horizontal (37%) inclinations. The results of the present study were closer a study by Oenning

et al. that reported 49.43% ERR associated with mesioangular ILTM on CBCT [12]. Other studies supported the results of this study regarding the higher frequency of ERR in mesially inclined third molars [8,12]. These findings could be related to the eruptive forces of mesially inclined impacted third molars and probability of more contact area with second molars. However, the relationship between impaction depth and ERR has been inconsistently reported in the literature. Our findings revealed a significant tendency of class C (36.2%) and B (30%) impactions for ERR, while Wang et al. [17] reported more ERR in class A and C, and Oenning et al. [12] showed a higher frequency of ERR in class A and B impactions. This discrepancy, as well as lower frequencies of ERR reported in other CBCT studies [8,17], could be due to differences in study inclusion criteria, sample size, definition of ERR and its complicating resemblances to proximal caries, particularly in partially erupted third molars. According to the current study data, 26% of second molars and 13.4% of third molars showed carious lesions; distal caries of the second molars were the most common pathos evaluated in the present study after ERR. Al-Khateeb et al. [7] reported similar findings regarding the prevalence of caries on the third molar (13.6%). Our findings of distal caries on the second molar were higher than some studies that reported frequencies of 7.9% [7], 12.6% [3], and 17.2% [26]. Our findings were similar to those reported by Ozec et al. (20%) [27]. However, several studies reported higher frequencies of 42% [28] and 52% [24]. The results of this study revealed higher frequencies of impaction depth in class A and B. This finding supported previous studies [3, 24,26], which found classes A and B more afflicted with distal caries on the second molar. This variation in findings must be due to a number of factors. First, the aforementioned studies, except for one [24], used less precise two-dimensional modalities compared to CBCT [19,20]. This frequency could be affected by oral hygiene as well as the eruption status of the third molar. We excluded cases with multiple restorations or carious lesions to minimize the effect of oral hygiene. Hence, the distal caries of the second molar could be related to the third molar position more so than the potentially higher risk for caries. However, it is not accurate to place the blame completely on the status of the third molars. In terms of the enlarged FS, the results of this study showed a relatively low frequency of 2.4%. Chu et al. [2] Guven et al. [29] and Patil et al. [30] reported the incidence of cystic/tumoral transformation of the FS to be as low as 1%, 3.1%, and 3.4%, respectively. These findings supported reports by other studies on cyst formation around an impacted third molar [29,31]. However, these studies were not exactly comparable to this study, due to the use of panoramic radiography and the different criteria used to define the enlargement. In the present study, we have defined the pathologic FS, according to White et al. [32] as an area radiographically larger than 5 mm in diameter. Others defined it as 2, 2.5, or 4 mm in diameter or utilized pathological evaluation as the criteria. Dentigerous or follicular cysts, compared to other cystic lesions, have more potential for ERR on adjacent teeth. Therefore, it is expected that FS size may be a defining factor and possibly have a direct effect on the extent of ERR of the adjacent teeth. However, the present study did not support this expectation. The results of the current study revealed that almost none of the enlarged FS, except for one, had an association with ERR on the adjacent second molar. This finding suggested that ERR mostly occurred by direct contact of the second and third molars rather than through the enlargement of dental follicle. This result reinforced the findings of Ericson et al. [33] which concluded that the ERR of maxillary incisors was most probably due to direct contact with canine in its eruption course rather than the dental follicle. To the extent of our knowledge, the present study used the largest sample size and variety of conditions evaluated among CBCT studies of the pathoses associated with the third molar. However, since the cases were selected from the CBCT images taken for pre-surgical evaluation, it might not be an ideal representation of the entire population. In addition, we did not assume the length of impaction period as a factor, which might cause some bias in the results of pathoses associated with impaction. We suggest that additional studies should be conducted to consider these factors.

Conclusions

Due to the prevalence of pathoses related to

ILTMs and high potential for inducing ERR in the second molars; we encourage dental professionals to consider prophylactic removal of these teeth, especially those with mesioangular or horizontal impactions.

Acknowledgments

The authors thank the Vice-Chancellery of Research, Shiraz University of Medical Sciences, for supporting this research (Grant# 9504). This manuscript has been extracted from the DDS Thesis of Dr. Sadegh Jozari, which was conducted under the supervision of Dr. Najmeh Movahhedian and the advisory of Dr. Shoaleh Shahidi. The authors would like to express their gratitude to Dr. Mehrdad Vossoughi of the Center for Research Improvement of the School of Dentistry for the statistical analysis and Ms. Marziyeh Setayesh for improving the use of English in this paper.

Conflict of Interest: None declared

Refrences

1. Tamimi D, ElSaid K. Cone beam computed tomography in the assessment of dental impactions. Seminars in Orthodontics 2009; 15:57-62.

2. Chu FC, Li TK, Lui VK, et al. Prevalence of impacted teeth and associated pathologies-a radiographic study of the Hong Kong Chinese population. Hong Kong Med J. 2003; 9:158-163.

3. Polat HB, Özan F, Kara Is, et al. Prevalence of commonly found pathoses associated with mandibular impacted third molars based on panoramic radiographs in Turkish population. Oral Surg Oral Med Oral Pathol Oral Radiol Endod. 2008; 105:41-47.

4. Richards D. Management of unerupted and impacted third molar teeth. A National Clinical Guideline. Evidence-Based Dentistry. 2000; 2:44-46.

5. Dodson TB. Surveillance as a management strategy for retained third molars: Is it desirable? J Oral Maxillofac Surg. 2012;70:20-24.

6. Mettes TG, Nienhuijs ME, van der Sanden WJ, et al. Interventions for treating asymptomatic impacted wisdom teeth in adolescents and adults. Cochrane Database Syst Rev. 2005; 18:CD003879

7. Al-Khateeb TH, Bataineh AB. Pathology associated with impacted mandibular third molars in a group of Jordanians. J Oral Maxillofac Surg. 2006; 64:1598-1602.

8. Oenning AC, Neves FS, Alencar PN, et al. External root resorption of the second molar associated with third molar impaction: comparison of panoramic radiography and cone beam computed tomography. J Oral Maxillofac Surg. 2014; 72:1444-1455.

9. Haney E, Gansky SA, Lee JS, et al. Comparative analysis of traditional radiographs and cone-beam computed tomography volumetric images in the diagnosis and treatment planning of maxillary impacted canines. Am J Orthod Dentofacial Orthop. 2010;137:590-597.

10. Pauwels R, Beinsberger J, Collaert B, et al. Effective dose range for dental cone beam computed tomography scanners. Eur J Radiol. 2012; 81:267-271.

11. Miracle AC, Mukherji SK. Conebeam CT of the head and neck, part 1: physical principles. AJNR Am J Neuroradiol. 2009; 30:1088-1095.

12. Oenning AC, Melo SL, Groppo FC, et al. Mesial Inclination of Impacted Third Molars and Its Propensity to Stimulate External Root Resorption in Second Molars—A Cone-Beam Computed Tomographic Evaluation. J Oral Maxillofac Surg. 2015;73:379-386.

13. Akarslan ZZ, Kocabay C. Assessment of the associated symptoms, pathologies, positions and angulations of bilateral occurring mandibular third molars: Is there any similarity? Oral Surg Oral Med Oral Pathol Oral Radiol Endod. 2009;108:26-32.

14. Zamiri B, Shahidi SH, Shoeleh S. Assessment of Anatomical Relationship between Impacted Lower Third Molar Tooth and Mandibular Canal in Panoramic View of Men and Women between Ages 20-70 Years Old. J Dent (Shiraz). 2003;4:29-38.

15. Pell GJ, Gregory B. Impacted mandibular third molars: classification and modified techniques for removal. Dent Digest 1933; 39:330-338.

16. Winter GB. Principles of exodontia as applied to the impacted mandibular third molar: a complete treatise on the operative technic with clinical diagnoses and radiographic interpretations. American medical book company; 1926.

17. Wang D, He X, Wang Y, et al. External root resorption of the second molar associated with mesially and horizontally impacted mandibular third molar: evidence from cone beam computed tomography. Clin Oral Investig. 2017;21:1335-1342.

18. The Management of Impacted Third Molar Teeth [Internet]. Illinois: American Association of Oral and Maxillofacial Surgeons. c 2017. Available from: https://www.aaoms.org/docs/practice_resources/clinical_resources/impacted_third_molars.pdf

19. Charuakkra A, Prapayasatok S, Janhom A, et al. Diagnostic performance of cone-beam computed tomography on detection of mechanically-created artificial secondary caries. Imaging Sci Dent. 2011;41 :143-150.

20. Kayipmaz S, Sezgin ÖS, Saricaoğlu ST, et al. An in vitro comparison of diagnostic abilities of conventional radiography, storage phosphor, and cone beam computed tomography to determine occlusal and approximal caries. Eur J Radiol. 2011; 80:478-482.

21. Shahidi S, Zamiri B, Bronoosh P. Comparison of panoramic radiography with cone beam CT in predicting the relationship of the mandibular third molar roots to the alveolar canal. Imaging Sci Dent. 2013; 43:105-109.

22. Alqerban A, Jacobs R, Souza PC, et al. In-vitro comparison of 2 cone-beam computed tomography systems and panoramic imaging for detecting simulated canine impaction-induced external root resorption in maxillary lateral incisors. Am J Orthod Dentofacial Orthop. 2009;136:764. e1-11.

23. Alqerban A, Jacobs R, Fieuws S, et al. Comparison of two cone beam computed tomographic systems versus panoramic imaging for localization of impacted maxillary canines and detection of root resorption. Eur J Orthod. 2011; 33:93-102.

24. Kang F, Huang C, Sah MK, et al. Effect of Eruption Status of the Mandibular Third Molar

on Distal Caries in the Adjacent Second Molar. J Oral Maxillofac Surg. 2016; 74:684-692.

25. Tyndall DA, Rathore S. Cone-beam CT diagnostic applications: caries, periodontal bone assessment, and endodontic applications. Dent Clin North Am. 2008; 52 :825-841.

26. Chang SW, Shin SY, Kum KY, et al. Correlation study between distal caries in the mandibular second molar and the eruption status of the mandibular third molar in the Korean population. Oral Surg Oral Med Oral Pathol Oral Radiol Endod. 2009; 108:838-843.

27. Ozeç I, Hergüner Siso S, Taşdemir U, et al. Prevalence and factors affecting the formation of second molar distal caries in a Turkish population. Int J Oral Maxillofac Surg. 2009; 38:1279-1282.

28. Allen RT, Witherow H, Collyer J, et al. The mesioangular third molar–to extract or not to extract? Analysis of 776 consecutive third molars. Br Dent J . 2009; 206:E23.

29. Güven O, KeskIn A, Akal ÜK. The incidence of cysts and tumors around impacted third molars. Int J Oral Maxillofac Surg. 2000; 29:131-135.

30. Patil S, Halgatti V, Khandelwal S, et al. Prevalence of cysts and tumors around the retained and unerupted third molars in the Indian population. J Oral Biol Craniofac Res. 2014; 4:82-87.

31. Lysell L, Rohlin M. A study of indications used for removal of the mandibular third molar. Int J Oral Maxillofac Surg. 1988; 17:161-164.

32. White SC, Pharoah MJ. Oral radiology: principles and interpretation(7nd edn): Elsevier Health Sciences 2014:696.

33. Ericson S, Bjerklin K, Falahat B. Does the canine dental follicle cause resorption of permanent incisor roots? A computed tomographic study of erupting maxillary canines. Angle orthod. 2002; 72:95-104.

2

An In vitro Analysis of the Effects of Iron Sulfate and Iron Acetate on *Streptococcus mutans*

Lavaee Fª; Ghapanchi Jᵇ; Motamedifar Mᶜ*; Sorourian Sᵈ

ª Assistant Professor, Oral and Dental Disease Research Center, School of Dentistry, Shiraz University of Medical Sciences, Shiraz, Iran
ᵇ Associate Professor, Oral and Maxillofacial Medicine Department, School of Dentistry, Shiraz University of Medical Sciences, Shiraz, Iran
ᶜ Professor, HIV/AIDS Research Center, Institute of Health, Shiraz University of Medical Sciences, Shiraz, Iran & Department of Bacteriology and Virology, School of Medicine, Shiraz University of Medical Sciences, Shiraz, Iran
ᵈ Undergraduate Student, Student Research Committee, School of Dentistry, Shiraz University of Medical Sciences, Shiraz, Iran

---

ARTICLE INFO

Key words:
Iron sulfate
Iron acetate
Streptococcus mutans

Corresponding Author:
Mohammad Motamedifar
Professor, HIV/AIDS
Research Center, Institute of
Health, Shiraz University of
Medical Sciences, Shiraz,
Iran & Department of
Bacteriology and Virology,
School of Medicine, Shiraz
University of Medical
Sciences, Shiraz, Iran
Email: motamedm@sums.
ac.ir

Abstract

Statement of problem: Dental caries is a common infectious disease induced by *Streptococcus mutans (S. mutans)*.

Objectives: Due to the high incidence rate of dental caries and iron deficiency in the Iranian population, we have conducted this study to analyze the effects of iron acetate and iron sulfate on controlling the growth of *S. mutans*.

Materials and Methods: In this in vitro study, we evaluated the antibacterial effects of iron sulfate and iron acetate on *S. mutans* by the disk diffusion method, minimum inhibitory concentration (MIC), and minimum bactericidal concentration (MBC). The results were compared to those for 0.2% chlorhexidine and penicillin as the controls.

Results: Iron sulfate had higher MIC and MBC values compared to penicillin and chlorhexidine (P<0.001). Iron acetate MIC and MBC values did not significantly differ with penicillin and chlorhexidine. The iron sulfate inhibition zones at the 25 and 50 µg/mL doses were more than those of iron acetate.

Conclusions: Iron sulfate and iron acetate solutions can inhibit the growth of *S. mutans*. Hence, different compounds that contain iron salts such as toothpastes, mouth washes, and food supplements can be produced to prevent dental caries and iron deficiency.

Introduction

Dental caries is a common infectious disease that results from mineralized tissue dissolution by cariogenic bacteria. *Streptococcus mutans (S. mutans)* is a common cariogenic bacterium [1]. This gram positive, non-mobile, anaerobic bacterium can produce acid and ferment food remnants, which result in teeth structure demineralization [1]. This bacterium attaches itself to the tooth's surface with its outer cell polysaccharide [2,3]. The iron concentration in people's saliva depends on their diet and physiologic lactoferrin levels. According to previous studies, iron appears to affect the aggregation and attachment of bacteria to the tooth's surface; hence, iron can impact the development or prevention of dental caries [4-7]. Dunning *et al.* discovered the anti-caries effects of the iron ion [8]. In 2001, Devulaplle *et al.* concluded that iron ions inhibit glycosyltransferase enzyme (GTF) produced by *S. mutans* [9]. There are different methods to prevent dental caries such as oral hygiene, dental floss, fluoride gels, fissure sealants, and mouthwashes [10]. In recent years, evaluation of antibacterial effects of different ions has been proposed as new complimentary and substitute methods to prevent caries. This study aims to analyze iron acetate and iron sulfate on *S. mutans* growth in vitro.

Materials and Methods

We prepared a standard strain of *S. mutans* (ATCC 35668, PTCC 1683), obtained from the Iranian Organization for Science and Technology, Tehran, Iran. We prepared iron sulfate (Sigma Chemical Co.) and iron acetate (Sigma Chemical Co.) solutions at concentrations of 6.25, 12.5, 25, and 50 µg/mL. The prepared concentrations were sterilized by autoclave. In order to determine the antimicrobial effect of iron sulfate and iron acetate on *S. mutans*, we used the disk diffusion technique [11]. A bacterial suspension of *S. mutans* was adjusted to 0.5 McFarland turbidity (1.5x108cfu/mL) in normal saline, after which it was cultured in blood agar for 24 hours. The bacterial suspension was applied with a sterile cotton swab on Muller Hinton agar (MHA, Merck, Germany) with 5% sheep blood. Then, 20 µL of either the iron sulfate concentration or iron acetate were applied to sterile,

air-dried paper disks (Padtan Teb, Iran). The positive controls were 10 unit penicillin disks (Mast, UK) and dried plain paper disks that contained 20 µL of 0.2% chlorhexidine. We incubated the plates at 37°C for 24 hours and subsequently measured the inhibition zones in millimeters. The broth dilution method was used to determine the minimum inhibitory concentration (MIC) and minimum bactericidal concentration (MBC) of iron sulfate and iron acetate. We added 100 µL of brain heart infusion broth (BHI, Hi-Media, India) to each well of 96-well microtiter plates. Then, 100 µL of the stock solutions were added to the wells in sequential order (final concentrations: 4.8-250 µg/mL). The well that only contained BHI medium was the negative control. The positive control wells were penicillin and 0.2% chlorhexidine, and a well that contained BHI and bacterial suspension. The microwell plates were incubated at 37°C in a 5% $CO2$ incubator for 24 hours. The first well that inhibited bacterial growth was considered to be the MIC. We also cultured 10 µL of the well contents without any bacterial growth on blood agar to evaluate the MBC. The plates were incubated for 24 hours at 37°C in a 5% $CO2$ incubator. The least concentration that did not show any *S. mutans* colony formation on the agar was considered to be the MBC. These evaluations were rendered twice with a one-week interval. SPSS™ software, version 18.0 (IBM Corp., Armonk, NY, USA) was used for statistical analysis. Non-parametric Kruskal-Wallis and Mann Whitney tests were used to compare different groups. $P<0.05$ was considered statistically significant.

Results

We used the disk diffusion method to determine the inhibitory ability of the studied solution on *S. mutans* growth. There was no inhibition zone observed at the 6.25 µg/mL concentration of iron sulfate and at 12.5 µg/mL of iron acetate. At 25 µg/mL of iron sulfate, the inhibition zone (7.07±5 mm) did not statistically differ from the inhibition zone for iron acetate (7.87±5.5 mm; $P>0.05$). However, the inhibition zone for 50 µg/mL iron sulfate (15±4.24 mm) was more than the inhibition zone for iron acetate (11.31±8 mm). This finding showed a more potent inhibitory effect of iron sulfate ($P<0.05$) at that concentration. The 0.2% chlorhexidine solution (control) had an inhibitory zone of 16.5 mm, which was significantly higher than the iron sulfate and iron acetate groups (P<0.05). Table 1 shows the mean MIC and MBC of the studied salt solutions in comparison with penicillin and 0.2% chlorhexidine. We observed a significantly greater MIC of iron sulfate (P<0.001), which indicated that iron sulfate had less antibacterial properties compared to iron acetate, penicillin, and 0.2% chlorhexidine. This finding showed the anti-S. mutans activity of this salt relative to penicillin and 0.2% chlorhexidine. The 0.2% chlorhexidine had a statistically higher MIC than penicillin (P=0.009). Iron sulfate had a significantly higher MBC compared to the other groups (P<0.001). According to the MIC and MBC results, iron sulfate showed the lowest inhibitory effect. Iron acetate had a more comparable inhibitory effect on S. mutans. Penicillin MBC was significantly higher compared to 0.2% chlorhexidine (P=0.009; Table 1).

Table 1: Mean MIC and MBC of the studied salt solutions in comparison with penicillin and chlorhexidine

Groups	MIC (µg/mL)	MBC (µg/mL)
Iron sulfate	586	1172
Iron acetate	108	234.4
Penicillin	1.3	2.7
Chlorhexidine	0.95	1.95

MIC= Minimum inhibitory concentration
MBC= Minimum bactericidal concentration

Discussion

In this study, we evaluated the antibacterial effects of different concentrations of iron sulfate and iron acetate. Iron sulfate inhibited S. mutans at higher concentrations compared to iron acetate. However, the inhibition zones for iron sulfate and iron acetate solutions were approximately the same. These salts have shown no significant differences in comparison with 0.2% chlorhexidine and penicillin, as the controls. In the disc diffusion method, one of the effective factors for production of an inhibitory zone

is diffusion of salt solutions in the agar. Hence, it seems that the decreased solubility of iron acetate in saline and lack of its proper diffusion in agar could be the reason for the smaller zone of inhibition. The findings of this study were similar to previous studies that reported the inhibitory effect of iron salts on S. mutans growth. However, those studies were conducted under different conditions and different concentrations. Berlutti et al. reported that a concentration of $Fe3+$ lower than 0.1 µM caused aggregation and proliferation of S. mutans. Concentrations higher than 1 µM showed no effect [6]. These findings confirmed our results with $Fe2+$; however, Berlutti et al. have tested the effects of $Fe3+$ salts on bovine teeth. We believe that the results of this study might be more accurate. Unlike $Fe3+$, $Fe2+$ is not harmful for humans and does not change to $Fe3+$. In addition, vitamin C can be prescribed along with $Fe2+$ion [12]. A study conducted by Dunnin et al. has shown that 10 mM of $Fe2+$ was more effective than $Fe3+$ and had bactericidal effects at a pH of 7-8 [8].Our results supported the findings of an in vitro study conducted by Al Shalan et al., in which they observed the effect of 4 iron supplements on dental carries. The process of demineralization and cavity induction on teeth was observed during 60 days under in vitro conditions. With the exception of ferrous, all other supplements that contained iron ion had significant inhibitory effects on cariogenesis [13]. A study by Alves KM. et al in 2011 reported that ferrous sulfate decreased demineralization, but did not allow re-mineralization [14]. Eskandari et al. also confirmed that ferrous sulfate supplements could not cause enamel demineralization [15]. Another study revealed that an iron solution could decrease enamel surface microhardness and wear in the dentin; hence, loss of dental structure could be controlled by rinsing the mouth with the iron solution, especially after erosive trauma [16]. Pecharki et al. showed that iron ion reduced the sucrose potential of cariogenesis by decreasing the population of S. mutans in dental biofilm [17]. Ribeiro et al. in a study on the anticariogenesis mechanism of iron ion, reached the conclusion that iron, like chlorhexidine and sodium fluoride, decreased demineralization of the enamel. This effect was achieved by reducing the bacterial population rather than inhibition of glucosyltransferase enzyme [18]. In order to eliminate the confounding factors, the present experiment was repeated 3 times with

2 different iron salts. These studies evaluated the effects of iron ion on demineralization, cariogenesis, enamel, and dentin surface microhardness. We could not compare those results with the details of the present study methodology. The previous studies reported inhibition of cariogenesis by the effects of different aspects of the cariogenesis processes.There are several prescriptions to reduce the oral microbial count that have both positive points and adverse effects. Chlorhexidine mouthwash has a wide range of antibacterial properties. It is prescribed to decrease the level of oral bacteria, especially before and after oral surgery, and for periodontal diseases. The adverse effects of this product, as with other oral hygiene products, include teeth discoloration and dental stain accumulation. It can also cause severe hypersensitivity reactions. If swallowed, chlorhexidine can cause stomach inflammation, bradycardia, cyanosis, and ultimately liver damage. Chlorhexidine gluconate is not prescribed for children under the age of 18. This product can affect taste for up to 4 hours after use [19-21]. On the other hand, the use of antibiotics for an extended period can cause antibacterial resistance; thus, it seems to be of benefit to investigate new antimicrobial agents [2,3]. In the present study, we did not have access to pure chlorhexidine powder. Thus, we used the mouthwash as a replacement, which could justify its lower MIC and MBC in comparison to chlorhexidine. Another limitation was the use of citric acid as the solvent due to the low solubility of iron acetate in water. The use of this acid might affect the antibacterial effects of this salt. The authors suggest that additional experiments should be conducted on other, more water soluble iron salts, or in combination with other salts that do not have antagonistic effects at different concentrations, or on other cariogenic bacteria. Finally, this study should be conducted as an in vivo experiment.

Conclusions

In this in vitro study, iron sulfate and iron acetate inhibited the growth of *S. mutans* as a dental cariogenic bacterium. Although the antibacterial effects of the iron salts were lower than chlorhexidine, we suggest an in vivo study to determine the effects of these solutions. Several products that contain iron salts, such as toothpastes, mouthwashes, and food supplements can be developed in order to take advantage of the antibacterial properties of the iron salts.

Acknowledgments

The authors would like to express their appreciation to the Vice-Chancellor of Shiraz University of Medical Sciences for supporting this research (grant # 8794120). This manuscript is based on the thesis written by Dr. Sahar Sorourian. The authors also thank Dr. Mehrdad Vosough of the Center for Research Improvement of the School of Dentistry for assistance with the statistical analysis. The authors wish to thank Mr. H. Argasi at the Research Consultation Center (RCC) at Shiraz University of Medical Sciences for his invaluable assistance in editing this manuscript.

Conflict of Interest: None declared.

References

1. Pitts NB, Zero DT, Marsh PD, *et al.* Dental caries. Nature reviews Disease primers. 2017;3:17030.
2. Ghapanchi J, Lavaee F, Moattari A, *et al.* The antibacterial effect of four mouthwashes against Streptococcus mutans and Escherichia coli. J Pak Med Assoc. 2015;65:350-3.
3. Ghapanchi J, Bazargani A, Zariean A, *et al.* Evaluation of the Anti-Streptococcus mutans Potential of Petroselinum crispum, an in vitro Study. European Journal of Medicinal Plants.2016;15:1-8.
4. Rezazadeh F, Bazargani A, Roozbeh-Shahroodi J, *et al.* Comparison of oral Lactobacillus and Streptococcus mutans between diabetic dialysis patients with non-diabetic dialysis patients and healthy people. J Renal Inj Prev.2016;5:148-152.
5. Lavaee F, Faez K , Faez K , *et al.* Antimicrobial and antibiofilm activity of silver, titanium dioxide and iron nano particles. Am J Dent. 2016;29:315-20.
6. Berlutti F, Ajello M, Bosso P, *et al.* Both lactoferrin and iron influence aggregation and biofilm formation in Streptococcus mutans. Biometals . 2004;17:271-8.
7. Shumi W, Lim J, Nam SW, *et al.* Fluorescence imaging of the spatial distribution of ferric ions over biofilms formed by Streptococcus mutans under microfluidic conditions. Biochip J.

2009;3:119-24.

8. Dunning JC, Ma Y, Marquis RE. Anaerobic killing of oral streptococci by reduced, transition metal cations.Appl Environ microbiol. 1998;64:27-33.

9. Devulapalle KS, Mooser G. Glucosyltransferase inactivation reduces dental caries. J Dent Res. 2001;80:466-9.

10. Moshaveri nia M, Golfeshan F, Sabzghabaie M. Evaluation of the relationship between the secretion of ABO blood groups antigens in saliva and DMFS caries index. Sadra medical sciences journal. 2013; 1; 253-64.

11. Motamedifar M, Khosropanah H, Dabiri S. Antimicrobial Activity of Peganum Harmala L. on Streptococcus mutans Compared to 0.2% Chlorhexidine. J Dent (Shiraz). 2016;17:213-218.

12. Albokordi M, MahmodianA, EstehghaghiR, et al. Study of the Effect of Simultaneous Iron, Zinc and Folic Acid Supplementation With or Without Vitamin A and C on Hemoglobin Levels of Teenaged Girl Students in Shahinshahr City. Journal of Medical Science University of ShahisSadoghi. 2007;16:14-23.

13. Al-Shalan TA. In vitro cariostatic effects of various iron supplements on the initiation of dental caries. Saudi Dent J. 2009;21:117-22.

14. Alves KM, Franco KS, Sassaki KT, et al. Effect of iron on enamel demineralization and remineralization in vitro. Arch Oral Biol. 2011;56:1192-1198.

15. Eskndari T, Motamedi far M, Hekmat far S, et al. The effect of three iron drop on the hardness of primary teeth in cariogenic circumstance. Journal of Dental Faculty of ShahidBeheshti Medica Science University. 2011;30:275-82.

16. Sales-Peres SH, Pessan JP, Buzalaf MA. Effect of an iron mouthrinse on enamel and dentine erosion subjected or not to abrasion: an in situ/ex vivo study. Arch Oral Biol. 2007;52:128-32.

17. Pecharki GD, Cury JA, PaesLeme AF, et al. Efect of Sucrose Containing Iron(II) on Dental Biofilm and Enamel Demineralization in situ. Caries Res .2005; 39:123-9.

18. Ribeiro CC, Ccahuana-Vásquez RA, Carmo CD. et al. The effect of iron on Streptococcus mutans biofilm and on enamel demineralization. Braz Oral Res. 2012;26:300-5 .

19. Kaur P, Singh H, Khatri A, et al. Evaluation and comparison of short term side effects of 0.2% and 0.12%. chlorhexidine mouthwash. JAMDSR. 2015;3:26-28.

20. Poorshahidi S, Davarmanesh M, Rezazadeh F, et al. In vitro inhibitory effects of Chlorhexidine and Persica mouthwashes on HSV-1 compared with acyclovir. J Isfahan Dent Sch. 2011;7:59-67.

21. Pourshahidi S, Rezazadeh F, Motamedifar M, et al. In Vitro Comparative Study on Antiherpetic Effect of Chlorhexidine and Persica Mouthwashes with Acyclovir. J Basic Applied Scien. 2012;8:286-90.

3

In vitro Investigation of Hydro-alcoholic Extract of Helichrysum leucocephalum on the Inhibition of *Streptococcus mutans* Growth

Motamedifar M[a*]; Nozari A[b]; Azhdari Ghasrodashti E[c]

[a]Department of Bacteriology, Shiraz Medical School & Shiraz HIV/AIDS Research Center, Institute of Health, Shiraz University of Medical Sciences, Shiraz, Iran
[b]Department of Pediatric Dentistry, School of Dentistry, Shiraz University of Medical Sciences, Shiraz, Iran
[c]Student Research Committee, School of Dentistry, Shiraz University of Medical Sciences, Shiraz, Iran

ARTICLE INFO

Key words:
Antimicrobial
Helichrysum leucocephalum
Streptococcus mutans

Corresponding Author:
Mohammad Motamedifar
Department of Bacteriology,
Shiraz Medical School,
Shiraz University of Medical
Sciences, Shiraz, Iran.
Email: motamedm@sums.ac.ir

Abstract

Statement of Problem: Indiscriminate use of antibacterial agents increases the antibiotic resistance, which consequently necessitates seeking alternatives such as herbal remedies.

Objectives: The aim of this study was to evaluate the antimicrobial effect of hydroalcoholic extract of *Helichrysum leucocephalum* (*H.leucocephalum*) on *Streptococcus mutans* (*S. mutans*) growth as a major cause of dental caries.

Materials and Methods: In this study, hydroalcoholic extract of *H. leucocephalum* was prepared. The antibacterial effects, minimal inhibitory concentration (MIC), and minimal bactericidal concentration (MBC) of hydroalcoholic extract of *H. leucocephalum* and penicillin were assessed. Agar well diffusion method and micro broth dilution assay were used on bacterial suspension adjusted to a 0.5 McFarland standard (equivalent to 1.5×10^8 CFU/mL).Each test was repeated four times to minimize lab errors.

Results: In this study, the inhibitory zone of hydroalcoholic extract of *H.leucocephalum* in concentration of 100 mg/mL was 34±0.1 mm and for penicillin was 10 mm. The MIC and MBC of *H.leucocephalum* hydroalcoholic extract were 5.6±6.25, 21.6±6.25 mg/mL, respectively.

Conclusions: Hydroalcoholic extract of *H. leucocephalum* have antibacterial effect on *S.mutans* at a concentration of 12.5mg/mL, indicating possible application of this extract in prevention of dental caries; however, future researches are necessary.

Introduction

Dental caries or tooth decay is one of the most important infective diseases of people in the world with multifactorial etiology. A wide group mixture of microorganisms including *S.mutans* has a great role in dental caries [1].

S.mutans is recognized to be a highly cariogenic microorganism in humans [2]. It is gram-positive cocci and encapsulated bacterium that adheres to the enamel surface and produces different glucans and acidificate dental plaque. The presence of these glucans is critical in the development of dental caries [3]. One approach to decrease the incidence of dental caries is to develop therapeutic agents with antimicrobial and/or anti adherent properties to inhibit the bacterial proliferation on the tooth surface.

The rising use for herbal drugs have so far directed the consideration of pharmaceutical scientists towards medicinal plants as traditional sources of drugs for the treatment of different diseases [4]. Among various families of plants studied, the genus *Helichrysum* of *Asteraceae* family deserves some noticeable interests. It is one of the largest genera in the family *Asteraceae* includes around 600 species [5,6]. *Helichrysum* is known as the "immortal, everlasting flower". The distribution of 19 species in Iran, growing on the mountainous area with clay soil, calcareous rocks, dry slopes and steppe areas is reported [7]. The *Helichrysum* oil inhibits microbial growth and protects the body against a long list of febrile microbial infections. *Helichrysum leucocephalum (H. leucocephalum)*, one of the six endemic species of the country is the subject of this study. *Helichrysum* species have been so far demonstrated to have diverse therapeutic properties such as hepato-protective, anti-allergic, antichlorotic, anti-diarrheal and antidiabetic effects. These remarkable properties in *Helichrysum* species is attributed to the presence of flavonoids as their principal constituents [8]. This plant is also used in folk medicine for the treatment of kidney stone and gall bladder disorders [9]. Various studies clearly indicated antidiabetic, antioxidant, anti-lipid peroxidation and antimicrobial effect of other *Helichrysum* species; however, there is not any published report on anti-microbial effect of *H. leucocephalum* on

S. mutans [10,11].The aim of this study was to evaluate the antimicrobial effect of hydroalcoholic extract of *H. leucocephalum* on *S.mutans* growth as a major pathogen of dental caries.

Materials and Methods

This experimental study was done in Department of Bacteriology and Virology of Shiraz University of Medical Sciences, Shiraz, Iran. Standard strain of *S. mutans* (ATCC 35668) was purchased from Iranian Research Organization for Science and Technology, Tehran, Iran.

Different parts of *H. leucocephalum* were collected from areas around Shiraz, Fars province, Iran, 2017. Herbal number of the plant was proved and a voucher number (PM937) was received from Shiraz school of pharmacy. All parts of the plant were dried at room temperature for 2 weeks. Then were ground into a fine powder. Hydroalcoholic extract was processed by percolation (about 72h). The plant powder (200g) was extracted with hydroalcoholic solution (70% and 96%, 500mL) using a percolator. The extract was concentrated in rotary evaporator to separate alcoholic part and then, it was kept in refrigerator until used [12].

Agar well diffusion technique was used to assess the antimicrobial effect of hydroalcoholic extract of *H.leucocephalum* on *S. mutans* growth. First, *S. mutans* was cultured in blood agar for 24 hours. Then, a bacterial suspension with 0.5 McFarland turbidity (1.5×10^8 cfu/mL) was adjusted in brain heart infusion (BHI) broth (Merck, Germany). By using a sterile cotton swab, the bacterial suspension was applied on Muller Hinton agar (MHA, Merck, Germany) with 5% blood sheep. The holes were prepared by using Cork borer in MHA (6mm in diameter and 4mm in height with 25mm distance). Each well was filled by 100μL of different concentrations of hydroalcoholic extract of *H.leucocephalum* (3.125-50 mg/mL). One hole was filled with 10U/ml of penicillin as positive control. The plates were incubated at 37°C in 5% incubator for 24 hours. Finally, inhibition zones were measured in millimeter [13]. To determine the minimum inhibitory concentration (MIC) and minimum bactericidal concentration (MBC) of hydroalcoholic extract of *H.leucocephalum*, micro broth dilution method was used. First, 100μL of

BHI were added to each well of 96-well micro plates. Then, 100µL of highest concentration of extract (100 mg/mL) was added to the first well. Other wells were filled with two fold lower concentrations until the seventh well, respectively (3.125-50 mg/mL). One well contained just BHI medium as negative control and one of the wells contained BHI and bacterial suspension as the control with bacterium. The plates were incubated at 37°C in 5% CO2 incubator for 24 hours. The first well in those series that showed no sign of visible growth of bacteria was considered as MIC. The MBC was determined by culturing 10µL of contents of wells that did not show any sign of bacterial growth on blood agar. The plates were incubated for 24 hours at 37°C in 5% CO2 incubator. The least concentration that inhibited colony forming of *S. mutans* on agar was considered as MBC. All data were expressed as descriptive data by SPSS (mean and standard deviation) [14].

Results

The anti-bacterial effects of (3.125-50 mg/mL) concentrations of hydroalcoholic extract of *H.leucocephalum* and penicillin as a control group were tested by using well diffusion agar technique.

The results of this study showed that 100 mg/mL concentration of extract, which created zones with the mean diameter of 34±0.1 mm, had the highest antibacterial effect on *S. mutans* compared to other concentrations. The mean inhibition zones for 50 mg/mL were 21±0.10 mm and the lower concentrations could not inhibit the growth of *S.mutans*. The mean diameter of zones created by penicillin was 10 mm (Table 1).

MIC of the extract on *S. mutans* was 15.6±6.25

mg/mL and MBC was 21.6±6.25 mg/mL. MIC and MBC for penicillin were detected both 5 U/mL.

Discussion

There is a considerable interest in many kinds of plant essential and extracts as the antibiotic alternatives. The results of this study showed that *H.leucocephalum* extract could inhibit the growth of *S.mutans* as the most important microorganism involved in dental caries. Various medicinal and antimicrobial properties of this plant were studied in many investigations. Preliminary research evidenced bactericidal activity of *H. leucocephalum* extracts, as also reported that antimicrobial screening revealed higher degree of inhibition for essential oil of the aerial parts of *H. leucocephalum* against *Staphylococcus aureus* and *Escherichia coli* both with MIC value of 16µg/mL [15]. In the *Helichrysum compactum* species, the antimicrobial activity has been attributed to flavonoids and chemically related compound [16]. The data obtained in the present study on the specific activity of *H.leucocephalum* extracts against *S.mutans* are in agreement with the results previously reported for *Helichrysum italicum* by Nostro *et al.* [17] . Another in vivo study has shown that a regular daily rinsing with mouthwash containing *Helichrysum litoreum* ethanol extract could reduce on 50% of subjects the salivary levels of *S.mutans*, which are the most virulent cariogenic pathogens in the oral cavity [18]. Antioxidant activities have been previously detected in another *H. pseudoplicatum* Nab [19].

The antibacterial activity of *Helichrysum* phenolics including coumarates, benzofurans, pyrones, and heterodimeric phloroglucinols was evaluated in a

Table 1: The effect of hydroalcoholic extract of *H.leucocephalum* on *S. mutans* by agarwell diffusion method

Extract Concentration (mg/mL)	Inhibition zone Mean± Standard deviation (mm)
100	34 ± 0.1
50	21± 0.10
25	0
Penicillin (10 U/mL)	10

study showed potent antibacterial effect against multidrug-resistant *Staphylococcus aureus* isolates [20]. The essential oil of *H. arenarium* had a significant anti-yeast activity (P<0.05); therefore, it can be used as an antifungal agent in the food and pharmaceutical industries [21]. Using the same method (micro broth dilution) as the current study, the essential oil of *Helichrysum aureonitens* in South Africa indicated antimicrobial activity against gram positive and gram negative bacteria with MICs in the range of 2.500–0.039 mg /mL [22]. The results of another study indicated that the extract of *H. plicatum* had significant antimicrobial activity [23]. Inhibition potential of *H. buddleioides* extract was indicated on gram positive bacteria such as *Staphylococcus aureus* [24].

Concentrations of 100 and 50 mg/mL of the extract made inhibition zones of bacterial growth around the wells while other concentrations could not create inhibition zone. As evidenced, the hydroalcoholic extract of *H. leucocephalum* exhibits significant antimicrobial activity against *S.mutans* and therefore could be considered as a source of natural antimicrobial compounds, but studies are necessary.

Conclusions

The results of antibacterial assays in the current study might be helpful in developing useful products for inhibiting the progress of dental caries and pharmaceutical purposes. However, future researches are necessary.

Acknowledgments

The authors thank the vice-chancellery of Research Shiraz University of Medical Sciences, for supporting the research. Also the authors thank Dr Mehrdad Vosough from the Dental Research Development Center for the statistical analysis. This paper is extracted from a thesis by Dr. Elmira Azhdari Ghasrodashti.

Conflict of Interest: None declared.

References

1. Nishikawara F, Katsumura S, Ando A, *et al*. Correlation of cariogenic bacteria and dental caries in adults. Journal of Oral Science, 2006;48:245–51.

2. Loesche WJ, Syed SA. The predominant cultivable flora of carious plaque and carious dentine.Caries Research.1973;7:201–16.

3. Forssten SD, Björklund M, Ouwehand AC. Streptococcus mutans, caries and simulation models. Nutrients. 2010; 2: 290-298.

4. García AM, González LR, Rocha GN, *et al*. Mesquite Leaves (Prosopis laevigata), a natural resource with antioxidant capacity and cardioprotection potential. Ind Crops Prod. 2013; 44:336-42.

5. Albayrak S, Aksoy A, Sagdic O, et al. Phenolic compounds and antioxidant and antimicrobial properties of Helichrysum species collected from Eastern Anatolia. Turkey. Turk J Biol. 2010; 34:463-73.

6. Georgiadou E, Rechinger KH. Helichrysum in: Rechinger K.H. (ed.) Flora Iranica No. 1980 ;145:51-72.

7. Rajaei P, Mozaffarian V. A new species of Helichrysum (Asteraceae, Gnaphalieae) from Iran. Iran J Bot. 2016; 22:8-10.

8. Suzgec S, Mericli AH, Houghton PJ, *et al*. Flavonoids of Helichrysum compactum and Their Antioxidant and Antibacterial Activity. Fitoterapia. 2005; 76:269-72.

9. Erhan Eroglu H, Budak U, Hamzaoglu E, *et al*. In vitro Cytotoxic Effects of methanol extracts of six Helichrysum Taxa used in traditional medicine. Pak J Bot. 2010; 42:3229-37.

10. Czinner E, Hagymasi K, Blázovics A, *et al*. The in vitro Effect of Helichrysi flos on Microsomal Lipid Peroxidation. J Ethnopharmacol. 2001; 77:31-5.

11. Aslan M, Orhan DD, Orhan N, *et al*. In vivo antidiabetic and antioxidant potential of Helichrysum plicatum spp. Plicatum capitulums in streptozotocin-Induced-Diabetic Rats. J Ethnopharmacol. 2007; 109:54-9.

12. Korbekandi H, Chitsazi MR, Asghari G, *et al*. Green biosynthesis of silver nanoparticles using Quercus brantii (oak) leaves hydroalcoholic extract. Pharmaceutical Biology.2015;53:807-812.

13. Culp DJ, Robinson B, Parkkila S, *et al*. Oral

colonization by Streptococcus mutans and caries development is reduced upon deletion of carbonic anhydrase VI expression in saliva. Biochim Biophys Acta. 2011; 1812: 1567-1576.

14. Motamedifar M, Khosropanah H, Dabiri SH. Antimicrobial Activity of Peganum Harmala L. on Streptococcus mutans Compared to 0.2% Chlorhexidine. J Dent Shiraz Univ Med Sci.2016; 17: 213-218.

15. Farboodniay Jahromi MA, Dehshahri S, Forouzandeh Samani S. Volatile Composition, Antimicrobial and free radical scavenging activities of essential oil and total extract of Helichrysum leucocephalum Boiss. Trends in pharmaceutical sciences. 2017;3 :193-200.

16. ¨uzgec S, Mericli AH, Houghton PJ, *et al*.Flavonoids of Helichrysum compactum and their antioxidant and antibacterial activity. Fitoterapia. 2005 ;76: pp. 269– 272.

17. Nostro A, Cannatelli MA, Crisafi G, *et al*.Modifications of hydrophobicity, in vitro adherence and cellular aggregation of Streptococcus mutans by Helichrysum italicum extract. Letters in Applied Microbiology.2004;38:pp.423–427.

18. Gianmaria F Ferrazzano , Lia Roberto, Maria Rosaria Catania, et al. Screening and Scoring of Antimicrobial and Biological Activities of Italian Vulnerary Plants against Major Oral Pathogenic Bacteria. Evid Based Complement Alternat Med. 2013; 2013: 316280.

19. Ebrahimzadeh MA, Tavassoli A. Antioxidant properties of Helichrysum pseudoplicatum Nab. Pharm Biomed Res. 2015; 1:37-43.

20. Taglialatela-Scafati O, Pollastro F, Chianese G, *et al*. Antimicrobial phenolics and unusual glycerides from Helichrysum italicum subsp. microphyllum. J Nat Prod. 2013;76:346-53.

21. Davoudi Moghadam H, Mohamadi Sani A, Mehraban Sangatass M. Study of Antifungal activity of Helichrysum arenarium essential oil on growth of Candida albicans and Saccharomyces cereviciae.JFM 2014;1:31-38.

22. Yanil VV, Oyedeji OA, Grierson DS , *et al*. Chemical analysis and antimicrobial activity of essential oil extracted from Helichrysum aureonitens. South African Journal of Botany. 2005;71: 250–252.

23. Dubravka J. Bigović, Tatjana R. Stević, Teodora R. Janković, *et al*. Antimicrobial activity of Helichrysum plicatum DC. Hemijska Industrija.2017; 71:337-342.

24. Prashith Kekuda TR, Vinayaka KS, Sandeepa KH, *et al*. Cytotoxic and Antimicrobial Activity of Anaphalis lawii (Hook.f.) Gamble and Helichrysum buddleioides DC. EC MICROBIOLOGY. 2017;6:169-176.

4

Evaluation of Surface Microhardness of Silver and Zirconia Reinforced Glass-ionomers with and without Microhydroxyapatite

Sharafeddin F[a]; Azar MR[b]; Feizi N[c]; Salehi R[d*]

[a]Professor, Department of Operative Dentistry, Biomaterials Research Center, School of Dentistry, Shiraz University of Medical Sciences, Shiraz, Iran
[b]Associate Professor, Department of Endodontics, School of Dentistry, Shiraz University of Medical Sciences, Shiraz, Iran
[c]Postgraduate Student, Department of Operative Dentistry, School of Dentistry, Shiraz University of Medical Sciences, Shiraz, Iran
[d]Assistant Professor, Department of Operative Dentistry, School of Dentistry, Kashan University of Medical Sciences, Kashan, Iran

ARTICLE INFO

Key words:
Microhardness
Glass-ionomer
Zirconia-reinforced glass-ionomer
Silver-reinforced glass-ionomer
Microhydroxyapatite

Corresponding Author:
Raha Salehi
Assistant Professor,
Department of Operative Dentistry, School of Dentistry, Kashan University of Medical Sciences, Kashan, Iran
Email: raha.salehi.21@Gmail.com.

Abstract

Statement of problem: Hardness of restorative materials like glass-ionomer is an important factor in the longevity of restoration.

Objectives: The aim of this study was to evaluate the microhardness of glass-ionomer modified with different materials.

Materials and Methods: Sixty disk-shaped specimens were examined in six groups in this study, including conventional glass-ionomer (Shofu, Japan), zirconia-reinforced glass-ionomer (Zirconomer, Shofu, Kyoto, Japan), silver-reinforced glass-ionomer (HI-DENSE XP, Shofu, Kyoto, Japan) and mixture of these three types of glass-ionomer with 20 wt% of microhydroxyapatite (Sigma-Aldrich, St. Louis, USA). All the specimens were stored in deionized water for 24 hours. Then Vickers microhardness test was carried out and the results were analyzed by using two-way ANOVA test and paired t-test ($P<0.05$).

Results: Zirconia-reinforced glass-ionomer with microhydroxyapatite exhibited significantly higher microhardness in comparison with other groups ($P<0.001$). Conventional glass-ionomer with microhydroxyapatite showed the lowest microhardness ($P<0.001$). After incorporation of microhydroxyapatite in both conventional and silver-reinforced glass-ionomer groups, microhardness decreased significantly ($P<0.001$).The microhardness of top and bottom of all groups was significantly different. ($P<0.001$).

Conclusions: Incorporation of 20% microhydroxyapatite to zirconia-reinforced glass-ionomer can improve microhardness.

Introduction

Since the development of glass-ionomers in the early 1970s, its application in dentistry as a restorative material is inconceivable [1].

Direct bonding to tooth structure is one of the most important advantages of glass-ionomers [2]. Biocompatibility and anticariogenic action , due to the release of fluoride, are other unique properties of glass-ionomers [3].While certain drawbacks such as low mechanical properties limits its use,efforts have been made to overcome these shortcomings [4]. Addition of fillers like silver, gold, and stainless steel powders has been investigated [5, 6]. These reinforced glass-ionomers exhibit reduced abrasion, but they have poor aesthetics. Polyethylene fiber also enhanced the mechanical properties [7]. It appears incorporation of zinc does not change the properties significantly [8]. Nonoclay could improve the mechanical properties to some extent [9]. Zirconium and its oxide were used to improve the strength of glass-ionomers due to their good dimensional stability and toughness [10]. In order to introduce a more biocompatible restorative material, bioactive glass and hydroxyapatite were incorporated into glass-ionomers to replace damaged tissues [11-13] and their effect on mechanical properties of cement were investigated [14,15].Hydroxyapatite, the main mineral component of the tooth structure and bone, is a bioceramic containing calcium and phosphorus [16,17]. It was reported that many mechanical properties of glass-ionomer improved by mixing the powder with bioceramics [14, 18, 19]. It can enhance the flexural strength of the demineralized dentin by remineralization [20]. Zirconia fillers provide mechanical strength and dimensional stability. Therefore, incorporation of zirconia and hydroxyapatite into glass-ionomer can enhance both the mechanical properties and bioactivity of the cement [10, 21].The present study was conducted to determine surface microhardness of silver-reinforced and zirconia-reinforced glass-ionomer with and without microhydroxyapatite particles.

Materials and Methods

In this experimental study, 60 specimens were prepared from three types of glass-ionomers (Shofu, Kyoto, Japan) and hydroxyapatite (Sigma-Aldrich, St. Louis, USA) in 6 groups (n=10). The experimental groups were categorized based on the materials used as Group 1: Conventional glass-ionomer (GIC), Group 2: Conventional glass-ionomer with 20 wt% of hydroxyapatite (GIC+HA),Group 3: Silver-reinforced glass-ionomer (HI-DENSE XP), Group 4: Silver-reinforced glass-ionomer with 20 wt% of hydroxyapatite (HI-DENSE XP+HA),Group 5: Zirconia-reinforced glass-ionomer (Zirconomer), and Group 6: Zirconia-reinforced glass-ionomer with 20 wt% of hydroxyapatite (Zirconomer+HA). The test specimens were prepared using a cylindrical plastic mold with a diameter of 6 mm, and height of 2 mm. In the group 1, conventional glass-ionomers powder was mixed with the liquid on a clean cold glass slab with a plastic spatula according to manufacturer's instructions (powder-to-liquid ratio was 1:1). Mixing procedure ended in 25 seconds. The mold was placed on a Mylar strip and a glass plate. Then the mold was overfilled with this mixture; a Mylar strips was placed on the top surface and compressed between two glass plates. In the group 2, glass-ionomer powder and hydroxyapatite powder were weighed carefully using a weighing machine accurate to 0.0001 g (A&D, GR+360, Tokyo, Japan). Then 80% of glass powder and 20% of hydroxyapatite were mixed. To achieve a homogenous mixture, the mixing procedure was carried out using an amalgam capsule and an amalgamator (Ultramat2, SDI, Bayswater, Victoria, Australia). Then it was mixed with glass-ionomer liquid similar to that in the group 1. The procedures were carried out in the same manner. In the groups 3 and 4, the powder-to-liquid ratio was 2:1. All the procedure was similar to those in previous groups. In groups 5 and 6, the powder-to-liquid ratio was 2:1.

All the specimens were prepared at the room temperature and humidity. A layer of varnish (Hoffmann, Berlin, Germany) was applied on the surfaces of all the specimens. The bottom surfaces were marked with a dot. The specimens were stored in distilled water at room temperature for 24 hours, with specimens in each group being stored individually.

After 24 hours, both sides of each disk were

polished with polishing paper dicks (Poli-pro Disks, Premier Dental Products, Plymouthmeeting, Pennsylvania, USA), using a low-speed rotary instrument with air coolant. The microhardness test

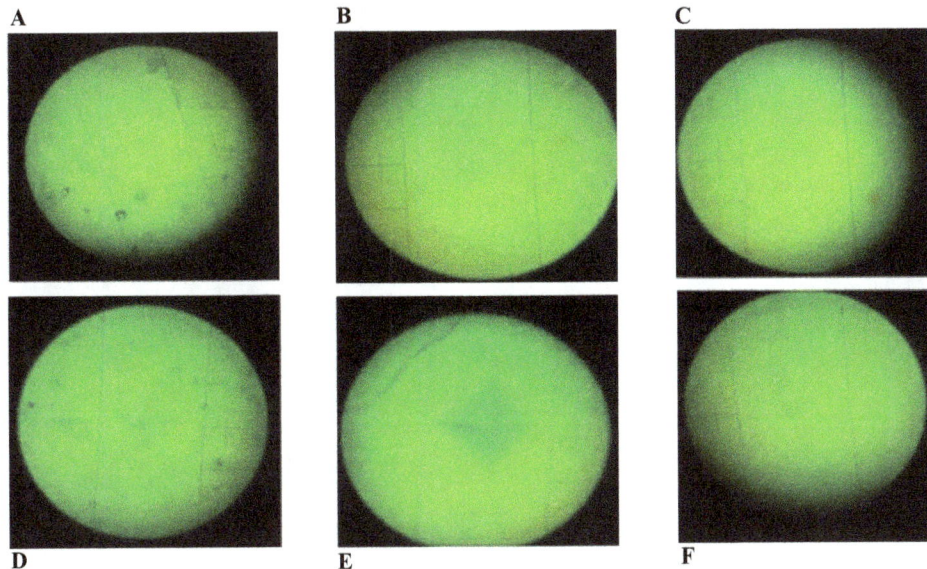

Figure1: Images of microhardness test of 6 experimental groups with stereomicroscope (40X). (A) Conventional glass-ionomer (B) Conventional glass-ionomer with hydroxyapatite (GIC+HA) (C) Silver-reinforced glass-ionomer (D) Silver-reinforced glass-ionomer with hydroxyapatite (E) Zirconia-reinforced glass-ionomer (Zirconomer) (F) Zirconia-reinforced glass-ionomer with hydroxyapatite

was performed with digital Vickers microhardness tester (MHV-1000Z, Sinowon, DongGuan, China) with a load of 300 gf in 15 seconds. Three Vickers tests were carried out on each surface (Figure1) and the mean value was calculated. Data were analyzed with SPSS. Two-way ANOVA and paired t-test were used.

Results

The mean microhardness (VHN) values of all the groups are presented in Table 1. The results showed that microhardness of conventional glass-ionomer and silver-reinforced glass-ionomer decreased due to the incorporation of microhydroxyapatite ($P<0.001$).In contrast, the microhardness of Zirconomer increased significantly after mixing with microhydroxyapatite ($P<0.001$).

The microhardness of the top and the bottom surfaces of the disks were analyzed with paired t-test. In all groups, the microhardness of the top and the bottom surfaces showed significant differences ($P<0.05$). The mean values are

presented in Table 1. Among all groups, Zirconomer with microhydroxyapatite (group 5) exhibited the highest values and the lowest values were recorded in conventional glass-ionomer with microhydroxyapatite (group 2).

Discussion

Hardness influences resistance to in-service scratching which compromises fatigue strength, leading to premature failure. It was reported that surface hardness of conventional glass-ionomer was higher than resin modified glass-ionomer[15]. Therefore, use of conventional glass-ionomer and its modifications can be more applicable. Hydroxyapatite is the main mineral component of tooth structure; therefore, incorporation of hydroxyapatite into glass-ionomer can affect some of its properties, including an increase in its fracture resistance [4].

Acris *et al.* [22] added hydroxyapatite to light-cured monomers and the results indicated that 50–60 wt% of hydroxyapatite enhanced Young's modulus and hardness. This large volume of hydroxyapatite was used because no other filler was used. In the present study smaller volume of microhydroxyapatite was mixed with glass powder (20 wt %) that was consistent with similar

Table 1: Mean ± SD of microhardness and P. Value the top and bottom surfaces in all groups(GIC: Glass ionomer cement, HA: Hydroxyapatite)

Group	Materials		Mean	P. Value
1	Conventional GIC	Top	40.739±1.078	
		Bottom	46.139±1.078	0.006
2	Conventional GIC+HA	Top	27.892±1.078	
		Bottom	33.291±1.078	0.007
3	Silver-reinforced GIC	Top	65.106±1.078	
		Bottom	70.506±1.078	0.001
4	Silver-reinforced GIC+ HA	Top	43.411±1.078	
		Bottom	48.810±1.078	0.01
5	Zirconomer	Top	48.817±1.078	
		Bottom	54.116±1.078	0.046
6	Zirconomer+HA	Top	67.660±1.078	
		Bottom	73.060±1.078	0.042

study. Improved mechanical behavior with apatite formation of hydroxyapatite in combination with release of ions from glass-ionomer can be advantageous. The results of a study by Mohammed and Raghd [14] showed that adding hydroxyapatite at a concentration of 15–20% resulted in optimal hardness. According to the results of our study, although hydroxyapatite has some benefits, it seems that a mixture of microhydroxyapatite and glass-ionomer has reduced microhardness. To achieve a uniform material, the powder should have the same particle size and structure. This can only be achieved by sintering the glass powder and hydroxyapatite. In the present study, we made efforts to produce a uniform mixture by mixing the powders using an amalgamator; however, some parts of the surface of the material could possibly be only hydroxyapatite or only glass-ionomer. It seems this factor accounts for the decrease in hardness of glass-ionomer and silver reinforced glass-ionomer.

Goenka et al. [16] reported that increasing hydroxyapatite up to 15 wt% in conventional glass-ionomer resulted in a decrease in the microhardness of the mixture. In the present study, the results were consistent with the reports of Goenka who showed a decrease in surface hardness. Yli Urpo et al. [23] reported that incorporation of bioactive glass into glass-ionomer decreased the mechanical properties of conventional glass-ionomer during immersion in deionized water.

It was reported that the microhardness of one type of silver-reinforced glass-ionomer was greater than that of conventional glass-ionomer, [24] but incorporation of microhydroxyapatite resulted in a decrease in surface microhardness to the range of conventional glass-ionomer, which might be attributed to lower microhardness of hydroxyapatite particles in comparison with silver particles. Furthermore, the concentration of hydroxyapatite might affect the mechanical properties. The volume of hydroxyapatite can change the amount of liquid that is needed to complete the reaction of particles. In the present study we used the same ratio as the manufacturer had suggested; therefore, it seems inadequate amount of liquid in the mixture can alter the mechanical properties.

Incorporation of zirconia into dental ceramics doubled their hardness; therefore, incorporation of zirconia into restorative glass-ionomer can enhance its microhardness [25]. In the present study, the microhardness of Zirconomer was higher in comparison with conventional glass-ionomer. Gu *et al.*[21] reported that microhardness of zirconia-reinforced glass-ionomer was 20% higher than the miracle mix but in the present study, the microhardness of Zirconomer was lower than that of silver-reinforced glass-ionomer. The microhardness of Zirconomer and metal-reinforced glass-ionomer is almost in the same range; hence, Zirconomer is preferred to metal-reinforced glass-ionomer due to its white color that is similar to tooth color.

In the current study, the results indicated that Zirconomer had a higher surface hardness after incorporation of microhydroxyapatite in comparison with other groups, consistent with a study of GU *et al.* [21] It seems that calcium ions of microhydroxyapatite, participating in the reaction of Zirconomer powder and liquid, alter the structure of the material, showing higher microhardness. Incorporation of nano- and micro-particles of silica could enhance the hardness of conventional glass-ionomer [26] but in the current study, incorporation of microhydroxyapatite decreased it. It seems that the size of the particles can affect the chemical reaction of the powder and liquid. Smaller particle size provides greater surface area that can alter the reaction. It seems even by using nano hydroxyapatite; it is possible to achieve higher microhardness values. Adequate mixing is also an important factor that affects the mechanical properties of the mixture. In the current study, the mixing time was the same as what was suggested by the manufacturer; however, subsequent to adding microhydroxyapatite, the mixing time might be changed. Therefore studies should determine the best mixing time.

In one study, it was reported that the microhardness of the top surface of resin-modified disks was higher than that of the bottom surface [27] but in the present study, in all the experimental groups the hardness of the bottom surfaces was higher than the top surface. Glass-ionomers used in this study were not light-cured; therefore, it seems presence of voids on the top surface can account for its lower microhardness. As the differences in all the groups were in the same pattern, it is more probable that the difference in the hardness of the top and the bottom surface was due to the better packing force, which compressed the material in the bottom surface.

Among all the materials used in this study, initial surface hardness of silver-reinforced glass-ionomer was higher but after incorporation of microhydroxyapatite, Zirconomer exhibited a great improvement. Further investigations should be carried out into other properties of the mixture of Zirconomer and hydroxyapatite. Zirconomer was introduced as white amalgam; therefore, the mechanical properties of the mixture of white amalgam with hydroxyapatite, with higher mechanical properties and mercury amalgam should be compared. May be, it can be a substitute for amalgam that aroused concerns about its mercury.

Nano-particles can affect the reaction due to their smaller size; hence, studies should be designed to evaluate the physical and mechanical properties of the mixture of nano hydroxyapatite particles and glass-ionomer.

Conclusions

Within the limitations of this study, it can be concluded that the incorporation of 20% concentration of microhydroxyapatite into Zirconomer can improve the surface microhardness. On the contrary, adding hydroxyapatite to conventional glass-ionomer and silver-reinforce glass-ionomer results in adverse effect.

Acknowledgments

This manuscript is based on a research project approved by the Biomaterial Research Center at the Shiraz School of Dentistry. The authors would like to thank the Biomaterial Research Center for testing specimens and Dr.Mohammad Salehi for the Statistical analysis. The authors deny any conflict of interests.

Conflict of Interest: None declared.

References

1. Sharafeddin F, Shoale S, Kowkabi M. Effects of Different Percentages of Microhydroxyapatite on Microhardness of Resin-modified Glass-ionomer and Zirconomer. J Clin Exp Dent. 2017;9:e805-811.

2. Sharafeddin F, Feizi N. Evaluation of the effect of adding micro-hydroxyapatite and nano-hydroxyapatite on the microleakage of conventional and resin-modified Glass-ionomer Cl V restorations. J Clin Exp Dent. 2017;9:e242-248.

3. Sharafeddin F, Choobineh MM. Assessment of the Shear Bond Strength between Nanofilled Composite Bonded to Glass-ionomer Cement Using Self-etch Adhesive with Different pHs and Total-Etch Adhesive. J Dent (Shiraz). 2016;17:1-6.

4. Sharafeddin F, Kowkabi M, Shoale S. Evaluation of the effect of home bleaching agents on surface microhardness of different glass-ionomer cements containing hydroxyapatite. J Clin Exp Dent. 2017;9:e1075-1080.

5. Lee JJ, Lee YK, Choi BJ, et al. Physical properties of resin-reinforced glass ionomer cement modified with micro and nano-hydroxyapatite. J Nanosci Nanotechnol. 2010;10:5270-6.

6. Moshaverinia A, Roohpour N, Chee WW, et al. A review of powder modifications in conventional glass-ionomer dental cements. Journal of Materials Chemistry. 2011;21:1319-28.

7. Sharafeddin F, Tondari A, Alavi A. The Effect of Adding Glass and Polyethylene Fibers on Flexural Strength of Three Types of Glass-Ionomer Cements. Research Journal of Biological Sciences. 2013;8:66-70.

8. Al-Angari SS, Hara AT, Chu TM, et al. Physicomechanical properties of a zinc-reinforced glass ionomer restorative material. Journal of oral science. 2014;56:11-6.

9. Fareed MA, Stamboulis A. Nanoclay addition to a conventional glass ionomer cements: Influence on physical properties. Eur J dent. 2014;8:456-63.

10. Gu YW, Yap AUJ, Cheang P, et al. Development of zirconia-glass ionomer cement composites. J non-cryst solids. 2005;351:508-14.

11. Efflandt SE, Magne P, Douglas WH, et al. Interaction between bioactive glasses and human dentin. J Mater Sci Mater Med. 2002;13:557-65.

12. Farooq I, Imran Z, Farooq U, et al. Bioactive glass: a material for the future. World J Dent. 2012;3:199-201.

13. Xie D, Zhao J, Weng Y, et al. Bioactive glass–ionomer cement with potential therapeutic function to dentin capping mineralization. Eur J oral sci. 2008;116:479-87.

14. R M,M RA. Assessment of diametral tensile strength and microhardness of glass-ionomer cement reinforced by different amounts of hydroxyapatite. J Bagh College of Dentistry. 2006;18:17-20.

15. Prabhakar AR, Jibi paul M, Basappa N. Comparative Evaluation of the Remineralizing Effects and Surface Microhardness of Glass Ionomer Cements Containing Bioactive Glass (S53P4): An in vitro Study. Int J Clin Pediatr Dent. 2010;3:69-77.

16. Goenka S, Balu R, Kumar TS. Effects of nanocrystalline calcium deficient hydroxyapatite incorporation in glass ionomer cements. J mech behav biomed mater. 2012;7:69-76.

17. Sharafeddin F, Moradian M, Motamedi M. Evaluation of Shear Bond Strength of Methacrylate- and Silorane-based Composite Resin Bonded to Resin-Modified Glass-ionomer Containing Micro- and Nano-hydroxyapatite. J Dent (Shiraz). 2016;17:142–148.

18. Khaghani M, Doostmohammadi A, Monshi A, et al. Effect of incorporating nano-particles of hydroxyapatite on bioactivity and compressive strength of dental glass-ionomer cements. Journal of Isfahan Dental School. 2013;8:593-605.

19. Arita K, Yamamoto A, Shinonaga Y, et al. Hydroxyapatite particle characteristics

influence the enhancement of the mechanical and chemical properties of conventional restorative glassionomer cement. Dent mater J. 2011;30:672-83.

20. Khoroushi M, Mousavinasab SM, Keshani F, *et al*. Effect of resin-modified glass ionomer containing bioactive glass on the flexural strength and morphology of demineralized dentin. Oper dent. 2013;38:E1-E10.

21. Gu YW, Yap AU, Cheang P, *et al*. Effects of incorporation of HA/ZrO 2 into glass ionomer cement (GIC). Biomaterials. 2005;26:713-20.

22. RW A, A L-M, M T, *et al*. Mechanical properties of visible light-cured resin reinforced with hydroxyapatite for dental restoration. Dent Mater. 2002;18:49-57.

23. Yli-Urpo H, Lassila LV, Närhi T,*et al*. Compressive strength and surface characterization of glass ionomer cements modified by particles of bioactive glass. Dental Materials. 2005;21:201-9.

24. Bala O, Arisu HD, Yikilgan I, *et al*. Evaluation of surface roughness and hardness of different glass ionomer cements. Eur J Dent. 2012;6:79-86.

25. Miyazaki T, Nakamura T, Matsumura H, *et al*. Current status of zirconia restoration. J Prosthodont Res. 2013;57:236-61.

26. Mabrouk M, Selim MM, Beherei H, *et al*. Effect of incorporation of nano bioactive silica into commercial Glass Ionomer Cement (GIC). J Genet Eng Biotechnol. 2012;10:113-9.

27. Bayindir YZ, Yildiz M. Surface hardness properties of resin-modified glass ionomer cements and polyacid-modified composite resins. J Contemp Dent Pract. 2004;5:42-9.

5

Evaluation of Compressive Strength and Sorption/Solubility of Four Luting Cements

Tavangar MS[a], Jafarpur D[b], Bagheri R[c*]

[a]Department of Dental Materials, School of Dentistry, Shiraz University of Medical Sciences, Shiraz, Iran
[b]Student Research Committee, School of Dentistry, Shiraz University of Medical Sciences, Shiraz, Iran
[c]Department of Dental Materials and Biomaterials Research Center, School of Dentistry, Shiraz University of Medical Sciences, Shiraz, Iran

ARTICLE INFO

Key words:
Compression Strength
Resin Luting Cements
Sorption/Solubility

Corresponding Author:
Rafat Bagheri
Department of Dental
Materials and Biomaterial
Research center, Shiraz
University of Medical
Sciences, Shiraz, Iran
Email: bagherir@sums.ac.ir,
Bagherir@unimelb.edu.au

Abstract

Statement of Problem: Compressive strength (CS) and sorption/solubility of the luting cements are two associated factors. Searching a correlation between sorption/solubility and compressive strength of various luting cements is required.

Objectives: To measure the water sorption/solubility, and compressive strength of three resin-based and one conventional glass ionomer (CGI) luting cement after 1 and 24 h of immersion in distilled water and to determine if there is any correlation between those properties found.

Materials and Methods: Four luting cements were investigated. For each material, 10 disc shaped specimens were prepared for measuring the sorption/solubility. The specimens were cured according to the manufacturer's instructions, and the sorption/solubility were measured in accordance with the ISO 4049's. For testing the compression strength, for each material 16 cylindrical specimens were prepared by insertion of cements into a stainless steel split mould. The specimens were cured, divided into groups of 8, and then stored in distilled water at $(37 \pm 1)°C$ for 1 and 24 h. The test was performed using the universal testing machine, the maximum load was recorded and CS was calculated. The data were analysed using SPSS software version 18. One-way ANOVA, *post-hoc* Tukey's test and Pearson's correlation coefficient were performed.

Results: G-CEM had the highest mean CS (153.60 ± 25.15) and CGI luting had the lowest CS (21.36 ± 5.37) ($p < 0.001$). After 24 h, mean CS values showed an increase for almost all materials except for RelyX™ U200 which showed a slight reduction. However, no statistically significant difference was founded (all $p > 0.05$). The lowest mean sorption/solubility value was for RelyX™ U200 and Panavia F, and the highest for CGI luting (all $p < 0.001$).

Conclusions: The compressive strength of all cements did not necessarily increase after 24 h and varied depending on the materials. There was a strong reverse correlation between sorption and CS values after both 1 and 24 h immersion. It may be practical for clinician to use those cements with the less sorption / solubility and more stable compression strength over time.

Introduction

Several categories of the luting cements are being used for cementation of direct or indirect restorations to the tooth structure [1]. Water based cements such as zinc phosphate and polycarboxylate cements have been used for a long time as the main luting agent for the cementation of restoration. Since 1972 [2] when it was introduced, glass ionomer cements have gained popularity due to their clinical advantages including fluoride release and their adhesion capabilities to the tooth structure [3]. However, poor early mechanical properties and moisture sensitivity are considered as disadvantages of these materials [4].

The resin luting cements are the latest type of luting agents for the cementation of indirect aesthetic restorations such as all-ceramic and porcelain veneers. Resin cements are classified into two types: conventional and self-adhesive resin luting cements. The self-adhesive resin luting cements (SARLC) have the ability to bond to the tooth structure and the internal surface of the restoration without using adhesive system. Resin luting cements are comprised of the same basic constituents as the composite restorative material but with lower concentration of filler particles with a variable amount of 55–70 W% [5]. Resin cements have advantages of colour stability, adhesion to dental structure and other materials, low water sorption and solubility, and better mechanical properties in comparison to traditional cements [6-8]. There are also major disadvantages, such as polymerization shrinkage [8].

Luting cements seal the interface of the indirect restoration and the prepared tooth surface; hence, the clinical success of the restoration depends on the mechanical and physical properties of the luting cements over the duration of the restoration [9]. These materials are subjected to forces of mastication and transferring the stresses from indirect restorations to the tooth structure. Therefore, it is necessary for luting cement to provide high strength in order to maintain the durability and success of the restorations [10,11].

In addition to the mechanical properties, other clinically related characteristics including dimensional stability and structural integrity should be considered for the selection of a durable luting agent [3]. To maintain the dimensional stability, luting cement should have adequate resistance to fracture and deterioration when exposed to the oral cavity fluids [1]. Water sorption and solubility may cause degradation of the cement, leading to disintegration in margin of the restorations. Clinically, loss of marginal integrity can cause unwanted consequences such as marginal leakage and discoloration, secondary caries, hypersensitivity, releasing toxic substances, and finally may result in debonding or the fracture of the restoration [3,12].

Previous studies reported comparable moisture sensitivity for the resin modified (RMGIC) with conventional glass ionomer cements [10]. Knobloch et al. [3] investigated sorption and solubility of 3 RMGICs and 3 resin cements reported that water sorption was significantly higher in all RMGICs as compared to resin cements, attributing it to the hydrophilic nature of HEMA in the composition of RMGICs [3]. Similarly, by evaluating the sorption and solubility of eight luting agents (two RMGICs and six resin cements) in distilled water and ethanol, Mese et al. found that RMGICs exhibited higher solubility and sorption as compared to resin cements [12].

Although the resin luting cement showed lower water sensitivity, the weakening of their mechanical properties has been reported after water storage [13]. Water is mainly absorbed by the polymer matrix, leading to hydrolytic degradation, debonding of the fillers, and matrix softening. When the resin matrix starts swelling because of water sorption, unreacted monomers and deboned fillers may leach out from the matrix. Consequently, moist conditions can decrease the final strength and increase the creep [12]. Örtengren et al. [14] studied the effect of 60 days of water sorption on the flexural strengths of two resin cements. Their findings showed that after water storage, resin cement revealed significantly lower flexural strength and higher deflection which may be explained by the plasticizing effect of water on the polymers.

Several studies have compared the mechanical properties, and water sorption / solubility of different classes of luting cements [11,12]. Yet, the correlation between water sorption and solubility of various categories of luting cements and their compressive strength has not been widely studied.

Therefore, the present study aimed to place various luting cements in distilled water and determine: 1) the effect of 1 and 24 h immersion on the compressive strength; 2) water sorption/solubility of those cements in accordance with the ISO 4049's; 3) if a correlation exists between the sorption/solubility and the compressive strength of the luting cements.

The null hypothesis is that the storage time does not affect compressive strength, or there is no correlation between the compressive strength and water sorption/solubility of the cements.

Materials and Methods

Four luting cements were investigated in this study, as shown in Table 1.

right angles to each other were made and the area (in square millimetres) was calculated by using the mean diameter. By measuring the thickness of the specimen at the centre of the specimen and at four equally spaced points on the circumference, the volume, V, was calculated in cubic millimetres as follows: $V = \pi \times (d/2)^2 \times h$, where $\pi = 3.14$, d is the mean diameter and h is the mean thickness of the specimen. The specimens of each material were immersed in distilled

Table 1: Description of the materials

Cement	Manufacturer	Type	LOT Number	Expiry date
RelyX™ U200 Automix syringe	3MESPE,St. Paul, MN, USA	SARLC	635906	2017-12
Panavia F 2 pastes	Kuraray Noritake Dental Inc., Okayama, Japan	CRLC	000035	2016-09-05
G-CEM Encapsulated	GC corporation, Tokyo Japan	SARLC	1307041	2016-07
CGI luting & lining cement Powder and liquid	GC corporation, Tokyo Japan	CGIC	1407171	2017-07

SARLC= Self Adhesive Resin Luting Cement, SGIC= Conventional Glass Ionomer luting Cement, CRLC= Conventional Resin Luting Cement.

Water sorption and Solubility test

For each material, 10 disc-shaped specimens of 10 ± 0.1mm of diameter and 1.0 ± 0.1mm of thickness were prepared. A polyethelyn mould was filled with the material according to the manufacturer's instructions. Then, the mould was sandwiched between two pieces of Mylar strip and pressed by two glass plates under hand pressure to remove the excess material. The light cured specimen were eradicated for the recommended exposure time trough Mylar strip using LED curing unit at a wavelength range of 440-480nm and an emitting light intensity of 1500 mW/cm^2 (Radii plus LED; SDI, Melbourne, Victoria, Australia). In accordance with the ISO 4049's instructions [15], the specimens were transferred to a desiccator (Labx Company, Ontario, Canada) containing freshly dried silica gel (SIGMA-ALDRICH, Taufkirchen, Germany) maintained at $(37\pm 1)°C$. After 22 h, the specimens were removed and transferred to a second desiccator maintained at $(23\pm1)°C$ for another 2 h.

After 24 h, the specimens were removed and weighed on an electronic balance (GR-3000, A & D CL Toshiba, Tokyo, Japan) to an accuracy of ± 0.1mg. This procedure was repeated every 24 h until a constant mass, m_1, was obtained. After the final drying, two measurements of the diameter at the

water at $(37\pm 1)°C$ for 7 d. After this time period, the specimens were removed, washed with distilled water, air dried and then weighed in one minute and recorded as m_2.

The specimens were reconditioned to a constant mass in the desiccator. The constant mass was recorded as m_3. The values for water sorption, Wsp , and solubility, Wsl, in $\mu g/mm^3$, was calculated using the following equations: $Wsl = (m_1 - m_3)/V$ and $Wsp = (m_2 - m_3)/V$ where m_1 is the conditioned mass prior to immersion in water; m_2 is the mass of the specimen after immersion in water for 7 d; m_3 is the mass of the reconditioned specimen (all in micrograms); and V is the volume of the specimen, in cubic millimetres.

Compression test

For each material, 16 cylindrical specimens of 4.0 mm in diameter and 8.0 mm long were prepared by insertion of cements into a stainless steel split mould. The light cure materials were cured according to the manufacturer's instruction by the same LED-curing unit mentioned above. The specimens were removed from the split mould and cured with the same exposure time on the opposite side and each lateral face. The specimens were divided into groups of 8

Table 2: Mean ± SD (MPa) of compressive strength for all luting cements analysed using Tukey's test

Luting cement	1 hour	24 hours	p value*
RelyX™ U200	138.50 ± 22.8 [A]	129.20 ± 19.92 [A]	0.59
Panavia F	110.07 ± 47.5 [A]	162.33 ± 22.00 [A]	0.31
G-CEM	153.60 ± 25.15 [A]	162.60 ± 18.48 [A]	0.65
CGI Luting	21.36 ± 5.37 [B]	30.50 ± 22.78 [B]	0.63

- In each column, mean values with different upper case letters show a significant difference (p value< 0.05).
*shows significance level of student's t test between two storage time in each material.

(n=8) and then stored in distilled water at (37 ± 1)°C for one and 24 h.

Following the storage, the compression strength test was performed using the universal testing machine (Zwick/Roll Z020, Zwick GmbH & Co, Germany) loaded at a crosshead speed of 0.5mm/min. The maximum load at specimen failure was recorded and compressive strength was calculated using the following formula: δ=F/S where F is the maximum load at the fracture point (N) and S is the surface area of the specimen (mm^2).

Data Analysis

The data were analysed using SPSS software version 18 (SPSS Inc., Chicago, IL, USA). One-way ANOVA was used to compare different variables between the materials, and *post-hoc* Tukey's test was performed to show significant differences in subgroup comparisons. Student's *t* test was used to show significant differences between the two storage times for compressive strength of each material. Correlations between sorption/solubility and compressive strength were assessed using Pearson's correlation coefficient. *p* value of < 0.05 was considered to be statistically

Table 3: Mean ± SD ($\mu g/mm^3$) of sorption and solubility for all luting cements analysed using Tukey's test

Luting cements	Sorption	Solubility
RelyX™ U200	23.61 ± 1.59[A]	1.23 ± 0.83[A]
Panavia F	24.10 ± 6.87[A]	8.40 ± 4.28[AB]
G-CEM	38.90 ± 4.59[B]	17.29 ± 9.55[BC]
CGI Luting	76.20 ± 6.17[C]	27.97 ± 2.11[C]

- In each column, mean values with different upper case letters show a significant difference (p value< 0.05).
(p < 0.05).

significant.

Results

As shown in Table 2, after 1 h of immersion in distilled water, the highest mean CS value was observed for G-CEM (153.6 ± 25.15), followed by RelyX™ U200 (138.5 ± 22.8) and Panavia F (110.07 ± 47.5). CGI luting showed the lowest mean CS (21.36 ± 5.37) (p < 0.001). After 24 h, mean CS values were numerically but not statistically raised for all the cements except for RelyX™ U200 which showed a slight reduction. After 24 h, CS values for Panavia F increased as high as G-CEM with the following order: G-CEM=Panavia F > RelyX™ U200 > CGI luting.

Table 3 compares the water sorption and solubility of all tested cements. The lowest mean sorption value was for RelyX™ U200 (23.6 ± 1.59) and Panavia F (24.10 ± 6.87). The highest mean sorption value was for CGI luting (76.20 ± 6.17) (p < 0.001). The lowest mean solubility value was found to be for RelyX™ U200 and Panavia F followed by G-CEM, and CGI luting, respectively (p < 0.001).

There was a strong reverse correlation between sorption and CS values after both 1 and 24 h of immersion (r = -0.702, p = 0.002; and r = -0.775, p < 0.001, respectively). Solubility showed a moderate reverse correlation with CS values after 1 h (r = -0.530, p = 0.035) and no significant correlation after 24 h (r = -0.409, p = 0.116).

Discussion

Compressive strength and sorption/solubility are correlated factors which enhance the longevity of bonded restorations when they are in an optimum level. A high compressive strength of the luting cements enables them to withstand masticatory forces in the mouth and increases the fracture resistance of the restoration, especially in brittle materials such as ceramics [15].

In this experiment, compressive strength and water sorption/solubility of two self- adhesive resin luting cements (SARLC), one conventional resin luting cement (CRLC), and one conventional glass ionomer (CGI) luting were examined and compared. In general, CGI luting exhibited significantly lower compressive strength and higher water sorption / solubility than both SARLC and CRLC. Comparison of the resin cements showed that CRLC had a lower strength than SARLC but it showed a comparable or less water sorption / solubility.

As shown in Table 2, compressive strength of all materials showed an increase after 24 h of immersion in distilled water except for RelyX™ U200 which revealed a slight decrease after 24 h. The increase in the materials' strength after 24 h can be related to their setting reaction. For glass ionomer cements, after mixing, the calcium polycarboxylate is formed in the first few minutes while the aluminum polycarboxylate, which improves the mechanical properties of the cement, takes at least 24 hours or even longer to be formed [16-18].

Likewise, for resin-based materials, polymerization and maturation take 24 h to be completed. Therefore, the mechanical properties of these materials are expected to be improved significantly after 24 hours. In the present study, one of the SARLC (RelyX™ U200) had a slight reduction from ≈138 to ≈129 MPa while the other one (G-CEM) had a slight increase from ≈153 to ≈162 MPa. The CRLC, Panavia F, showed the lowest compressive strength (≈110 MPa) among resin-based cements after 1 h of setting while after 24 h of setting, it had a remarkable increase (≈162 MPa) that was equal to the highest value for G-CEM.

These results suggest that the growth in the luting cements' strength is not directly dependent on the period of 24 h of setting. The effect of 24 h of immersion in distilled water on the compressive strength of the resin cements varied depending on the materials. Some materials showed a slight reduction and some others significant increase in strength after 24 h of immersion. This result is in agreement with that of a previous study [19].

A previous study [19] evaluating the shear punch strength of resin cements reported a reduction of strength for almost all SARLCs after one week, one month and even more after three months of immersion in distilled water. While Panavia F with HEMA

content in their composition showed an increase after one-week of immersion, it has been concluded that the HEMA could be a major factor in the reinforcement or stiffness of the polymer system [20].

It has been shown [21] that the water sorption of a SARLC (Maxcem) was significantly higher than a CRLC (Panavia F). It has also been hypothesized that the significant decrease in the strength of SARLC might be related to its greater water sorption than CRLC [19]. However, the results of our study did not prove this claim. The water sorption / solubility of the tested luting cements followed the following trend: RelyX™ U200 < Panavia F < G-CEM < CGI luting.

This result reveals that although G-CEM had the greatest water sorption/ solubility among other resin-based cements, did not drop the strength but also exhibited the highest strength value either after 1 or 24 h of immersion in water. On the other hands, RelyX™ U200 with the least sorption and solubility exhibited the lowest strength after 24 h of immersion. In other words, G-CEM with higher strength than RelyX™ U200 had higher water sorption and solubility. Hence, it is speculated that having a high water sorption/solubility does not necessarily decrease the compressive strength of resin luting cements. But, some factors other than sorption/solubility, such as polimerization, mode of curing (dual- or self-cure), and degree of conversion (%DC) might have a great influence on the strength [22] or sorption/ solubility [23] of the resin luting cements.

Factors that may affect polymerization include cement film thickness, opacity, and translucency of both the cement and restoration. Properly cured resin cement will exhibit high compressive and flexural strengths and less solubility in the oral fluids. The mixing method of the resin cement is also an important clinical factor that improves the performance of the resin cement [22]. Although resin cements are insoluble in oral fluids, being resins, they absorb water. Due to water sorption, the flexural strength of the resin cements is decreased [24]. The flexural strength affected by the thickness of the cement, the greater decrease occurred in the greater film thickness of the cement because it makes the cement unable to scatter stresses from masticatory function between the tooth and restoration. Therefore, keeping the resin cement layers to a thin layer minimizes the plasticizing effect in the resin cements [25].

In the present study, Panavia F (a dual-cure luting cement) showed significantly less sorption/solubility than G-CEM (a light cure luting cement) which can be due to their different mode of curing. A recent study [23] investigated the effect of curing mode on the surface energy and sorption/solubility of SARLC and CRLC and found a greater sorption/solubility values for SARLC than the CRLC. The author concluded that the degree of conversion (%DC) was negatively correlated with the sorption/solubility values. Dual curing is shown to reduce the sorption and/or solubility in comparison with self-curing by increasing %DC [23].

The convention glass ionomer used in this study (CGI Lutin) exhibited the lowest strength and the highest sorption and solubility. It is well known that water has an important role in the glass ionomer cement. It contributes to the transportation of calcium and aluminum cations, reacting with the polyacid to form a polyacrylate matrix [26]. During the early stage of maturation, moisture contamination leads to loss of components, decrease of physical properties and loss of translucency [27]. After hardening, desiccation and loss of water results in the inadequacy of the reactions and surface crazing [28]. Therefore, it is expected to absorb and lose water easily.

Conclusions

Within the limitations of this study, the following conclusions were drawn. In general, most of the cements showed an increase in the compressive strength after 24 h immersion in comparison with the 1 h immersion except for RelyX™ U200 that had a slight decrease. RelyX™ U200 and Panavia F, revealed the lowest sorption / solubility and CGI luting the highest. There was a strong reverse correlation between sorption and CS values after both 1 and 24 h immersion. Based on the results of this study, it is speculated that it may be practical for clinician to use those cements with the less sorption / solubility and more stable compression strength over time.

Acknowledgments

The authors would like to thank the Vice Chancellor for Research Affairs of Shiraz University of Medical Sciences for financial support of the research.

Conflict of Interest: None declared.

References

1. Giti R, Vojdani M, Abduo J, et al. The Comparison of Sorption and Solubility Behavior of Four Different Resin Luting Cements in Different Storage Media. J Dent (Shiraz). 2016;17:91-97.

2. Wilson AD, Kent BE. A new translucent cement for dentistry. The glass ionomer cement. Br Dent J. 1972;132:133-135.

3. Knobloch LA, Kerby RE, McMillen K, et al. Solubility and sorption of resin-based luting cements. Oper Dent. 2000;25:434-440.

4. Bagheri R, Taha NA, Azar MR, et al. Effect of G-Coat Plus on the mechanical properties of glass-ionomer cements. Aust Dent J. 2013;58:448-453.

5. Simon JF, Darnell LA. Consideration for proper selection of dental cements. Compend Contin Educ Dent. 2012;33:28–36.

6. Rueggeberg FA, Caughman WF. The influence of light exposure on polymerization of dual-cure resin cements. Oper Dent. 1993;18:48–55.

7. Suzuki S, Minami H. Evaluation of toothbrush and generalized wear of luting materials. Am J Dent. 2005;18:311-317.

8. Kumbuloglu O, Lassila LV, User A, et al. A study of the physical and chemical properties of four resin composite luting cements. Int J Prosthodont. 2004;17:357-363.

9. Radovic I, Monticelli F, Goracci C, et al. Self-adhesive resin cements: a literature review. J Adhes Dent. 2008;10:251-258.

10. Patil SG, Sajjan MS, Patil R. The effect of temperature on compressive and tensile strengths of commonly used luting cements: an in vitro study. J Int Oral Health. 2015;7:13-19.

11. Li ZC, White SN. Mechanical properties of dental luting cements. J Prosthet Dent. 1999;81:597-609.

12. Mese A, Burrow MF, Tyas MJ. Sorption and solubility of luting cements in different solutions. Dent Mater J. 2008;27:702-709.

13. Azar MR, Bagheri R, Burrow MF. Effect of storage media and time on the fracture toughness of resin-based luting cements. Aust Dent J. 2012;57:349-354.

14. Ortengren U, Elgh U, Spasenoska V, et al. Water sorption and flexural properties of a composite resin cement. Int J Prosthodont. 2000;13:141-147.

15. ISO 4049:2000 (E). Dentistry-polymer-based filling, restorative and luting materials; 7.12 Water sorption and solubility. International Organization for Standardization; 2000. Available

at: https://www.iso.org/standard/23041.html

16. Powers JM, Farah JW, O'Keefe KL, *et al*. Guide to all-ceramic bonding. Available from: http://www.Kuraraydental.com/guides/-item/guide-to-all-ceramic-bonding: 2013.

17. Oilo G. Early erosion of dental cements. Eur J Oral Sci. 1984;92:539-543.

18. Pearson GJ, Atkinson AS. Long-term flexural strength of glassionomer cements. Biomaterials. 1991;12:658-660.

19. Williams JA, Billington RW. Changes in compressive strength of glass-ionomer restorative materials with respect to time periods of 24 h to months. J Oral Rehabil. 1991;18:163-168.

20. Bagheri R, Mese A, Burrow MF , *et al*. Comparison of the effect of storage media on shear punch strength of resin luting cements. J Dent. 2010;38:820-827.

21. Fano L, Fano V, Ma W, *et al*. Hydrolytic degradation and cracks in resin-modified glass-ionomer cements. J Biomed Mater Res B Appl Biomater. 2004;69:87-93.

22. Nakamura T, Wakabayashi K, Kinuta S, *et al*. Mechanical properties of new self-adhesive resin-based cement. J Prosthodont Res.

2010;54:59-64.

23. Hyun-Jin Kim, Rafat Bagheri, Young Kyung Kim, Jun Sik Son, Tae-Yub Kwon. Influence of Curing Mode on the Surface Energy and Sorption/Solubility of Dental Self-Adhesive Resin Cements. Materials (Basel). 2017 Feb; 10: 129.

24. McCabe JF, Walls AW. Applied dental materials. 9th Edition. Blackwell: Oxford, UK; 2008. p. 274-285..

25. Oysaed H, Ruyter IE. Composites for use in posterior teeth: mechanical properties tested under dry and wet conditions. J Biomed Mater Res. 1986;20:261-271.

26. Ferracane JL, Berge HX, Condon JR. In vitro aging of dental composites in water – effect of degree of conversion, filler volume, and filler/matrix coupling. J Biomed Mater Res. 1998;42:465-472.

27. Wilson AD, McLean JW. Glass-ionomer cement. 1th edition. Chicago: Quintessence Publ Co.; 1988. p. 30-33

28. Phillips S, Bishop BM. An in vitro study of the effect of moisture on glass ionomer cement. Quintessence Int. 1985;16:175-177.

6

Assessment of the Mandibular Canal and Mental Foramen Variations Using Cone Beam Computed Tomography

Ghapanchi J[a]; Zangoei Boushehri M[b]; Haghnegahdar AA[c]; Nayyrain SH[d]; Shakibasefat H[e]; Paknahad M[f*]

[a]Associated Professor, Department of Oral and Maxillofacial Medicine, School of Dentistry, Shiraz University of Medical Sciences, Shiraz, Iran
[b]Oral and Maxillofacial Radiologist, Shiraz, Iran
[c]Assistant Professor, Department of Oral and Maxillofacial Radiology, School of Dentistry, Shiraz University of Medical Sciences, Shiraz, Iran
[d]Under graduate Student, Shiraz University of Medical Sciences, International Branch, Shiraz, Iran
[e]Postgrduate student, Department of oral and maxillofacial medicine, School of Dentistry , Shiraz University of Medical Sciences, Iran
[f]Assistant Professor, Oral and Dental Disease Research Center, Department of Oral and Maxillofacial Radiology, School of Dentistry, Shiraz University of Medical Sciences, Shiraz, Iran

ARTICLE INFO

Key words:
Cone Beam Computed Tomography (CBCT)
Mandibular Canal
Mental foramen

Corresponding Author:
Maryam Paknahad
Oral Radiology Department,
Shiraz Dental School,
Ghasrodasht Street, Shiraz Iran
Email: paknahadmaryam@
yahoo.com

Abstract

Statement of the Problem: It is crucial to have sufficient knowledge about inferior alveolar canal variations in mandibular surgeries. Anatomic imaging of the mandibular canal prior to surgical procedures such as implant placement and sagittal split osteotomy is essential for achieving the best results and confronting minimal complications.

Objectives: The aim of this study was to determine normal variations of the mandibular canal and mental foramen in a selected Iranian population.

Material and methods: This cross-sectional study was conducted on 334 cone beam computed tomography (CBCT) of patients , comprising of 119 males and 215 females , aged between 15-75 years (mean age, 45 ± 7.5 years). The prevalence of anterior loop, the level of mandibular canal cortication, and mental foramen variations were recorded on CBCT images.

Results: Statistical analysis showed no significant differences in the prevalence of the anterior loop and mental foramen variations in both sides regarding the age and gender ($p>0.05$). Anterior loop was detected in 90.5% of cases, while accessory mandibular canals were observed in 4.6% of the patients. More than one mental foramen was detected in 5 (4.2%) men and 17 (7.9%) women in the right side and in the left side; this was detected in 11(9.2%) men and 10 (4.7%) women. No significant differences were found in the number of mental foramen regarding to gender and age in both sides ($p>0.05$). A non-significant relationship was observed between the age groups, the gender, and the prevalence of accessory canals. Moreover, statistical analysis did not demonstrate a significant relationship between gender and mandibular canal cortication in both sides.

Conclusions: This study demonstrated that there were numerous anatomical variations of the mandibular canal, mental foramen and, anterior loop.

Introduction

The inferior alveolar canal transmits the inferior alveolar nerve and vessels supplying the mandibular teeth and adjacent structures. It is a hollow space surrounded by bony tissue extending from the mandibular foramen posteriorly toward the mental foramen anteriorly [1]. Knowledge about the accurate position and course of the mandibular canal within the mandible and identifying the anatomical variations are very important for preventing potential complications such as neurosensory disturbances that may occur during surgical dental procedures such as endodontic therapy and implant placement [2]. Injury to inferior alveolar nerve may occur frequently due to the proximity of the lower first and second molar roots to the inferior alveolar canal during extraction of these teeth [3]. Paresthesia of the inferior alveolar nerve after obturation of the teeth during endodontic treatment was also reported [4]. In previous studies, different imaging modalities have been applied for assessment of the normal variation of the anatomy of the mandibular canal including conventional radiographs [1, 5, 6], computed tomography (CT) [7-10] and cone beam computed tomography (CBCT) [11-15]. Conventional radiographs have several limitations including limited reproducibility, magnification and distortion [9]. These techniques only represent two- dimensional (2D) position of the canal and do not demonstrate the buccolingual position of the canal [16]. CBCT is a new accurate modality for three-dimensional (3D) reconstruction of the imaging of dental and maxillofacial structures without any superimposition or magnification [17-20]. A few studies have evaluated the anatomic variations of the mandibular canal and mental foramen using CBCT [21-24]. The purpose of the present study was to evaluate the variations of the mandibular canal and mental foramen in a selected Iranian population using CBCT.

Materials and Methods

The present study was approved by the Institutional Review Board. This cross-sectional study was conducted on CBCT images of 334 patients (119 males and 215 females) aged between 15-75 years (mean age, 45±7.5 years) who were referred to a private oral and maxillofacial radiology center for various reasons from 2012 to 2016. Patients with maxillofacial deformities, pathologic conditions or positive history of fracture or any previous manipulation, which could change the position of inferior alveolar canal, were excluded. All images were taken by Planmeca Promax 3D MID (Helsinki/ Finland). The adjusted scan parameters were 60- 90 KVp and 1 -14 mA depending on the size of the patients. The exposure time was 14 seconds, effective exposure time was 2–6 seconds, and voxel size was 150μm. The CBCTs were analyzed by an oral and maxillofacial radiologist on LG LED computer viewer (E2042C, Korea) using Romexis viewer software. The prevalence of anterior loop, the accessory canals, the level of corticalization of the mandibular canal, and the mental foramen variations were identified in cross-sectional and axial views. Statistical analyses were carried out using SPSS 18 (SPSS, Chicago, IL, USA). Fisher exact test was used to analyze the relationship between age and recorded items. Pearson Chi-square at the significance level of p<0.05 was used to evaluate the relationship between gender and the anatomical variations of the inferior alveolar canal.

Results

The prevalence of the anterior loop regarding gender in the left and right side is presented in Table 1. There were no significant differences in the prevalence of anterior loop regarding gender in both sides of the mandible. The prevalence of the number of mental foramen in the left and right sides is presented in Table 2. Single right mental foramens were found in 114 (95.8%) men and 198 (92.1%) women. More than one foramen (Figure 1) was detected in 5 (4.2%) men and 17 (7.9%)

Table 1: The prevalence of anterior loop regarding gender in the left and right sides

Side	Gender Male	Female	P-value
Left	108(90.8%)	194(90.2%)	0.876
Right	107(89.9%)	196 (91.2%)	0.707

Table 2: The anatomic variation of the mental foramen in the left and right sides

	Mental foramen		
Side	Solitary	Double	More than 2
Left	313(93.7%)	18(5.4%)	3(0.9%)
Right	312(93.4%)	16 (4.8%)	6(1.8%)

women. Solitary left mental foramen was detected in 108 (90.8%) men and 205 (95.3%) women. More than one foramen was detected in 11(9.2%) men and 10 (4.7%) women. No significant differences were found in the anatomic variation of mental foramen regarding to gender in the left (p=0.228) and right sides (p=0.191). 285 patients (93.1%) of 15-45 years old group and 29 (96.7%) of older group had one mental foramen on the right side. On the left side, 285 images (93.8%) of the15-45-year-old group and 28(93.3%) of the older group had single mental foramen. Statistical analysis did not show a significant relationship between age and the frequency of mental foramen on the right (p=0.451) and left sides (p=0.929). The incidence of accessory canals in the right and left sides regarding to gender is presented in Table 3.A non-significant relationship was also found between gender and prevalence of accessory canal on the right side (Table 3). A total of 304 patients (91%) were 15-45 (group1) years old and 30 cases (9%) were more than 45 years old (group 2). The accessory canals were not found in 288 (94.7%) patients in the 15-45-year-old group and 28 (93.3%) of the older group. A non-significant relationship was observed between the age groups and prevalence of accessory canals (p=0.745). The

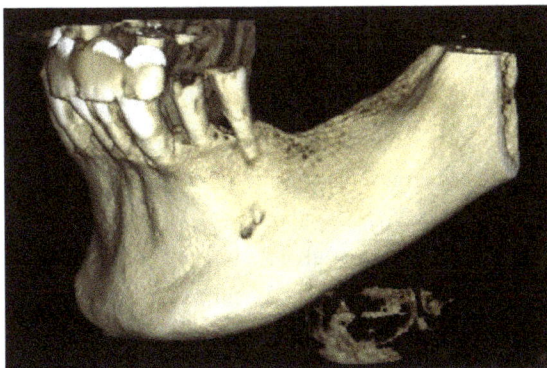

Figure 1: Double mental foramen in a sample patient

upper and lower cortication of the right mandibular canal were detected in 42 (35.3%) males and 58 (27%) females, and lower or upper cortication in 42 (35.3%) male and 71 (33%) females and in 7 men (5.9%) and 16 women (7.4%) in some instances. Upper and lower cortication on the left side was observed in 47 men (39.5%) and 62 (28.8%) women. Lower or upper cortication was detected in 34 (26.8%) males and 68 (31.6%) females, and finally in 27 (22.7%) male and 64 (29.8%) female no cortication was detected. Statistical analysis did not demonstrate a significant relationship between gender and mandibular canal cortication on the right (p=0.232) and left sides (p=0.228).

Table 3: The prevalence of accessory canals regarding gender in the left and right sides

	Gender		
Side	Male	Female	P-value
Left	4 (3.4%)	14 (6.5%)	0.222
Right	6 (5%)	12 (5.6%)	0.834

Discussion

The present study provided information about the variations in the mandibular neurovascularization that must be identified to decrease the potential risk for hemorrhages and neural disturbances during surgical procedures such as implant placement and orthognathic surgeries. Verification of the existence of accessory mental foramina is important for prevention of accessory nerve damage with subsequent neurosensory impairment during periapical surgery and anesthetic applications [25, 26]. In the current research, the results showed that 12.8% of patients had accessory mental foramina that were higher than previous reports. In previous studies, the accessory mental foramen was observed in 9.2% [22], 3% [27], 6.5% [26], 7% of patients [23] in CBCT images. This variation in the prevalence of accessory mental foramen in studies, which used the same detection method (CBCT), may be due to the difference in the sample size and the racial variation of the patients studied. To avoid injuring the mental nerve, it is essential to evaluate whether an anterior loop of the mental nerve or the incisive canal lies mesial to it [28]. Apostolakis *et al.* showed that an anterior loop could be identified in 48% of the cases with a mean length of 0.89 mm (0-5.7) [21]. In this study, the anterior loop was found in a large number of the images (on right side of 303 and left side of 302 patients).

Powcharoen and Chinkrua suggested that the absence of mandibular canal cortication has high sensitivity and specificity for predicting intraoperative IAN exposure during third molar surgery [29]. In this research, mandibular canal cortication was the prominent finding in most of the cases. Corticalization of the mandibular canal was observed in 59% of hemimandibles in the study by de Oliveira-Santos *et al.* [24]. No cortication was seen on the left sides of 27.2% patients and right side of 29.3% ones. Large variations exist in the size of mandibular accessory foramina. They may be as small as 0.1 mm or reach a width of more than 1.5 mm and often resemble the original foramina in size. Smaller foramina have seldom been measured because they are indistinguishable from the normal porous appearance. Furthermore, variations also exist in relation to their number. Some mandibles may have none, while in rare instances in one mandible up to 100 foramina were observed. Most studies agree that the majority of foramina are concentrated in the posterior areas of the mandible and to a lesser degree in the symphysis, and are much more frequent on the internal than the external surface of the mandible [30]. The incidences of accessory canals in the retromolar area of the right side were 4.8% (16 cases) and 4.5% (15 cases) in the left side (Figure 2). The frequency of retromolar canal (RMC) in CBCT images has been reported to be 8.5% in Korean, 28.1% in Turkish [31] and 52% (37% of sides) in the Japanese populations [32]. Previous studies suggested that panoramic radiograph is not a suitable imaging modality for assessment of RMC because of the superimposition of various structures over the area. CBCT images provide 3D images without any superimpositions and with higher resolution. Moreover, von Arx *et al.* reported a prevalence of 25.6% of RMC in CBCT and showed that among 31 RMC observed in CBCT, panoramic radiographs were able to identify just 7 cases (5.7% of samples) [33]. Similarly, Muinelo-Lorenzo *et al.* [34] demonstrated that only 32.5%

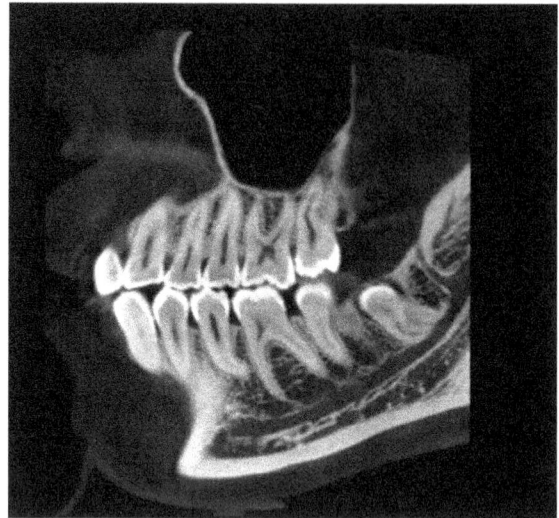

Figure 2: Retromolar accessory canal in a sample patient

of RMFs detected on CBCT images were found on panoramic radiographs. Furthermore, Sisman *et al.* found 253 RMC (26.7%) on 947 sides of CBCT images while only 29 RMC were seen on panoramic radiographs (3.1%) [35].

Conclusions

This study showed that that there were numerous anatomical variations in the normal anatomy of the mandibular canal and the mental foramen. Dentists should be familiar with these variations in order to prevent treatment complications. CBCT provides an effective tool for pre-surgical evaluation of the neurovascular structures and its variations.

Conflict of Interest: None declared.

References

1. Ylikontiola L, Moberg K, Huumonen S, *et al.* Comparison of three radiographic methods used to locate the mandibular canal in the buccolingual direction before bilateral sagittal split osteotomy. Oral Surg Oral Med Oral Pathol Oral Radiol Endod. 2002;93:736-42.
2. Saralaya V, Narayana K. The relative position of the inferior alveolar nerve in cadaveric hemi-mandibles. Eur J Anat. 2005;9:49-53.
3. Kipp DP, Goldstein BH, Weiss WW Jr. Dysesthesia after mandibular third molar surgery: a retrospective study and analysis of

1,377 surgical procedures. J Am Dent Assoc. 1980;100:185-92.

4. Brodin P. Neurotoxic and analgesic effects of root canal cements and pulp-protecting dental materials. Dent Traumatol. 1988;4:1-11.

5. Klinge B, Petersson A, Maly P. Location of the mandibular canal: comparison of macroscopic findings, conventional radiography, and computed tomography. Int J Oral Maxillofac Implants. 1988;4:327-32.

6. Liu T, Xia B, Gu Z. Inferior alveolar canal course: a radiographic study. Clin Oral Implants Res. 2009;20:1212-8.

7. Yoshioka I, Tanaka T, Khanal A, et al. Relationship between inferior alveolar nerve canal position at mandibular second molar in patients with prognathism and possible occurrence of neurosensory disturbance after sagittal split ramus osteotomy. J Oral Maxillofac Surg. 2010;68:3022-7.

8. Yoshioka I, Tanaka T, Habu M, et al. Effect of bone quality and position of the inferior alveolar nerve canal in continuous, long-term, neurosensory disturbance after sagittal split ramus osteotomy. J Craniomaxillofac Surg. 2012;40:e178-e83.

9. Yu IH, Wong YK. Evaluation of mandibular anatomy related to sagittal split ramus osteotomy using 3-dimensional computed tomography scan images. Int J Oral Maxillofac Surg. 2008;37:521-8.

10. Wittwer G, Adeyemo WL, Beinemann J, et al. Evaluation of risk of injury to the inferior alveolar nerve with classical sagittal split osteotomy technique and proposed alternative surgical techniques using computer-assisted surgery. Int J Oral Maxillofac Surg. 2012;41:79-86.

11. Huang CS, Syu JJ, Ko EW, et al. Quantitative evaluation of cortical bone thickness in mandibular prognathic patients with neurosensory disturbance after bilateral sagittal split osteotomy. J Oral Maxillofac Surg. 2013;71:2153. e1-. e10.

12. Angel JS, Mincer HH, Chaudhry J, et al. Cone-beam Computed Tomography for Analyzing Variations in Inferior Alveolar Canal Location in Adults in Relation to Age and Sex. J Forensic Sci. 2011;56:216-9.

13. Balaji SM, Krishnaswamy NR, Kumar SM, et al. Inferior alveolar nerve canal position among South Indians: A cone beam computed tomographic pilot study. Ann Maxillofac Surg. 2012;2:51-55.

14. Adibi S, Paknahad M. Comparison of cone-beam computed tomography and osteometric examination in preoperative assessment of the proximity of the mandibular canal to the apices of the teeth. Br J Oral Maxillofac Surg. 2017;55:246-250.

15. Khorshidi H, Raoofi S, Ghapanchi J, et al. Cone Beam Computed Tomographic Analysis of the Course and Position of Mandibular Canal. J Maxillofac Oral Surg. 2017;16:306-311.

16. Simonton JD, Azevedo B, Schindler WG, et al. Age-and gender-related differences in the position of the inferior alveolar nerve by using cone beam computed tomography. J Endod. 2009;35:944-9.

17. Shahidi S, Vojdani M, Paknahad M. Correlation between articular eminence steepness measured with cone-beam computed tomography and clinical dysfunction index in patients with temporomandibular joint dysfunction. Oral Surg Oral Med Oral Pathol Oral Radiol. 2013;116:91-7.

18. Paknahad M, Shahidi S. Association between mandibular condylar position and clinical dysfunction index. J Craniomaxill Surg. 2015;43:432-6.

19. Paknahad M, Shahidi S, Akhlaghian M, et al. Is Mandibular Fossa Morphology and Articular Eminence Inclination Associated with Temporomandibular Dysfunction? J Dent(shiraz). 2016;17:134-141.

20. Paknahad M, Shahidi S, Abbaszade H. Correlation between condylar position and different sagittal skeletal facial types. J Orofac Orthop. 2016;77:350-6.

21. Apostolakis D, Brown JE. The anterior loop of the inferior alveolar nerve: prevalence, measurement of its length and a recommendation for interforaminal implant installation based on cone beam CT imaging. Clin Oral Implants Res. 2012;23:1022-30.

22. Oliveira-Santos C, Souza PH, De Azambuja Berti-Couto S, et al. Characterisation of

additional mental foramina through cone beam computed tomography. J Oral Rehabil. 2011;38:595-600.

23. Naitoh M, Hiraiwa Y, Aimiya H, *et al.* Accessory mental foramen assessment using cone-beam computed tomography. Oral Surg Oral Med Oral Pathol Oral Radiol Endod. 2009;107:289-94.

24. de Oliveira-Santos C, Souza PH, de Azambuja Berti-Couto S, *et al.* Assessment of variations of the mandibular canal through cone beam computed tomography. Clin Oral Investig. 2012;16:387-93.

25. Katakami K, Mishima A, Shiozaki K, *et al.* Characteristics of accessory mental foramina observed on limited cone-beam computed tomography images. J Endod. 2008;34:1441-5.

26. Kalender A, Orhan K, Aksoy U. Evaluation of the mental foramen and accessory mental foramen in Turkish patients using cone-beam computed tomography images reconstructed from a volumetric rendering program. Clin Anat. 2012;25:584-92.

27. Imada TS, Fernandes LM, Centurion BS, *et al.* Accessory mental foramina: prevalence, position and diameter assessed by cone-beam computed tomography and digital panoramic radiographs. Clin Oral Implants Res. 2014;25:e94-9.

28. Rosa MB, Sotto-Maior BS, Machado Vde C, *et al.* Retrospective study of the anterior loop of the inferior alveolar nerve and the incisive canal using cone beam computed tomography. Int J Oral Maxillofac Implants. 2013;28:388-

92.

29. Powcharoen W, Chinkrua C. Cone beam computed tomographic assessment of mandibular canal as predictors of intraoperative nerve exposure after third molar surgery. Int J Oral Maxillofac Surg. 2015;44:e125.

30. Haveman CW, Tebo HG. Posterior accessory foramina of the human mandible. J Prosthet Dent. 1976;35:462-8.

31. Orhan K, Aksoy S, Bilecenoglu B, *et al.* Evaluation of bifid mandibular canals with cone-beam computed tomography in a Turkish adult population: a retrospective study. Surg Radiol Anat. 2011;33:501-7.

32. Kawai T, Asaumi R, Sato I, *et al.* Observation of the retromolar foramen and canal of the mandible: a CBCT and macroscopic study. Oral Radiol. 2012;28:10-4.

33. Von Arx T, Hänni A, Sendi P, *et al.* Radiographic study of the mandibular retromolar canal: an anatomic structure with clinical importance. J Endod. 2011;37:1630-5.

34. Muinelo-Lorenzo J, Suárez-Quintanilla J, Fernández-Alonso A, *et al.* Descriptive study of the bifid mandibular canals and retromolar foramina: cone beam CT vs panoramic radiography. Dentomaxillofac Radiol. 2014;43:20140090.

35. Sisman Y, Ercan-Sekerci A, Payveren-Arıkan M, *et al.* Diagnostic accuracy of cone-beam CT compared with panoramic images in predicting retromolar canal during extraction of impacted mandibular third molars. Med oral Patol oral Cir Bucal. 2015;20:e74-e81.

7

Recent Advances and Future Perspectives for Reinforcement of Poly(methyl methacrylate) Denture Base Materials

Abdulrazzaq Naji S[a]; Jafarzadeh Kashi T[b]; Behroozibakhsh M[c*]; Hajizamani H[d]; Habibzadeh S[e]

[a]Ph.D Student , Foundation of Technical Education, College of Health and Medical Technology, Baghdad, Iraq and Department of Dental Biomaterials, School of Dentistry, International Campus, Tehran University of Medical Sciences, Tehran, Iran
[b]Associate professor , Iranian Tissue Bank and Research Center, Department of Dental Biomaterials, School of Dentistry, Tehran University of Medical Sciences, Tehran, Iran
[c]Assistant professor, Research Center for Science and Technology in Medicine, Department of Dental Biomaterials, School of Dentistry, Tehran University of Medical Sciences, Tehran, Iran
[d]Ph.D Student, Research Center for Science and Technology in Medicine, Department of Dental Biomaterials, School of Dentistry, Tehran University of Medical Sciences, Tehran, Iran
[e]Assistant Professor, Department of Prosthodontics, Tehran University of Medical Sciences, International Campus, School of Dentistry, Tehran, Iran

ARTICLE INFO

Key words:
Denture base materials
Poly(methyl methacrylate)
Reinforcement

Corresponding Author:
Marjan Behroozibakhsh
Assistant professor, Department of Dental Biomaterials, School of Dentistry, Tehran University of Medical Sciences, Tehran, Iran
Email: behroozibakhsh@tums.ac.ir

Abstract

Poly(methyl methacrylate) (PMMA) is the most common material used to fabricate complete and partial dentures. Despite its desirable properties, it cannot fulfill all mechanical requirements of prosthesis. Flexural fatigue due to repeated masticatory and high-impact forces caused by dropping are the main causes of denture fractures. In the past, different reinforcing agents such as rubbers, macro fibers, and fillers have been employed to improve the mechanical properties of denture base resins. Development of Nano dentistry has introduced new approaches for reinforcement of dental materials. Interest in nanostructure materials is driven by their high surface area to volume ratio, which enhances interfacial interaction and specific new biological, physical, and chemical properties. Researchers to reinforce PMMA resins have used Nanoparticles (Nps) which were comprised of silver, Titania (TiO_2), zirconia (ZrO_2), alumina, and ceramic. Although different reports describe the use of nanofiber and nanotubes in dental composites, few studies have evaluated the reinforcement potential of nanofiber and nanotubes in PMMA denture base resins. The current article aims to review the different attempts to enhance the mechanical properties of denture base materials. We also focus on recent advances and potential future developments for reinforcement of the PMMA acrylic resins.

Introduction

Poly(methyl methacrylate)(PMMA)was introduced in 1937 by Wright [1]. PMMA has been extensively used as a denture base material because of its desirable properties. Satisfying aesthetics, ease of processing, durability, chemical stability, light weight, and acceptable cost are some of the favorable properties. Despite these characteristics, the denture base materials do not have sufficient mechanical properties for every intended purpose. Flexural fatigue due to repeated masticatory forces and high-impact forces caused by dropping the prosthesis are the main intraoral and extraoral causes of denture fractures, respectively [2]. Flexural fatigue occurs consequent to repeated flexing and can be described as growth and propagation of microcracks in the stress concentration areas [3]. Midline fractures, which are a common problem for patients who wear maxillary complete dentures, usually occur due to cyclic deformation consequent to flexural fatigue. A survey by Darbar et al.[4] has reported that 29% of failures in dentures occurred at the midline labial frenum. Impact failures usually happen as a result of accidental dropping during cleaning, coughing or sneezing, or sudden strokes to the denture [3]. Therefore, the ability of a denture base material to withstand crack propagation and impact forces is an important factor which affects its performance. Hence, there is a need for enhancement of the mechanical properties of PMMA based materials to achieve stronger and more fracture-resistant dentures [5]. Chemical modification and the addition of some fibers, fillers, and rubberlike substances are different methods introduced to improve the mechanical properties of PMMA-based materials. [3] Here, we provide a general background about different attempts to improve the mechanical properties of denture base materials, and review recent advances and potential future developments for reinforcement of the PMMA acrylic resins.

Discussion

Rubbers, fibers and fillers

In this section, we review different attempts that have been launched during past decades to improve the mechanical properties of denture base resins.

Rubbers, different fibers, and fillers are some additives employed to reinforce dental resins. In addition, we mention the latest advances for each reinforcing agent.

Rubber reinforced poly(methyl methacrylate) (PMMA)

Adequate impact strength and fracture toughness are 2 of the most important requirements for denture based resins. One of the main drawbacks of PMMA denture bases is low fracture toughness; thus, the conventional denture base polymers are susceptible to breakage with high mastication forces and during accidents. Many studies have been performed to evaluate the toughness and mechanisms of toughness improvement in rubber-modified acrylic polymers [6, 7]. In rubber-reinforced polymers, the resin matrix is filled with a rubbery particle which has a modulus of elasticity lower than that of the polymer matrix and a higher Poisson's ratio than the matrix. Therefore the reinforced polymer will have a lower modulus and a higher Poisson's ratio compared to the unmodified polymer. The most significant advantage of this modification is an increase in toughness as well as ultimate elongation in comparison with the relatively brittle resin acrylic material [8]. In this structure, the rate of crack propagation through the PMMA will decelerate at the interface of the rubber and resin since the rubber reinforced resins can absorb greater amounts of energy compared to the unmodified resins. One problem of these reinforced dentures is increased flexibility due to low Young's modulus [3].Rodford [6, 7] has described the development of high impact strength denture base materials using butadiene-styrene rubber. Butadiene-styrene is a low molecular weight rubber (15-35 000), which has the advantage of up to 30% incorporation in PMMA without excessive increase in viscosity. This polymer contains reactive (acrylate) end groups which facilitate grafting to the PMMA.Alhareb et al. [9, 10] have suggested that nitrile butadiene rubber (NBR) particles and treated ceramic fillers could improve impact and fracture resistance of heat-polymerized PMMA denture base resins. This research concluded that the optimum addition of the filler in the polymer matrix was 7.5% NBR together with 2.5% Al_2O_3(Alumina)/2.5% YSZ(Yttria-stabilized zirconia). They proposed that in cases that need high impact strength and fracture toughness, reinforcement of PMMA denture base by NBR with ceramic fillers could be the best choice for removable prosthodontics.

Fibers

Polymer fiber composites are materials composed of a polymer matrix and a reinforcement fiber, which is the stronger Constituent of the composite. In a polymer fiber composite, the fibers are embedded in a polymer matrix. The polymer matrix forms a continuous phase that surrounds the fibers; thus, the applied loads are transferred from the polymer matrix to the fibers. One of the most important factors that affect the strength of the composite is proper adhesion of the fibers to the polymer matrix. This adhesion makes it possible to transfer the stresses from the matrix to the fibers. The stiffness of the fibers is an important characteristic for strengthening of brittle materials like denture base resins. Impregnation of the fibers into the polymer matrix is another important factor which affects the strength of the fiber reinforced composite [11]. In some studies, reinforcement of denture PMMA resin has failed due to the stress concentrations around the embedded fibers. This phenomenon often happens as the result of poor distribution of the reinforced fibers and bad adhesion between resin matrix and fibers. Nylon fibers are one of the fibers used as a reinforcing agent for PMMA due to their resistance to shock and frequent stressing, high resistance to abrasion and creep, elastic memory, and cyclic stress conductivity [12]. Larson *et al.* have reported the use of carbon fibers to improve the strength of denture bases [13]. Carbon fiber is applied in many studies to improve the mechanical properties of the matrix because of its inherent high strength and optimal combination of the carbon fibers and matrix [14]. Mainly, carbon fibers have been used to enhance fatigue and impact strength [15]. Despite good mechanical properties, cytotoxicity of carbon fibers is problematic [15]. Moderate cytotoxicity has been determined by Özen *et al.* [16] for heat-polymerized acrylic resin reinforced with both glass and carbon fiber. The aramid fibers, which have high resistance to impact forces, are another agent for reinforcing denture base materials. They have excellent wettability compared to carbon fibers

and do not need treatment by a coupling agent. Biological evaluations have shown no evidence for any cyto-genotoxic effects of aramid fibers [17]. Disadvantages of these fibers include their yellow hue and poor adhesion to acrylic resin materials. It is also reported that the rough surfaces of materials reinforced with aramid fibers are difficult to polish as the result of exposed fibers at the surface of the material [18]. Recently, a novel botryoidal aramid fiber reinforcement of a PMMA resin was introduced by Xinye *et al.* [19]. In this research, they achieved a homogeneous fiber distribution in the resin matrix by separation of each fiber via grafting of microspheres to aramid fibers. The researchers proposed that this new approach could successfully improve the mechanical properties of fiber reinforced composites along with acceptable safety in vitro. However, they suggested that more experimentation would be required to fully evaluate the long-term mechanical performance and biocompatibility of this novel composite in vivo. Glass fibers have been considered as reinforcing materials for denture base resins because of their excellent aesthetics, superior strength, and good biocompatibility [20]. Jaikumar *et al.* [21] found that higher flexural strength of the acrylic resin specimens reinforced with glass fibers compared to high impact denture base resins. The same results were reported by Hamouda *et al.* in 2014 [22]. Unalan *et al.* [23] stated that the form of glass fiber could affect the transverse strength of reinforced denture base resins. They obtained the highest transverse strength in samples reinforced with chopped strand mat form. Vallittu *et al.* [24] evaluated the effect of fiber concentration on fracture resistance of acrylic resin and observed better enhancement in fracture resistance of resin-modified materials at higher concentrations of glass fibers. Sang-Hui *et al.* [25] evaluated the effects of glass fiber mesh with different amount of fibers and various structures on the mechanical properties of dentures. They concluded that the content of the glass fiber mesh was more important than the structure, and determined that between 4.35 and 4.73 vol% was the most effective concentration. Nagakura *et al.* [26] reported that the flexural modulus of glass-fiber-reinforced thermoplastics (GFRTPs) use in removable partial dentures (RPDs) increased from 1.75 to 7.42 GPa with increased glass fiber content from 0 to 50 mass%, such that the flexural strength and modulus of GFRTP with a fiber content of 50 mass% were 3.9 and 4.2 times, respectively, of unreinforced polypropylene. The position of glass fibers in resin matrix could also affect the mechanical properties. It has been reported that placing the fibers normal to the loading force could enhance the mechanical properties [27]. Goguta et al. [28] reported that impact strength of PMMA reinforced with stick glass fibers significantly increased when stick fibers were placed parallel to the long axis of the specimen and perpendicularly to the force direction. The mechanical properties of PMMA reinforced with glass fibers also depends on good adhesion between fibers and the resin matrix. In order to achieve better adhesion, glass fibers are treated with silane coupling agent before loading into the resin matrix. Several studies have reported that the reinforced resins with silane-treated fibers have higher transverse strength and fracture resistance than acrylics that have untreated glass fibers [29, 30].

Fillers

Metals in various forms such as wires, plates, and fillers have been incorporated into PMMA to improve thermal conductivity and radiopacity, as well as mechanical properties. One of the disadvantages of PMMA is its low thermal conductivity. The high thermal conductivity of denture bases leads to improved tissue health, a better sense of taste, and reduction of the foreign body feeling of dentures. Various studies have added metal fillers to improve the thermal conductivity of acrylic resins [31, 32]. The reinforcement of polymers used in dentistry with metal strengtheners has been considered by many researchers. [31-33] One of the drawbacks of metal fillers is that they do not chemically bond to resins. Different efforts have been made to enhance the adhesion between the metal to resin matrix such as silanization, sandblasting, and metal adhesive resins [3]. The incorporation of metals as a reinforcement agent into PMMA have limited value because of the negative effects on esthetics, stress concentration, and minor influence of metal wires on flexural fatigue resistance [3]. Ceramic fillers are also incorporated as reinforcing fillers in PMMA denture base resins. Silicon dioxide (SiO_2), commonly used reinforcing filler in dental materials,

has been used as filler in elastomers and composite resins. However, McNally et al. [34] reported that the addition of untreated and surface treated silica could not be recommended as a reinforcing agent for denture base resins. Hydroxyapatite (HA), $Ca_{10}(PO_4)_6(OH)_2$, is another filler employed in different dental materials. Incorporation of HA fillers into PMMA resin has resulted in supe¬rior mechanical properties including flexural strength and modulus [35]. However, the mechanical properties of PMMA reinforced with HA could be limited because of the incompatibility between the PMMA and HA. Modification of the composite has been proposed to improve the interfacial interaction between the HA filler and PMMA [36, 37]. Tham et al. [37] suggested that the silane coupling agent [3-methacryloxypropyltrimethoxy silane (γ-MPS)] could significantly enhance the mechanical and thermal properties of the PMMA/HA composite due to enhanced adhesion between HA particles and the resin matrix. Reinforcement of denture base resins using mica has also been proposed in some studies [38]. Muscovite mica, a hydrated silicate, is the most common type of mica. It is predominately white. Muscovite mica is commonly employed for reinforcement of polymers. Incorporation of mica into polymeric matrix increases stiffness, strength, scratch resistance, dimensional stability, and lowers the coefficient of linear thermal expansion. [39]. Unalan et al. have evaluated the effects of different ratios of silanized mica filler on the surface hardness of a denture tooth material and obtained the best surface hardness value by the addition of 10% mica and 10% glass to the denture teeth material [40].

Nanoscaled reinforcement materials

The concept of nanotechnology was first introduced in 1959 by Feynman. Since then, nanotechnology has been widely used in many applications, including medical sciences, and plays an important role in diagnosis, treatment, and regenerative medicine [41]. A nanomaterial is an object, which at least one of its dimensions is at the nanometer scale (approximately 1 to 100 nm). Nanomaterials are categorized according to dimension – those with all 3 dimensions less than 100 nm [nanoparticles (Nps) and quantum dots]; those that have 2 dimensions less than 100 nm (nanotubes, nanofibers, and nanowires); and those that have one dimension less than 100 nm (thin films, layers, and coatings) [42]. The development of nanodentistry has led to nearly perfect oral health by the use of nanomaterials and biotechnologies, including nanorobots and tissue engineering. New opportunities in the field of dentistry include local anesthesia, treatment of dentin hypersensitivity, use of nanomaterials in preventive dentistry, and use of different nanofillers and nanofibers in composites to achieve better esthetics and mechanical properties [43]. Here, we focus on new applications of nanomaterials for reinforcement of PMMA dental base materials.

Nanofillers

Recently, researchers have proposed the incorporation of nanofillers for reinforcement of denture base resins. Size, shape, surface area, concentration, and dispersion of nanofillers into resin matrix all affect the mechanical properties of the filler/resin composite. Alumina NPs, zirconia (ZrO_2) NPs, titania (TiO_2) NPs, silver NPs, gold NPs, Pt NPs, HA NPs, SiO_2 NPs, and nanoclay particles are among the fillers that have been introduced to enhance the mechanical properties of denture base acrylics [35]. Here, we focus on some of the most common reinforced nanofillers that have been used for prosthodontics approaches. Silver Nps have been considered due to their distinctive physical, chemical, and biological properties, including high electrical and thermal conductivity, chemical stability, and non-linear optical behavior. It has been reported that silver Nps exhibit broad-spectrum bactericidal and fungicidal activities at very low concentrations [44]. Controversial results have been reported about the influence of silver NPs on the mechanical properties of denture base resins. [45, 46]. More studies should be conducted to evaluate the effects of different concentrations of silver Nps on various types of acrylic resins. The benefit of antibacterial properties of silver Nps has not been wiped out by the adverse effect on the mechanical properties of the denture base material. Modification of polymers with nanoscaled TiO_2 have also been of interest with researchers because of its unique properties. Pleasing color, high biocompatibility, excellent mechanical properties, low cost, high stability, and appropriate antimicrobial effects are among the

desirable properties which make TiO_2 a favorable additive for biomaterials [47]. TiO_2 Nps have been used as an additive to improve both mechanical and antibacterial properties of different dental materials [48]. TiO_2 exhibits great oxidizing power under UV radiation, and can decompose organic materials and bacteria. It has been reported that powdered TiO_2 can kill Streptococcus mutans, Escherichia coli, and Candida albicans [49].Controversial results have been reported by different researchers about the effect of TiO_2 Nps on mechanical properties of acrylic resins [50, 51]. Good wettability between fillers and the matrix is an important factor in order to improve the composite's properties. It has been shown that incorporation of silanized TiO_2 NPs in PMMA resin matrix increases the impact strength, transverse strength, and surface hardness of the resin [50, 52]. Different attempts have made to add ZrO_2 Nps to PMMA denture base material to improve the mechanical properties. Gad et al. [53] reported higher transverse strength in reinforced samples with ZrO_2 Nps compared to unreinforced repaired resin. They suggested that ZrO_2 Nps might be considered as a new approach for denture base repair. Asopa et al. [54] reported similar results with significantly higher transverse strength in the reinforced specimens that used ZrO_2 Nps compared to the control group. In their study, incorporation of ZrO_2 Nps into resin matrix adversely affected the impact strength and surface hardness. Ahmed et al. [55] also reported enhanced flexural strength, fracture toughness, and hardness in heat-polymerized acrylic modified by the addition of zirconium oxide nanofillers. The improved mechanical properties could be attributed to particle sizes of the ZrO_2 Nps. Also, the phase transformation of ZrO_2 from tetragonal to monoclinic absorbs the energy of crack propagation in a procedure called transformation toughening. Good distribution and surface treatment such as silanization of nano-size particles may affect their reinforcing effect [53]. It has been proposed that Nps have to be distributed evenly within the resin matrix; otherwise, they may adversely affect the mechanical properties of the resin composite at higher concentrations of added fillers due to the agglomeration of ZrO_2 Nps [53, 56].

Nanofibers

Different reports have described the nanofiber-reinforced effect in dental composites [57, 58]. Based on our findings, few studies have evaluated the reinforcement potential of nanofibers in PMMA denture base resins. Glass nanofibers, HA nanofibers, fibrillar silicate, and polymeric nanofibers have been introduced for reinforcement of dental materials [59]. It has been suggested that extreme reduction in fiber diameter size to the nanometer scale causes improvements in strength, modulus, and toughness. Fibers are the preferred reinforced materials compared to particles since they can provide a larger area for load transfer and promote toughening mechanisms such as fiber bridging and fiber pullout (Figure 1) [60]. One of the limitations for the use of nanofibers as a reinforcing agent is their incomplete wetting by resin, which compromises strength as the result of air inclusion and voids [61]. Another drawback of nanofibers is inadequate dispersion into the resin matrix that leads to the creation of bundles. These bundles may even act as defects and adversely influence the mechanical properties of the resin matrix and resultant composite [62]. Glass nanofibers are among the nanofibers introduced in the field of dentistry. Amorphous SiO_2 (glass) is used in commercially available dental composites because most requirements of dental composites could be obtained by the addition of appropriate amounts of glass. In addition, the refractive index of glass approximates that of dental resins and consequently gives a translucent appearance to the dental composite, which is similar to the structure of human teeth. Conventionally, dental resin composites are modified with glass particles that

range from tens of nanometers to several microns. Despite these properties, the mechanical properties of the glass particle reinforced composites are not adequate for use in large stress-bearing areas. The electrospun glass nanofibers are expected to improve the mechanical properties of dental resins considerably more than micron-scaled glass particles/fibers. The nano-scaled glass fibers have desired properties of small fiber diameter, large aspect ratio, and high mechanical properties. When a micro-crack in the dental resin matrix is formed under an applied stress across the crack planes, the thin and long nano-scaled glass fibers remain intact and support the applied load. Therefore, crack propagation is inhibited by the fibers with simultaneous reinforcement of the matrix. In comparison with micron-sized glass fibers, the glass nanofibers are over 10-times thinner and contain significant surface Si–OH groups that can readily interact with different silane coupling agents. Consequently, the interfacial bonding between the resin matrix and the nanoscaled silanized glass fiber can be extremely powerful [59, 63].HA is another reinforcing agent used in forms of particles and fibers in numerous dental materials due to its mineral releasing effect, biocompatibility, and strength [64, 65]. Mechanical performances of dental resins could be reinforced using inorganic fibers such as HA nanofibers. Good dispersion of HA nanofibers into a resin matrix at low mass can significantly improve the mechanical properties of the composite, while a higher mass fraction of the nanofibers cannot effectively reinforce the resin due to the formation

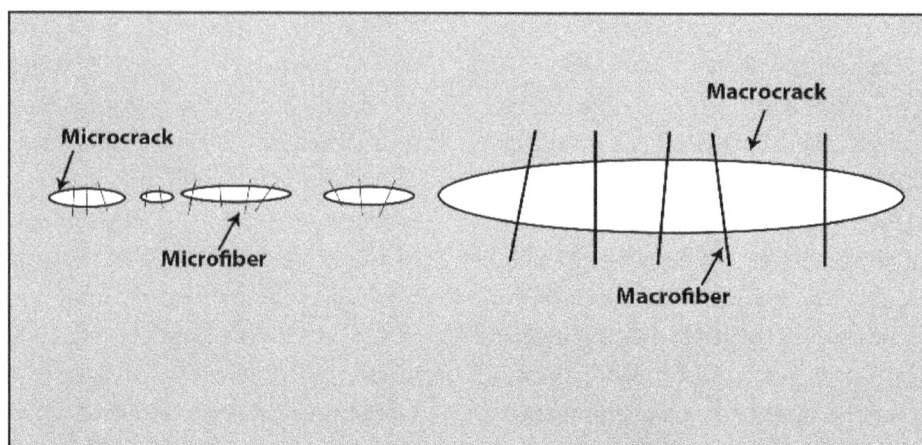

Figure 1: Fiber bridging of micro and macro fibers across micro- and macrocracks

of bundles that may even serve as defects. Chen eta al. have reported that good dispersion of HA nanofibers could be obtained by surface treating of nanofibers with glyoxylic acid (GA) [62]. In another attempt, Fong used nylon 6 nanofiber to reinforce dental restorative resin composites and obtained higher mechanical properties in reinforced samples. This study suggested that when a heavy force was imposed on the composite, the existent nanofibers effectively deflected the crack due to the powerful linking force between the nylon 6 nanofibers and resin matrix. When the crack broke away from the nylon 6 nanofibers, a large number of fracture lines were created on the fracture surface that caused tremendous energy consumption during the fracture [66]. A core-shell structure of a polyacrylonitrile (PAN) and PMMA nanofibers is also used as a reinforcing agent for Bisphenol A Glycidyl Methacrylate (BisGMA) dental resins [67]. In this core-shell structure the PMMA is located in the shell and surrounded by a dental resin matrix. After curing, liner PMMA chains become interpenetrated and entangled with the cross-linked resin matrix network and produce a strong nano interface linking force with strong interfacial adhesion between nanofibers and resin matrix, which would consequently enhance the mechanical properties of the resultant composite [59].It has been reported that incorporation of PAN nanofibers into BisGMA, Triethylene glycol dimethacrylate (TEGDMA) resin blends increased the toughness of the material. This toughening effect depended on the resin monomer solution composition and nanofiber/resin ratio [68].

Nanotubes

The introduction of nano-scale material offers new, promising additives for improvement of the mechanical properties of dental composites because of their high surface area to volume ratio. This property increases the interfacial interaction between nano materials with the resin matrix and consequently induces the specific biological, physical, and chemical properties in resin composites. In terms of high surface area, nanotubes consist of long cylinders with a hollow cavity at their center. They exhibit increased surface area compared with Nps. The aspect ratio of nanotubes is usually more than 10 and it can reach up to several thousand [69]. It is reported that the open-ended tubular structure of the nanotubes may allow the methyl methacrylate monomer to enter into the tubes by capillary action and undergo polymerization. Thus, the higher degree of cross-linking leads to increased load transfer within the nanotube-resin composite. The acrylic resins modified with nanotubes may exhibit considerably higher mechanical properties than the conventional ones. Crack bridging in the tubular structure of nanotubes by fiber pullout from the matrix has been reported in some studies as the main reason for improvement of the mechanical properties of modified resin acrylics [70].Carbon nanotubes (CNTs), ZrO_2 nanotubes, TiO_2 nanotubes, and halloysite nanotubes (HNT) are among the nanotubes used for reinforcement of dental materials.CNTs are the most well-known nanotubes that have been introduced to reinforce materials. CNTs are strong, resilient, and lightweight. They have excellent mechanical and electrical properties [71] and are classified into 2 main types according to the structure of the CNTs – single-walled and multi-walled (Figure 2) [72]. Studies have shown superior mechanical properties in CNT modified polymer-based composites compared to unmodified composites. In addition to

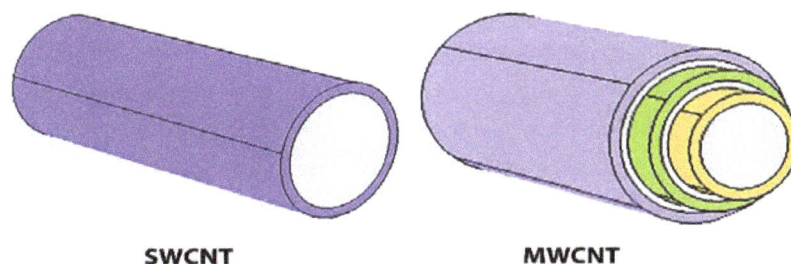

SWCNT   MWCNT

Figure 2: Schematic representation of single-walled and multi-walled carbon nanotubes (CNTs)

the high intrinsic strength and moduli, CNTs can transfer the stress 10 times more than conventional additives [73]. Single-walled CNTs can be used as promising agents to reinforce dental resins due to their ultrahigh specific surface area and exceptional physical performances. The bent single-walled CNTs can recover their original shape on strain release without direct fracture [74]. The reinforcing effect of CNTs may be restricted because of weak interfacial adhesion with the resin matrix as well as the tendency of nanotubes for agglomeration, which causes poor distribution throughout the matrix. The atomically smooth surface of the nanotubes reduces the linking force between the nanotubes and the resin matrix, which limits load transfer from the resin matrix to the nanotube [75]. Hence, good dispersion and enhancement of linking forces between nanotubes and the resin matrix are 2 main factors that affect the reinforcing effect of CNTs. Sonication, chemical modification, surfactant treatment, solution casting, in situ polymerization of monomers, and the combination of these are methods have been introduced to enhance the dispersion of CNTs [76, 77]. Zhang *et al*. [77] modified single-walled carbon nanotubes (SWCNTs) with nano-SiO_2. They observed good levels of dispersion and improved flexural strength in the modified resin composite. Wang *et al*.[72] reinforced PMMA denture base material with 0.5 wt%, 1 wt%, and 2 wt% of multiwalled CNTs and dispersed them with sonication. Their results showed improved flexural strength by the addition of 0.5% and 1% multi-walled carbon nanotubes (MWCNTs) into the PMMA resin, but not for the 2% MWCNTs modified group due to improper dispersion of MWCNTs throughout the matrix. They concluded that MWCNTs adversely affected the fatigue resistance of PMMA resins, particularly with higher concentrations of MWCNTs. HNT has a tubular structure with 2 layers of aluminosilicate (Al2Si2O5(OH)4•2H2O) [78]. Abundance, easy purification, safety, biocompatibility, and ease of handling are advantages of halloysite [59, 79]. The chemical characteristic of the outer surface of HNTs is close to SiO_2, whereas the inner surface approximates Al_2O_3. Nano-sized crystals of HNTs have high mechanical properties. Separation of HNTs in halloysites and dispersing them evenly throughout the resin matrix is simple. The HNT can

be completely split in the existence of polar solvents and mechanical agitation. Because of the presence of a rich Si–OH group on the outer layer of the HNTs, a very strong interfacial linking force can be produced between the silanized halloysite and resin matrix [59]. Reham evaluated the mechanical properties of PMMA resin modified with HNT and concluded that incorporation of low percentages of HNTs into PMMA resin significantly increased the hardness values, whereas the flexural strength and Young's modulus did not significantly improve [80]. Recently, ZrO_2 nanotubes have been greatly used in optoelectronic devices, biomedical materials, and industrial catalysts due to their distinctive pore structures and large specific surface area. It is reported that the untreated ZrO_2 nanotubes have a better reinforcing effect compared to those treated with a silane coupling agent. ZrO_2 nanotubes have unique long tubular structures. When the untreated ZrO_2 nanotubes are mixed with PMMA resin matrix, the chains of the polymer form a three-dimensional network with added nanotubes without any bonding effect. Hence, under an applied force, the polymer chain can slip along the nanotube axis and, consequently, bending stress and bending displacement may improve. On the other hand, the silane coupling agent can play a connective role between the polymer chains and the ZrO_2 nanotubes to prevent the polymer from sliding over the surface of the nanotubes. This would reduce the reinforcing effect of the nanotubes [81].The TiO_2 nanotubes (TNTs) have been considered in medicine due to their high-specific surface area, photocatalytic property, and ion-exchangeability. The tubular form of TiO_2 has a surface area of 250 m²/g that results from the internal and external surfaces, and the surfaces between the layers of the walls, which vary from 2 to 10. The surface area of TNTs is approximately 5 times that of the Nps [69]. Recently, TNTs have been considered for different biological applications such as drug delivery, bio-scaffolds, titanium-based implants, and reinforcement of resin composites. Byrne *et al*. [82] reported improved Young's modulus and strength of modified polystyrene with functionalized TNTs. Porras *et al*. [83] also described improved mechanical properties of polyethylene oxide/chitosan composite reinforced with synthesized TNTs. Improvement of mechanical properties of resin based cement reinforced with TNTs was also reported by Khaled *et al.* [84] In another attempt, Dafar *et al.*[85] evaluated the mechanical properties of flowable dental resin composites reinforced with TNTs, and reported improved fracture toughness and Young's modulus in the experimental resin composite.Recently, Abdulrazzaq Naji *et al.* incorporated 2.5 wt% and 5 wt% TNTs into the PMMA denture base material and evaluated the fracture toughness, flexural strength, and microhardness of modified denture base resins. They observed significant enhancement in all evaluated mechanical properties. The researchers noted that these improved mechanical properties were a linear function of the concentration of added TNTs [86].

Conclusions

In this review, we provided a general background about the efforts to enhance the mechanical properties of denture base materials and relevant new aspects. Rubbers, different macro fibers, metallic, and ceramic fillers have been used for decades as reinforcing agents for PMMA denture base resins. The concept of nanotechnology presents a new era for reinforcement of materials because of the high surface area to volume ratio and the specific biological, physical, and chemical properties of nanomaterials. Nps that include silver Nps, TiO_2 Nps, ZrO_2 Nps, alumina Nps, and ceramic Nps have been employed to improve the mechanical properties of denture base resins. Recently, nanofibers and nanotubes have been introduced to reinforce dental materials. Nanofibers/tubes with higher surface area to volume ratio than Nps provide higher mechanical properties of reinforced composites compared to Nps.Different mechanisms have been presented for the reinforcing effect of nanofibers/tubes. A larger surface area can provide a larger area for load transfer and facilitate toughening mechanisms such as fiber/tube bridging and fiber/tube pullout. Higher degrees of cross-linking due to the incorporation of monomers into hollow parts of nanotubes have been suggested to reinforce nanotubes. Uniform dispersion and complete wetting of the nanofibers/tubes are 2 important factors that affect the reinforcing effect of nanofibers/tubes.

Further studies have to be conducted on using nanofiber/tubes in PMMA denture base resins in order to evaluate the reinforcing mechanism of these additives. The use of nanofibers/tubes may offer a new approach for reinforcement of PMMA resins and possibly be considered as promising reinforcing agents for denture base resin materials in the future.

Conflict of Interest: None declared

Refrences

1. Peyton FA. History of resins in dentistry. Dent Clin North Am. 1975;19:211-22.

2. Wiskott HW, Nicholls JI, Belser UC. Stress fatigue: basic principles and prosthodontic implications. Int J Prosthodont. 1995;8:105-16.

3. Jagger DC, Harrison A, Jandt KD. The reinforcement of dentures. J Oral Rehabil. 1999;26:185-94.

4. Darbar UR, Huggett R, Harrison A. Denture fracture--a survey. Br Dent J. 1994;176:342-5.

5. Zappini G, Kammann A, Wachter W. Comparison of fracture tests of denture base materials. J Prosthet Dent. 2003;90:578-85

6. Rodford R. The development of high impact strength denture-base materials. J Dent. 1986;14:214-7.

7. Rodford RA. Further development and evaluation of high impact strength denture base materials. J Dent. 1990;18:151-7.

8. Broutman LJ, Panizza G. Micromechanics studies of rubber-reinforced glassy polymers. Int J Polym Mater. 1971;1:95-109.

9. Alhareb AO, Akil HM, Ahmad ZA. Mechanical Properties of PMMA Denture Base Reinforced by Nitrile Rubber Particles with Al_2O_3/YSZ Fillers. Procedia Manufacturing. 2015;2:301-6.

10. Alhareb AO, Akil HM, Ahmad ZA. Impact strength, fracture toughness and hardness improvement of PMMA denture base through addition of nitrile rubber/ceramic fillers. Saudi J Dent Res. 2016;8:26-34.

11. Vallittu PK. A review of fiber-reinforced denture base resins. J Prosthodont. 1996;5:270-6.

12. Kohli S, Bhatia S. Polyamides in dentistry. International Journal of Scientific Study. 2013;1:20-5.

13. Larson WR, Dixon DL, Aquilino SA, *et al.* The effect of carbon graphite fiber reinforcentent on the strength of provisional crown and fixed partial denture resins. J Prosthet Dent. 1991;66:816-20.

14. Zheng J, Xiao Yu, Gong T, *et al.* Fabrication and characterization of a novel carbon fiber-reinforced calcium phosphate silicate bone cement with potential osteo-inductivity. Biomed Mater. 2015;11:015003.

15. Alla RK, Sajjan S, Alluri VR, *et al.* Influence of fiber reinforcement on the properties of denture base resins. Journal of Biomaterials and Nanobiotechnology. 2013;4:91-97.

16. Özen J, Sipahi C, ÇAĞLAR A, *et al.* In vitro cytotoxity of glass and carbon fiber-reinforced heat-polymerized acrylic resin denture base material. Tur J Med Sci. 2006;36:121-6.

17. Henderson JD Jr, Mullarky RH, Ryan DE. Tissue biocompatibility of kevlar aramid fibers and polymethylmethacrylate, composites in rabbits. J Biomed Mater Res. 1987;21:59-64.

18. Grave AM, Chandler HD, Wolfaardt JF. Denture base acrylic reinforced with high modulus fibre. Dent Mater. 1985;1:185-7.

19. He X, Qu Y, Peng J, *et al.* A novel botryoidal aramid fiber reinforcement of a PMMA resin for a restorative biomaterial. Biomater Sci. 2017;5:808-16.

20. Kumar G, Nigam A, Naeem A, *et al.* Reinforcing Heat-cured Poly-methyl-methacrylate Resins using Fibers of Glass, Polyaramid, and Nylon: An in vitro Study. J Contemp Dent Pract. 2016;17:948-52.

21. Jaikumar RA, Karthigeyan S, Ali SA, *et al.* Comparison of flexural strength in three types of denture base resins: An in vitro study. J Pharm Bioallied Sci. 2015;7:S461-4.

22. Hamouda IM, Beyari MM. Addition of glass fibers and titanium dioxide nanoparticles to the acrylic resin denture base material: comparative study with the conventional and high impact types. Oral Health Dent Manag. 2014;13:107-12.

23. Unalan F, Dikbas I, Gurbuz O. Transverse Strength of Poly-Methylmethacrylate Reinforced with Different Forms and Concentrations of E-Glass Fibres. OHDMBSC. 2010;9:144-147.

24. Vallittu PK, Lassila VP, Lappalainen R. Acrylic resin-fiber composite--Part I: The effect of fiber concentration on fracture resistance. J Prosthet Dent. 1994;71:607-12.

25. Yu SH, Cho HW, Oh S, *et al.* Effects of glass fiber mesh with different fiber content and structures on the compressive properties of complete dentures. J Prosthet Dent. 2015;113:636-44.

26. Nagakura M, Tanimoto Y, Nishiyama N. Fabrication and physical properties of glass-fiber-reinforced thermoplastics for non-metal-clasp dentures. J Biomed Mater Res B Appl Biomater. 2017;105:2254-2260.

27. Galan D, Lynch E. The effect of reinforcing fibres in denture acrylics. J Ir Dent Assoc. 1989;35:109-13.

28. Goguta L, Marsavina L, Bratu D, *et al.* Impact strength of acrylic heat curing denture base resin reinforced with E-glass fibers. TMJ. 2006;56:88-91.

29. Vallittu P. Curing of a silane coupling agent and its effect on the transverse strength of autopolymerizing polymethylmethacrylate—glass fibre composite. J Oral Rehabil. 1997;24:124-30.

30. Prasad AH, Kalavathy, Mohammed HS. Effect of Glass Fiber And Silane Treated Glass Fiber Reinforcement On Impact Strength Of Maxillary Complete Denture. Annals and Essences of Dentistry. 2011;3:7-12.

31. Sehajpal SB, Sood VK. Effect of metal fillers on some physical properties of acrylic resin. J Prosthet Dent. 1989;61:746-51.

32. Yadav P, Mittal R, Sood VK, *et al.* Effect of incorporation of silane-treated silver and aluminum microparticles on strength and thermal conductivity of PMMA. J Prosthodont. 2012;21:546-51.

33. Zhang X, Zhang X, Zhu B, *et al.* Mechanical and thermal properties of denture PMMA reinforced with silanized aluminum borate whiskers. Dent Mater J. 2012;31:903-8.

34. Mc Nally L, O'sullivan DJ, Jagger DC. An in vitro investigation of the effect of the addition of untreated and surface treated silica on the transverse and impact strength of poly (methyl methacrylate) acrylic resin. Biomed Mater Eng. 2006;16:93-100.

35. Gad MM, Fouda SM, Al-Harbi FA, *et al.* PMMA denture base material enhancement: a review of fiber, filler, and nanofiller addition. Int J Nanomedicine. 2017;12:3801-12.

36. Pan Y, Liu F, Xu D, *et al*. Novel acrylic resin denture base with enhanced mechanical properties by the incorporation of PMMA-modified hydroxyapatite. Progress in Natural Science: Materials International. 2013;23:89-93.

37. Tham WL, Chow WS, Mohd Ishak ZA. Simulated body fluid and water absorption effects on poly (methyl methacrylate)/hydroxyapatite denture base composites. Express Polym Lett. 2010;4:517-28.

38. Mansour MM, Wagner WC, Chu TM. Effect of mica reinforcement on the flexural strength and microhardness of polymethyl methacrylate denture resin. J Prosthodont. 2013;22:179-83.

39. Shepherd PD, Golemba FJ, Maine FW. Mica as a Reinforcement for Plastics. ACS Publications.1974;134:41-51.

40. Unalan F, Gurbuz O, Nihan N, *et al*. Effect of mica as filler on wear of denture teeth polymethylmethacrylate (PMMA) resin. Balkan Journal of Stomatology. 2007;11:133-137.

41. Grumezescu AM. Nanobiomaterials in Dentistry Applications of Nanobiomaterials. 1st. USA: Elsevier; 2016. p.498.

42. Luisa F, Duncan S. European Commission. NANOTECHNOLOGIES: Principles, Applications, Implications and Hands-on Activities. Luxembourg: Office for Official Publications of the European Communities; 2012. p.406.

43. Hoshika S, Nagano F, Tanaka T, *et al*. Expansion of nanotechnology for dentistry: effect of colloidal platinum nanoparticles on dentin adhesion mediated by 4-META/MMA-TBB. J Adhes Dent. 2011;13:411-6.

44. Sivakumar I, Arunachalam KS, Sajjan S, *et al*. Incorporation of antimicrobial macromolecules in acrylic denture base resins: a research composition and update. J Prosthodont. 2014;23:284-90.

45. Ghaffari T, Hamedi-Rad F. Effect of Silver Nano-particles on Tensile Strength of Acrylic Resins. J Dent Res Dent Clin Dent Prospects. 2015;9:40-3.

46. Sodagar A, Kassaee MZ, Akhavan A, *et al*. Effect of silver nano particles on flexural strength of acrylic resins. J Prosthodont Res. 2012;56:120-4.

47. Chatterjee A. Properties improvement of PMMA using nano TiO_2. J Appl Polym Sci. 2010;118:2890–7.

48. Elsaka SE, Hamouda IM, Swain MV. Titanium dioxide nanoparticles addition to a conventional glass-ionomer restorative: influence on physical and antibacterial properties. J Dent. 2011;39:589-98.

49. Matsubayashi Y, Sugawara T, Kuroda S, *et al*. Studies on the bactericidal effects of titanium dioxide for the utilization of medical material. IEICE Technical Report. 2005;12:21-24.

50. Sodagar A, Bahador A, Khalil S, *et al*. The effect of TiO_2 and SiO_2 nanoparticles on flexural strength of poly (methyl methacrylate) acrylic resins. J Prosthodont Res. 2013;57:15-9.

51. Harini P, Mohamed K, Padmanabhan TV. Effect of Titanium dioxide nanoparticles on the flexural strength of polymethylmethacrylate: an in vitro study. Indian J Dent Res. 2014;25:459-63.

52. Alwan SA, Alameer SS. The effect of the addition of silanized Nano titania fillers on some physical and mechanical properties of heat cured acrylic denture base materials. J BCD. 2015;27:86-91.

53. Gad M, ArRejaie AS, Abdel-Halim MS, *et al*. The Reinforcement Effect of Nano-Zirconia on the Transverse Strength of Repaired Acrylic Denture Base. Int J Dent. 2016;2016:7094056.

54. Asopa V, Suresh S, Khandelwal M, *et al*. A comparative evaluation of properties of zirconia reinforced high impact acrylic resin with that of high impact acrylic resin. Saudi J Dent Res. 2015;6:146-51.

55. Ahmed MA, Ebrahim MI. Effect of zirconium oxide nano-fillers addition on the flexural strength, fracture toughness, and hardness of heat-polymerized acrylic resin. WJNScE. 2014;4:50-57.

56. Gad MM, Rahoma A, Al-Thobity AM, *et al*. Influence of incorporation of ZrO_2 nanoparticles on the repair strength of polymethyl methacrylate denture bases. Int J Nanomedicine. 2016;11:5633-43.

57. Uyar T, Cokeliler D. The Improvement of Dental Composite Properties with Electromagnetically Aligned Nanofiber. MRS Proceedings. 2014; 1685:u06-12.

58. Uyar T, Cokeliler D, Dogan M, *et al*. Electrospun nanofiber reinforcement of dental composites with electromagnetic alignment approach. Mater Sci Eng C Mater Biol Appl. 2016;62:762-70.

59. Li X, Liu W, Sun L, *et al*. Resin composites

reinforced by nanoscaled fibers or tubes for dental regeneration. Biomed Res Int. 2014;2014:542958.

60. Chen L, Yu Q, Wang Y, *et al*. BisGMA/TEGDMA dental composite containing high aspect-ratio hydroxyapatite nanofibers. Dent Mater. 2011;27:1187-95.

61. Boyd SA, Su B, Sandy JR, *et al*. Cellulose nanofibre mesh for use in dental materials. Coatings. 2012;2:120-37.

62. Chen L, Xu C, Wang Y, *et al*. BisGMA/TEGDMA dental nanocomposites containing glyoxylic acid-modified high-aspect ratio hydroxyapatite nanofibers with enhanced dispersion. Biomed Mater. 2012;7:045014.

63. Gao Y, Sagi S, Zhang L, *et al*. Electrospun nano-scaled glass fiber reinforcement of bis-GMA/TEGDMA dental composites. J Appl Polym Sci. 2008;110:2063-70.

64. Arcis RW, Lopez-Macipe A, Toledano M, *et al*. Mechanical properties of visible light-cured resins reinforced with hydroxyapatite for dental restoration. Dent Mater. 2002;18:49-57.

65. Cucuruz AT, Andronescu E, Ficai A, *et al*. Synthesis and characterization of new composite materials based on poly(methacrylic acid) and hydroxyapatite with applications in dentistry. Int J Pharm. 2016;510:516-23.

66. Fong H. Electrospun nylon 6 nanofiber reinforced BIS-GMA/TEGDMA dental restorative composite resins. Polymer. 2004;45:2427-32.

67. Cheng L, Zhou X, Zhong H, *et al*. NaF-loaded core–shell PAN–PMMA nanofibers as reinforcements for Bis-GMA/TEGDMA restorative resins. Mater Sci Eng C Mater Biol Appl. 2013;34:262-9.

68. Vidotti HA, Manso AP, Leung V, *et al*. Flexural properties of experimental nanofiber reinforced composite are affected by resin composition and nanofiber/resin ratio. Dent Mater. 2015;31:1132-41.

69. Bavykin DV, Walsh FC. Titanate and titania nanotubes: synthesis, properties and applications. Cambridge, UK: Royal Society of Chemistry; 2010. p. 154.

70. Khaled SM, Charpentier PA, Rizkalla AS. Synthesis and characterization of poly(methyl methacrylate)-based experimental bone cements reinforced with TiO_2-SrO nanotubes. Acta Biomater. 2010;6:3178-86.

71. Cadek M, Coleman JN, Barron V, *et al*. Morphological and mechanical properties of carbon-nanotube-reinforced semicrystalline and amorphous polymer composites. Appl Phys Lett. 2002;81:5123-5.

72. Wang R, Tao J, Yu B, *et al*. Characterization of multiwalled carbon nanotube-polymethyl methacrylate composite resins as denture base materials. J Prosthet Dent. 2014;111:318-26.

73. Harris PJ. Carbon nanotubes and related structures: new materials for the twenty-first century. AAPT. 2002;3:463-464.

74. Li X, Fan Y, Watari F. Current investigations into carbon nanotubes for biomedical application. Biomed Mater. 2010;5: 22001.

75. Hamouda IM. Current perspectives of nanoparticles in medical and dental biomaterials. J Biomed Res. 2012;26:143-51.

76. Chen J, Rao AM, Lyuksyutov S, *et al*. Dissolution of full-length single-walled carbon nanotubes. J Phys Chem B. 2001;105:2525-8.

77. Zhang F, Xia Y, Xu L, *et al*. Surface modification and microstructure of single-walled carbon nanotubes for dental resin-based composites. J Biomed Mater Res B Appl Biomater. 2008;86:90-7.

78. Joussein E, Petit S, Churchman J, *et al*. Halloysite clay minerals–a review. Clay minerals. 2005;40:383-426.

79. Vergaro V, Abdullayev E, Lvov YM, *et al*. Cytocompatibility and uptake of halloysite clay nanotubes. Biomacromolecules. 2010;11:820-6.

80. Abdallah RM. Evaluation of polymethyl methacrylate resin mechanical properties with incorporated halloysite nanotubes. J Adv Prosthodont. 2016;8:167-71.

81. Yu W, Wang X, Tang Q, *et al*. Reinforcement of denture base PMMA with ZrO 2 nanotubes. J Mech Behav Biomed Mater. 2014;32:192-7.

82. Byrne MT, McCarthy JE, Bent M, *et al*. Chemical functionalisation of titania nanotubes and their utilisation for the fabrication of reinforced polystyrene composites. J Mater Chem. 2007;17:2351-8.

83. Porras R, Bavykin DV, Zekonyte J, *et al*. Titanate nanotubes for reinforcement of a poly(ethylene oxide)/chitosan polymer matrix. Nanotechnology. 2016;27:195706.

84. Khaled S, Miron RJ, Hamilton DW, *et al.* Reinforcement of resin based cement with titania nanotubes. Dent Mater. 2010;26:169-78.

85. Dafar MO, Grol MW, Canham PB, *et al.* Reinforcement of flowable dental composites with titanium dioxide nanotubes. Dent Mater. 2016;32:817-26.

86. Abdulrazzaq Naji S, Behroozibakhsh M, Jafarzadeh Kashi TS, *et al.* Effects of incorporation of 2.5 and 5 wt% TiO_2 nanotubes on fracture toughness, flexural strength, and microhardness of denture base poly methyl methacrylate (PMMA). J Adv Prosthodont. Forthcoming.

8

Evaluation of Antibacterial Properties of Dental Adhesives Containing Metal Nanoparticles

Shafiei F [a*]; Ashnagar A [b] ; Ghavami-Lahiji M [c] ; Najafi F [d] ; Amin Marashi SM [e]

[a]Assistant professor, Department of Dental Biomaterials, School of Dentistry, Tehran University of Medical Sciences, Tehran, Iran
[b]Pharm-D, School of Pharmacy, Shahid Beheshti University of Medical Sciences, Tehran, Iran
[c]Ph.D. candidate for Dental Biomaterials, Research Center for Science and Technology in Medicine, Department of Dental Biomaterials, School of Dentistry, Tehran University of Medical Sciences, Tehran, Iran
[d]Assistant professor, Department of Resin and Additives, Institute for Color Science and Technology, Tehran, Iran
[e]Assistant professor, Department of Microbiology and Immunology, Alborz University of Medical Sciences, Karaj, Iran

ARTICLE INFO	Abstract
Key words: Dental adhesive Nanoparticle Antibacterial Silver Titanium dioxide	**Statement of problem:** Secondary dental caries is a common clinical finding in composite restoration. The development of a bactericidal dental adhesive provides a promising method to reduce the risk of secondary caries.

Statement of problem: Secondary dental caries is a common clinical finding in composite restoration. The development of a bactericidal dental adhesive provides a promising method to reduce the risk of secondary caries.

Objectives: This study aimed to assess the antibacterial activity of silver (Ag) and titanium dioxide (TiO_2) nanoparticles incorporated into an experimental dentin bonding agent formulation.

Materials and Methods: Ag and TiO_2 nanoparticles at 0.05, 0.1, 0.2, 0.5, and 1 wt% concentrations were incorporated into the adhesives. The suspensions were sonicated to ensure homogenous dispersion of nanoparticles in the adhesive system. Formulation was composed of acetone, 2,2-bis[4-(2-hydroxy-3-methacryloxypropoxy)phenyl]propane (Bis-GMA), 1,6-bis-[2-methacryloyloxyethyl carbonyl amino]-2,4,4-trimethylhexane (UDMA), trimethylolpropane trimethacrylate (TMPTMA), 2-hydroxyethyl methacrylate (HEMA), and photoinitiator, with polyvinylpyrrolidone (PVP) as the stabilizer. We counted the colony-forming units (CFU%) of two cariogenic bacteria, *Streptococcus mutans (S. mutans)* and *Lactobacillus acidophilus (L. acidophilus)*, that were exposed to the powdered light cured adhesive specimens. The effects of various concentrations of each nanoparticle were compared by one-way ANOVA, followed by the post hoc Bonferroni test.

Results: All samples exhibited definite antibacterial activity ($P<0.05$) compared to the control specimens. The Ag nanoparticle samples showed higher antibacterial properties compared to the TiO_2 nanoparticle samples. Increasing the concentration of nanoparticles resulted in significant differences in bactericidal properties, with the exception of 0.2 to 0.5 wt% Ag nanoparticle specimens exposed to *S. mutans* and the 0.2 to 0.5 wt% TiO_2 nanoparticle specimens exposed to *L. acidophilus*.

Conclusions: These metal-based nanoparticles exhibited dose-dependent bactericidal activities. The Ag nanoparticles had higher antibacterial activity compared to the TiO_2 nanoparticles. Incorporation of these nanoparticles into dental adhesives is a promising way to reduce the risk of secondary caries. However, further clinical evaluations should be performed.

Corresponding Author:
Farhad Shafiei
Department of Dental Biomaterials, School of Dentistry, Tehran University of Medical Sciences, North Kargar Avenue, Tehran 14174, Iran
Email: faradent@yahoo.com

Introduction

The basic mechanism behind tooth decay is demineralization attributed to acid produced by bacteria [1-3]. Carbohydrates metabolize to acid by cariogenic bacteria that exist in plaque such as *Streptococcus mutans (S. mutans) and Lactobacillus acidophilus (L. acidophilus)*. Thus, development of bonding agents and other restorative and preventive materials that have the capability to reduce bacterial activity at the tooth/composite interface can effectively decrease secondary caries [4-6].While the clinical performance of resin-based materials has greatly improved in terms of restoration aesthetics, durability, and bonding strength; recently, there is increased focus on the acquisition of antibacterial properties. Incorporation of soluble antimicrobial agents, such as chlorhexidine, in the resin matrix have been investigated [7]. The results have shown clear inhibition of bacteria, but the release kinetics is difficult to control and long-term effect is not expected. One of the advantages of adding a releasing agent is that the antibacterial effect can produce an impact beyond the area of the resinous material. However, frequently mechanical properties of the resin material are reduced [7]. Another strategy is to employ an antibacterial agent, which is immobilized in the resin matrix and not released. In this case, the antibacterial effect is limited to bacteria that directly contact the material. Antibacterial agents incorporated in adhesives [8, 9] and filler composites [10] have shown good bacterial inhibition. Among various metals, silver (Ag) has attracted significant attention due to its antibacterial effects [11-14]. One of the advantages of Ag over general antibiotics is that Ag has wide-spectrum antibacterial activity with very high efficiency and relatively low cytotoxicity [12]. Ag nanoparticles placed in a polymer matrix produce a large reservoir of Ag ions that can be released over time and provide a long-lasting antibacterial effect [15]. Titanium dioxide (TiO_2) is a bactericide and a biocompatible material with potential use in many applications. Bioactivity of this material can also be useful in closure of the gaps in the interface and remineralization of the adjacent tooth [16, 17]. We took into consideration the aforementioned problems and the increased need to develop an efficient and biocompatible dental adhesive

to inhibit secondary caries. First, we aimed to synthesize a dental bonding incorporated with metal Ag and TiO_2 nanoparticles, and subsequently assessed the antibacterial activities of the light-cured dental bonding by exposing them to *S. mutans and L. acidophilus*.

Materials and Methods

Adhesive preparation

Table 1 lists the information about the materials and their use. In order to prepare 10 g base formulation of dentine bonding agent, we used a magnetic stirrer to mix 1.4 g of 2,2-bis[4-(2-hydroxy-3-methacryloxypropoxy)phenyl] propane (Bis-GMA), 2.6 g of 2-hydroxyethyl methacrylate (HEMA), 0.8 g trimethylolpropane trimethacrylate (TMPTMA), 1.2 g of 1,6-bis-[2-methacryloyloxyethyl carbonyl amino]-2,4,4-trimethylhexane (UDMA), and 4 g of acetone. All weights were obtained by a laboratory scale (Sartorius AG, Germany) that had an accuracy of four decimal places. The mixture was mixed until homogenous. Then, we divided the base formulation into different containers and added the antibacterial nanoparticles at the following weight percentages: 0.05, 0.1, 0.2, 0.5, and 1 wt% to the mixture. We used Ag and TiO_2 spherical shaped nanoparticles that had a diameter of 20 nm and 99.9% purity. We added 0.5 wt% polyvinylpyrrolidone (PVP) to the mixture to avoid agglomeration of the nanoparticles. Direct sonication by a probe is the preferred method to disperse nanoparticles. Thus, in this study, we used ultrasound vibrations from an ultrasonic probe (UP400S - Hielscher Ultrasonics GmbH, Germany) with each mixture for 3 minutes, at 0.5 cycle with an amplitude of 60%. Then, 0.5 wt% photoinitiator (IRGACURE 819) and 0.1 wt% p-Methoxyphenol (PMP) were added to each bottle. After the addition of the photoinitiator, the mixing was continued with a magnetic stirrer in the dark at 40°C for 30 minutes. The samples were stored in a light resistant glass bottles to avoid pre-term light curing from the environment.

Uncured adhesives were used for particle size analysis. The 1 at% Ag and TiO_2 nanoparticle adhesives were sonicated using an ultrasonic probe for 30 seconds before insertion into the DLS (Zetasizer Nano, Malvern Instruments, UK) cuvettes. The results confirmed the presence of nano-sized particles in the resin. The nanoparticle-adhesives had an average polydispersity index (PDI) of 0.279 for Ag and 0.173 for TiO_2. This clearly indicated that the nanoparticle-adhesives were almost homogenous.

Shear bond strength test

We conducted a shear strength test to confirm the bonding properties of the newly synthesized adhesives. Commercial dental bonding (3M ESPE™ Single Bond™) was used as the control sample. A total of 18 dentinal samples were etched for 20 seconds with 37% commercial phosphoric acid, rinsed with distilled water, and slightly dried. Then, the prepared 1wt% Ag nanoparticle and TiO_2 nanoparticle dental adhesives were applied to the samples with a micro brush. After 15 seconds, a slight stream of air spray was used to ensure development of the resin tags. The adhesives were light cured for 40 seconds by a 400 mW/cm² intensity light curing unit (Coltolux 75, Coltene, Whaledent, NJ, USA). Then, we placed a plastic tube (diameter: 4 mm, height: 4mm) on the dentine surface and filled with dental resin composite (Shade A2, 3M ESPE™ Filtek™ Z250 universal restorative). The samples

Table 1: Materials used in the study

Materials	Manufacturer	Utilization
Nano silver (Ag)	US Research Nanomaterials	Filler
Nano Titanium dioxide (TiO_2)	Sigma- Aldrich	Filler
Acetone	Merck	Solvent
2,2-Bis[4-(2-hydroxy-3-methacryloxypropoxy)phenyl] propane (Bis-GMA)	Degussa	Adhesive monomer (di-methacrylate)
2-Hydroxyethyl methacrylate (HEMA)	Sigma- Aldrich	Hydrophilic monomer
1,6-bis-[2-methacryloyloxyethyl carbonyl amino]-2,4,4-trimethylhexane (UDMA)	Degussa	Adhesive monomer (di-methacrylate)
Trimethylolpropane trimethacrylate (TMPTMA)	Sigma- Aldrich	Adhesive monomer (tri-functional monomer)
Phenylbis(2,4,6-trimethylbenzoyl) phosphine oxide (IRGACURE 819)	Sigma- Aldrich	Photoinitiator
P-Methoxyphenol (PMP)	Merck	Inhibitor
Polyvinylpyrrolidone (PVP)	Sigma-Aldrich	Prevent agglomeration of nanoparticles

were cured for 40 seconds. After removing the plastic tube, 40 seconds were cured again to ensure complete polymerization. Then, the specimens were stored in distilled water for 24 hours at 37°C. Shear bond strength was measured by a Universal Testing Machine (UTM) (Santam, SMT-20, Iran). The chisel was attached to the upper arm of the UTM. The load was applied parallel to the dentin/ resin composite interface with a load cell of 20 kg (Bongshin Loadcell Co., Ltd., South Korea) at a crosshead speed of 0.5 mm/min until the specimens debonded.

Antibacterial assessment

We used a cylindrical stainless steel mold (diameter: 9 mm, height: 2 mm) to prepare the cured samples. The mold was placed on a cover glass. Then, uncured adhesive was injected into the mold by a 10 ml sterile syringe with a 0.22 µm syringe filter to ensure that probable agglomerated particles would not be present at the samples. Another cover glass was carefully placed on the mold such that no bubble was made in the adhesive. The samples were put in a vacuum oven (Ehret GmbH, Germany) for 30 minutes for complete evaporation of the acetone. The samples were cured for 60 seconds, 30 seconds per side. Then, the specimens were removed from the mold and kept in sterile surgical covers. All cured samples were ground by a laboratory universal grinder (Mortar Grinder PULVERISETTE 2, Fritsch). Powdered adhesive specimens were sterilized under a UV lamp (Laminar Flow UV Cabinet, JTLV C2, Iran) for 180 minutes. We used two cariogenic bacteria in this study – S. mutans (ATCC 35668) and L. acidophilus (ATCC 314). These bacteria were prepared from the microbial collection at Pasteur Institute of Iran, Tehran, Iran. We prepared 2.0 McFarland turbidity of each bacteria in sterile laboratory tubes. Turbidity was confirmed by a spectrophotometric (Biophotometer Plus, Eppendorf) assessment of optical density. We used two, 96-well microtiter plates for bacterial cultivation. Positive control wells consisted of culture medium plus bacterial solution. The powdered antibacterial-adhesives were placed into the wells. All wells were poured with 200 µl blood culture (Baharafshan, Iran) using a micropipette (Eppendorf Research). Then, 6.66 µl of the bacterial suspension was inserted into the designated wells. The microtiter plates were incubated for 24 hours at 37°C in CO_2 by placing both microtiter plates in an isolated jar that contained a lit candle. The flame extinguished when all of the oxygen was consumed. After 24 hours, 1 µl from each well was extracted and diluted in a sterile laboratory tube with 999 µl of physiologic serum. Then, 10 µl of each solution was removed with a micropipette and spread on the surface of the solid medium. We used sterilized chocolate agar medium to grow S. mutans and sterilized MRS agar medium for L. acidophilus. All plates were incubated for 24 hours at 37°C in CO_2. We counted the bacteria by determining the colony-forming unit (CFU%), as an estimate of viable bacteria.

Statistical analysis

Colony counts of the bacteria were standardized from 0%-100% based on the colony count of the control group. The effect of nanoparticle type and concentration for each bacteria was analyzed by two-way ANOVA. We took into consideration the significant interaction of the aforementioned factors and performed a comparison of the effects of each nanoparticle at various concentrations by one-way ANOVA, followed by the post hoc Bonferroni test. Nanoparticles were compared at each concentration by the independent t-test. Without adjustment for α error, the significance level was set at $P<0.05$.

Results

Shear strength test

The shear bond strength value confirmed that the specimens had bonding properties similar to

Table 2: Shear bond strength of commercial and two fabricated dental adhesive. Bond strength values are presented as MPa

Adhesive	Bond strength Mean ± SD (MPa)
Commercial, Single Bond (3M ESPE)	7.57 ± 0.1
Silver (Ag)-containing adhesive	7.58 ± 0.08
Titanium dioxide (TiO₂)-containing adhesive	7.55 ± 0.09

commercial adhesives (Table 2). The shear strength values of the specimens were similar to the control group; therefore, the specimens were considered for the antibacterial test.

Colony count test

We analyzed the interaction between concentration and nanoparticle by two-way ANOVA. The results indicated a significant interaction in both bacteria ($P<0.001$) as seen in Table 3. The number of the bacterial colonies was calculated. As described earlier, the colony counts were standardized concerning the control colony count. At 24 hours, the CFU% was approximately 500 for *L. acidophilus* for the control group. The Ag-adhesive had a gradual reduction in CFU% with increasing concentrations of Ag, as follows: 372 (0.05%), 340 (0.1%), 303 (0.2%), 185 (0.5%), and 130 (1%) for *L. acidophilus*. CFU% counts were approximately 320 for *S. mutans* in the control group. The Ag-containing adhesive also showed a gradual reduction in CFU% with increasing concentrations of Ag, as follows: 207 (0.05%), 183 (0.1%), 108 (0.2%), 104 (0.5%), and 51 (1%) for *S. mutans*. Mean and standard deviation (SD) of CFU% data is shown in Table 4. One-way ANOVA followed by Bonferroni analysis among different concentrations showed statistically significant differences ($P<0.05$), with the exception of two concentrations. There was no statistically significant difference between the 0.2 wt% and 0.5 wt% concentrations of the TiO$_2$ nanoparticle on *L.*

acidophilus ($P=0.068$). In addition, the difference between the 0.2 wt% and 0.5 wt% concentrations of the Ag nanoparticle on *S. mutans* was not statistically significant ($P=1.00$). We used the t-test to compare the effects of each concentration on CFU% between both nanoparticles. The results indicated a statistically significant difference between the two types of nanoparticle-adhesives at each concentration. Figure 1 shows the behavior of these nanoparticles concerning CFU% for *L. acidophilus* and *S. mutans*.

Discussion

Antimicrobial surfaces present a major challenge, particularly in dentistry, where bacterial biofilms tend to accumulate and propagate on solid surfaces. Resin composite restorations are more susceptible to secondary caries due to the increased tendency to colonize bacteria on their surfaces. Polymerization shrinkage of the resin composites makes the bonding interface the weakest area. Thus, the role of a dental adhesive is important. One way to address this problem is to design materials with antibacterial properties. Dental bonding agents, as an important and delicate player in the integrity of a composite restoration, can be suitable hosts for antibacterial materials. The current study has aimed to fabricate antibacterial adhesives and evaluate the antibacterial properties of various concentrations of two nanoparticles, TiO$_2$ and Ag, incorporated into an adhesive.

Table 3: Two-way ANOVA (5x2) to assess the interactions of the nanoparticles and concentrations

Bacteria	Source	F	P-value
Lactobacillus acidophilus (*L. acidophilus*)	Concentration	2143.13	<0.001
	Nanoparticle	986.60	<0.001
	Concentration* Nanoparticle	222.97	<0.001
Streptococcus mutans (*S. mutans*)	Concentration	1060.90	<0.001
	Nanoparticle	782.48	<0.001
	Concentration* Nanoparticle	30.99	<0.001

* simultaneous effect of two variables (concentration and nanoparticle) on the colony count of bacteria

Table 4: Colony counts of *L. acidophilus* and *S. mutans* in Ag and TiO_2 nanoparticle containing specimens

Bacteria	concentration	CFU% of Ag-containing adhesive Mean±SD	CFU% of TiO_2-containing adhesive Mean±SD
	0.05	73.80±0.71	80.02±1.19
	0.1	68.40±0.5	70.21±0.7
L. acidophilus	0.2	59.76±0.9	63.97±1.01
	0.5	36.92±0.87	66.86±1.05
	1	26.18±0.9	37.20±1.17
	0.05	64.28±1.35	92.029±1.29
	0.1	57.54±1.75	66.98±1.25
S. mutans	0.2	33.33±1.54	52.46±1.11
	0.5	32.80±1.66	44.16±1.66
	1	16.14±2.34	30.62±1.73

CFU= Colony-forming unit, Ag= Silver, TiO_2= Titanium dioxide, *L. acidophilus*= *Lactobacillus acidophilus*, *S. mutans*= *Streptococcus mutans*

Nanotechnology has been employed in many fields in recent years. Currently, nanoparticles are used for different physical, biomedical, and pharmaceutical applications. Metal-based nanoparticles have promising antibacterial properties. Among these materials, the Ag nanoparticle and TiO_2 nanoparticle have been investigated in numerous studies.

It has been reported that Ag is highly toxic to the majority of microorganisms [18, 19]. The nanoparticle form of Ag exhibits an increased bactericidal effect because of enhanced surface area exposure to the microorganisms [19]. However, the mechanism of action of Ag on microorganisms is not fully understood. It has been suggested that loss of ability to replicate DNA and/or changes in the bacterial cell wall occur after the application of Ag nanoparticles [20]. In addition, the photocatalysis properties of TiO_2 have been employed in many fields. Produced free radicals (HO• and O_2 •−) from TiO_2 following UV exposure, are known as reactive oxygen species (ROS). ROS are strong oxidants that have the capability to induce oxidative damage in the cell walls of microorganisms [21]. Studies have shown that TiO_2 has photocatalysis and bactericidal properties; however, the use for this capability has been less studied in dental adhesives.

It has shown good antibacterial property in resin composites; however, mechanical properties might decrease. Shirai *et al.* reported that after completion of UV radiation, the antimicrobial property of TiO_2 continued. This property could be employed as an adjunct treatment to eliminate residual bacteria after debridement [21]. The bioactivity of TiO_2 added to an adhesive was proven by Welch *et al.* with the formation of hydroxyl apatite at the surface. The advantages of this feature included closure of gaps between resin material and the tooth, as well as remineralization of the adjacent tooth [16]. Sun *et al.* reported that the mechanical properties and degree of conversion of the adhesive improved by the addition of the TiO_2 nanoparticle [22]. Dentinal tubules are reported to enhance bond strength with resinous materials due to formation of resin tags [16]. Dentinal tubules have diameters of approximately 1-2.5 µm [16, 23]. Therefore, we did not anticipate that our nanoparticle-containing adhesive would interfere with the bonding system. The nanoparticles were smaller than the dentinal tubules. The results of a preliminary study revealed that shear bond strength of the nanoparticle-containing adhesive was comparable to commercial counterparts. This finding agreed

A. *Lactobacillus acidophilus (L. acidophilus)*

B. *Streptococcus mutans (S. mutans)*

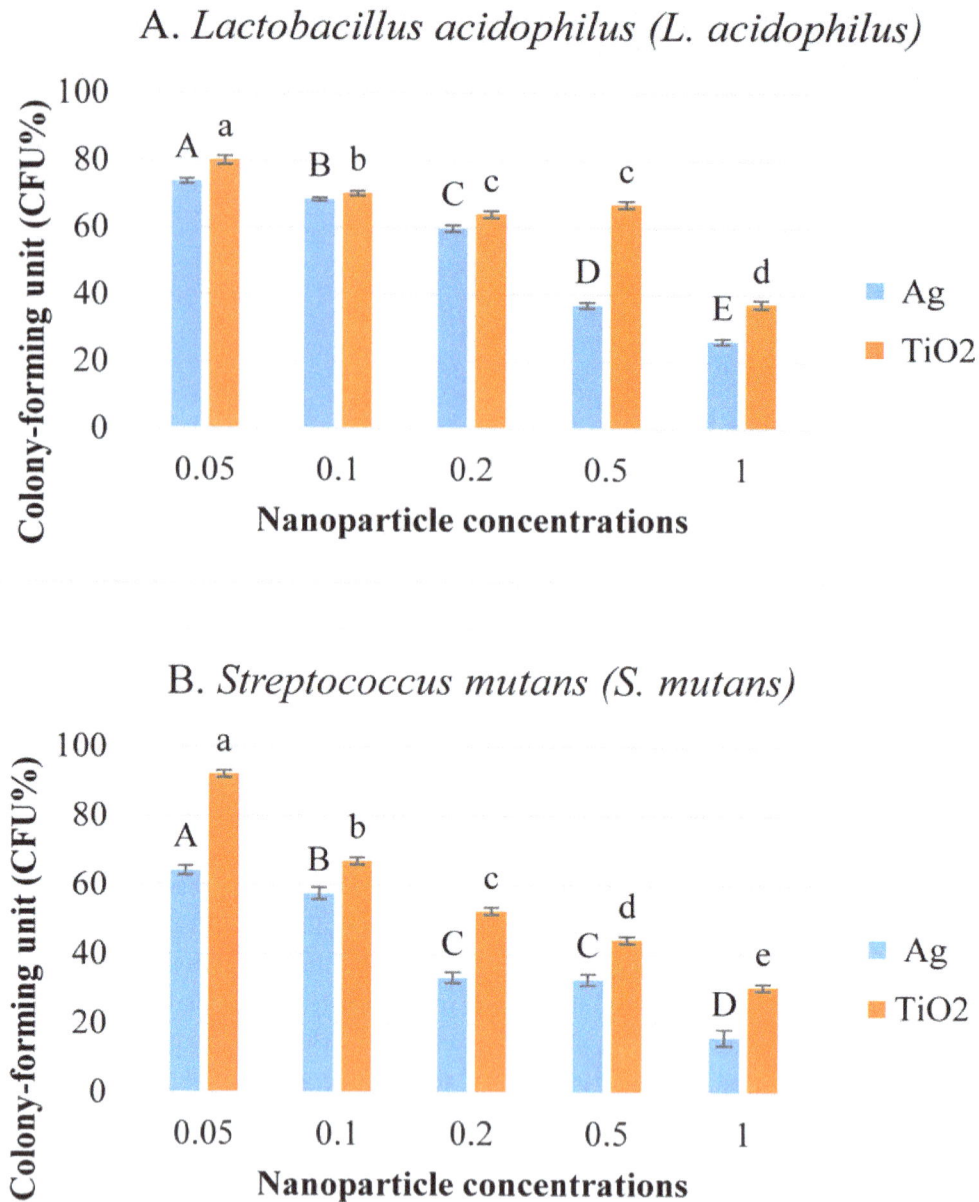

Figure 1: The effect of nanoparticle concentration on colony-forming unit (CFU%) in both *Lactobacillus acidophilus (L. acidophilus)* (A) and *Streptococcus mutans (S. mutans)* (B). Values marked by different capital and lowercase letters are significantly different in the silver (Ag) and titanium dioxide (TiO_2) groups (P<0.05)

with other studies [16, 24, 25] that added different nanoparticles to commercial adhesives and reported no reductions in shear bond strength. However, we synthesized antibacterial adhesives and the nanoparticle in our study was added to our experimental base formulation *et al.* [26] reported significant improvement in mechanical properties of synthetic dental adhesives, especially with incorporation of 0.1% and 0.2% diamond nanoparticles. No decrease in bond strength data might be explained by usage of the tri-functional monomer TMPTMA in our adhesive formulation.

According to Silva, replacement of triethylene glycol dimethacrylate (TEGDMA) with a cross-linker monomer (TMPTMA) improved the chemical-mechanical properties of adhesives [27]. Here, we used Ag and TiO_2 nanoparticles to develop an intrinsic bactericidal methacrylate based dental adhesive. Various concentrations of each of the incorporated nanoparticles were made to identify the effect of concentration on bactericidal properties of Ag and TiO_2. The results indicated that adhesive containing nanoparticles exhibited definite antibacterial properties. This bactericidal property was dose-dependent, which agreed with results reported by Degrazia *et al.* [28]. Each dosage had a statistically significant difference in CFU% compared to other concentrations, with the exception of the 0.2 wt% and 0.5 wt% Ag-containing samples in *S. mutans* and the 0.2 wt% and 0.5 wt% TiO$_2$-containing samples in *L. acidophilus*. This similarity should be noted when choosing the desired concentration because of the potential impact on mechanical properties while there would be no significant changes in bactericidal properties. We observed that the Ag nanoparticle specimens had a noticeably sharp drop in colonies from the 0.2 wt% to 0.5 wt% in *L. acidophilus* and from the 0.1 wt% to 0.2 wt% in *S. mutans* (Figure 1, Table 4). The TiO$_2$ nanoparticle specimens had a sharp drop in colonies from the 0.5 wt% to 1 wt% in *L. acidophilus*, whereas we observed that the CFUs of *S. mutans* followed an approximately regular pattern. The 1 wt% showed the highest antibacterial activity in both nanoparticles. The Ag particles had stronger bactericidal action against *S. mutans* and *L. acidophilus* compared to the TiO$_2$ particles. This difference was more noticeable with *S. mutans*, especially at the higher dosages. Cheng *et al.* [29] incorporated Ag nanoparticles into an amorphous calcium nanocomposite. They used 0.028 wt% nanoAg. [29]. The Ag containing specimens reduced approximately 15.2 CFU% compared to neat nanocomposite. This CFU% reduction was lower than our 0.05% Ag nanoparticle specimens that had a 35 CFU% reduction in *S. mutans*. This might be attributed to the higher amount of Ag used in our study. In addition, the methodology and antibacterial test differed between studies. Cheng *et al.* placed the bacteria on a large resin surface, whereas we immersed adhesive powder in the bacterial suspension. Welch *et al.* incorporated nano TiO$_2$ into a commercially available bonding agent to achieve a bioactive and bactericidal dental adhesive [16]. They reported that the antibacterial properties of the nano TiO$_2$ depended on UV irradiation time and were not concentration dependent. However, our results demonstrated that the bactericidal properties of the TiO$_2$ nanoparticle were concentration dependent. Welch *et al.* used *Staphylococcus epidermidis,* which is a part of the human skin's normal flora. The choice of this bacteria to assess bactericidal properties of a dental adhesive, which is faced with challenges from cariogenic bacteria seems irrelevant. In this study, we performed the CFU test to obtain preliminary information on the efficacy of the nanomaterial antibacterial agent. Considering the promising findings, further studies can be done with various microbial tests on these adhesives. We suggest assessing the effect of addition of these nanoparticles on the mechanical behavior of dental adhesive. Higher concentrations of these materials should be tested to obtain the highest bactericidal activity. Other nanoparticles such as zinc oxide (ZnO) might have antibacterial properties, supported by strong mechanical improvement.

Conclusions

We tentatively incorporated metal-based nanoparticles into a synthesized etch and rinse dental adhesive to assess antibacterial properties of the newly developed material on cariogenic bacteria. We found that these metal-based nanoparticle exhibited bactericidal activities in a dose-dependent manner without affecting shear bond strength. The Ag nanoparticles showed higher antibacterial activity compared to the TiO$_2$ nanoparticles. Incorporation of such materials into dental adhesives is a promising way to reduce the risk of secondary caries. However, further clinical evaluation should be performed.

Acknowledgements

This study was financially supported by a grant for scientific research (No. 92-03-69-23934) from Tehran University of Medical Sciences.

Conflict of Interest: None declared.

References

1. Featherstone JD. The continuum of dental caries—evidence for a dynamic disease process. J Dent Res. 2004;83:C39-C42.
2. Deng DM, Ten Cate JM. Demineralization of dentin by Streptococcus mutans biofilms grown in the constant depth film fermentor. Caries Res. 2003;38:54-61.
3. Totiam P, Gonzalez-Cabezas C, Fontana MR, *et*

al. A new in vitro model to study the relationship of gap size and secondary caries. Caries Res. 2007;41:467-73.

4. Chen C, Cheng L, Weir MD, *et al*. Primer containing dimethylaminododecyl methacrylate kills bacteria impregnated in human dentin blocks. Int J Oral Sci. 2016;8:239-245.

5. Ge Y, Wang S, Zhou X, *et al*. The use of quaternary ammonium to combat dental caries. Materials (Basel). 2015;8:3532-49.

6. Wang L, Li C, Weir MD, *et al*. Novel multifunctional dental bonding agent for class-V restorations to inhibit periodontal biofilms. RSC Advances. 2017;7:29004-14.

7. Imazato S, Kinomoto Y, Tarumi H, *et al*. Antibacterial activity and bonding characteristics of an adhesive resin containing antibacterial monomer MDPB. Dent Mater. 2003;19:313-9.

8. Ahn SJ, Lee SJ, Kook JK, *et al*. Experimental antimicrobial orthodontic adhesives using nanofillers and silver nanoparticles. Dent Mater. 2009;25:206-13.

9. Imazato S, Kuramoto A, Takahashi Y, *et al*. In vitro antibacterial effects of the dentin primer of Clearfil Protect Bond. Dent Mater. 2006;22:527-32.

10. Yoshida K, Tanagawa M, Atsuta M. Characterization and inhibitory effect of antibacterial dental resin composites incorporating silver-supported materials. J Biomed Mater Res. 1999;47:516-22.

11. Brunetto PS, Fromm KM. Antimicrobial coatings for implant surfaces. CHIMIA International Journal for Chemistry. 2008;62:249-52.

12. Slenters TV, Hauser-Gerspach I, Daniels AU, *et al*. Silver coordination compounds as light-stable, nano-structured and anti-bacterial coatings for dental implant and restorative materials. J Mater Chem. 2008;18:5359-62.

13. Lee HY, Park HK, Lee YM, *et al*. A practical procedure for producing silver nanocoated fabric and its antibacterial evaluation for biomedical applications. Chem Commun (Camb). 2007;28:2959-61.

14. Monteiro DR, Gorup LF, Takamiya AS, *et al*. The growing importance of materials that prevent microbial adhesion: antimicrobial effect of medical devices containing silver. Int J Antimicrob Agents. 2009;34:103-10.

15. Damm C, Münstedt H, Rösch A. Long-term antimicrobial polyamide 6/silver-nanocomposites. J Mater Sci. 2007;42:6067-73.

16. Welch K, Cai Y, Engqvist H, *et al*. Dental adhesives with bioactive and on-demand bactericidal properties. Dent Mater. 2010;26:491-9.

17. Heravi F, Ramezani M, Poosti M, *et al*. In vitro cytotoxicity assessment of an orthodontic composite containing titanium-dioxide nano-particles. J Dent Res Dent Clin Dent Prospects. 2013;7:192-198.

18. Morones JR, Elechiguerra JL, Camacho A, *et al*. The bactericidal effect of silver nanoparticles. Nanotechnology. 2005;16:2346-53.

19. Prabhu S, Poulose EK. Silver nanoparticles: mechanism of antimicrobial action, synthesis, medical applications, and toxicity effects. Int Nano Lett. 2012;2:32.

20. Feng QL, Wu J, Chen GQ, *et al*. A mechanistic study of the antibacterial effect of silver ions on Escherichia coli and Staphylococcus aureus. J Biomed Mater Res. 2000;52:662-8.

21. Shirai R, Miura T, Yoshida A, *et al*. Antimicrobial effect of titanium dioxide after ultraviolet irradiation against periodontal pathogen. Dent Mater J. 2016;35:511-6.

22. Sun J, Forster AM, Johnson PM, *et al*. Improving performance of dental resins by adding titanium dioxide nanoparticles. Dent Mater. 2011;27:972-82.

23. Parkinson CR, Sasov A. High-resolution non-destructive 3D interrogation of dentin using X-ray nanotomography. Dent Mater. 2008;24:773-7.

24. Melo MA, Cheng L, Zhang K, *et al*. Novel dental adhesives containing nanoparticles of silver and amorphous calcium phosphate. Dent Mater. 2013;29:199-210.

25. Zhang K, Melo MA, Cheng L, *et al*. Effect of quaternary ammonium and silver nanoparticle-containing adhesives on dentin bond strength and dental plaque microcosm biofilms. Dent Mater. 2012;28:842-52.

26. Ebadi Z, Atai M, Ebrahimi M. Mechanical and Anti-bacterial Properties of Dental Adhesive Containing Diamond Nanoparticles. Iran J Polym Sci Technol. 2011;24:121-31.

27. da SILVA EM, Miragaya L, Noronha-Filho JD, *et al*. Characterization of an experimental

resin composite organic matrix based on a tri-functional methacrylate monomer. Dent Mater J. 2016;35:159-65.

28. Degrazia FW, LEITUNE VCB, Garcia IM, *et al*. Effect of silver nanoparticles on the physicochemical and antimicrobial properties of an orthodontic adhesive. J Appl Oral Sci. 2016;24:404-10.

29. Cheng L, Weir MD, Xu HH, *et al*. Antibacterial amorphous calcium phosphate nanocomposites with a quaternary ammonium dimethacrylate and silver nanoparticles. Dent Mater. 2012;28:561-72.

9

Evaluation of Surface Characteristics of Denture Base Using Organic-Inorganic Hybrid Coating: An SEM Study

Jafari AA[a], Lotfi-Kamran MH[b], Ghafoorzadeh M[c], Shaddel SM[d*]

[a]Department of Medical Parasitology and Mycology, School of Medicine, Shahid Sadoughi University of Yazd Medical Sciences, Yazd, Iran

[b]Department of Prosthodontics, School of Dentistry, Shahid Sadoughi University of Yazd Medical Sciences, Yazd, Iran

[c]Paramedical School, Shahid Sadoughi University of Yazd Medical Sciences, Yazd, Iran

[d]Department of Prosthodontics, ShahidSadoughi University of Yazd Medical Sciences, Yazd, Iran

ARTICLE INFO

Key words:
Denture Base
Hybrid Coating
Surface Roughness
Scanning Electron Microscopy

Corresponding Author:
Sayed Mehrzad Shaddel
Department of Prosthodontics,
Shahid Sadoughi University
of Yazd Medical Sciences,
Yazd, Iran
Email: mehrzad1702@gmail.com

Abstract

Statement of Problem: Despite the numerous positive features of acrylic denture base, there are a number of undeniable associated disadvantages. The properties of denture base have been improved through various interventions including application of different types of filler and coatings.

Objectives: This study aimed to evaluate the surface roughness, thickness and coating quality of organic-inorganic coating on the denture base through scanning electron microscopy. Moreover, the colour change was evaluated visually.

Materials and Methods: The organic-inorganic hybrid coatings were prepared. Acrylic discs of 10×10 mm were fabricated. The test discs were dipped in the hybrid coating and cured. In order to evaluate the surface roughness and coating thickness, the surface and cross-section of the samples in both coated and control groups were subjected to scanning electron microscopy. The colour change and transparency were visually evaluated with naked eyes. The data were statistically analyzed by student's *t* test.

Results: The hybrid materials perfectly covered all the surfaces of acrylic resin and established proper thickness. The coated group seemed smoother and flatter than the control group; however, the difference was not statistically significant (for all parameters $p > 0.05$). It was quite a thin coating and no perceptible colour change was observed.

Conclusions: The hybrid coating maintained good binding, caused no noticeable discoloration, and thoroughly covered the acrylic resin surface with uniform delicate thickness. It also slightly improved the acrylic resin surface roughness.

Introduction

Among the several materials used for the denture bases, polymethyl methacrylate (PMMA) resins are the most favored ones [1]. They owe their popularity to their excellent working characteristics, pleasant physical and aesthetic properties, ease of fabrication, and cost-effectiveness [2]. Yet, like other denture base materials, there are some inherent limitations associated with PMMA resin which make it much different with an ideal denture base material [2,3].

When PMMA is polymerized, the compounds (monomers) of low molecular weight are converted (monomers) to polymers of high molecular weight [2,4]. Decreasing the processing temperature and time, results in increased residual monomer content within the processed denture base [2]. Its small size and hydrophilic nature causes the PMMA monomers to diffuse rapidly into the oral cavity and body [2,5], causing tissue irritation, hypersensitivity, or allergic reactions in some cases [4]. The mechanical properties and dimensional stability of dentures were found to be negatively influenced by the plasticizing effect of the excess monomer [6]. Meanwhile, a post-polymerization curing cycle is suggested to eliminate any remaining peroxides [7].

The surface-related features of denture-base materials including roughness, free energy, wettability, hydrophobicity, etc. are clinically important since they play roles in plaque accumulation and staining [1]. Surface roughness, particularly, affects the adhesion and retention of Candida Albicans [8]. Different species of Candida are opportunistic pathogens that reside in the oral cavity of even healthy individuals [9]. Candida biofilms contribute to the development and maintenance of denture stomatitis, which is known as the most common and clinically considerable lesion in denture wearers by virtue of their ability to adhere to acrylic resin [3].

The hybrid organic–inorganic materials are currently becoming so popular due to some particular features which promote them to the material of choice for a wide spectrum of technological applications [10]. Their employment in base resins may improve the colour stability and also reduce their water absorption and solubility, which can consequently extend the denture longevity [11].

At the molecular scale (nanometer), hybrid materials are composites comprised of two components [12], one of which is usually inorganic and the other is organic in nature. Accordingly, hybrids are different from the traditional composites whose components are at the macroscopic level (micrometer to millimeter) [12]. The material that is mixed at the microscopic level is generally so homogeneous that its properties are either between the two original phases or beyond the original one [13].

Interestingly, hybrids of adjustable characteristics can be designed or engineered for particular applications, based on the nature of their components [11,14]. Through the convenient process of sol–gel, hybrid materials can be prepared in the form of powders, monoliths or coatings. In this method, the chemical composition of the hybrid can be highly controlled at low temperature and large area processing [12].

Hybrid materials can be employed in decorative coatings in which the organic dyes are embedded in hybrid coatings. They are also used in scratch-resistant coatings that have hydrophobic or anti-fogging properties. Moreover, hybrids are employed in devices with nanocomposite base for electronic and optoelectronic applications (e.g. light-emitting diodes, photodiodes, solar cells, gas sensors and field effect transistors) [15].

In construction industry, the hybrids are included in fire retardant materials. In dentistry, they are used in nanocomposite-based dental filling materials. Likewise, they are used in proton conducting membranes of fuel cells, antistatic/anti-reflection coatings, as corrosion protection, porous hybrid materials, and antibacterial properties [12,15]. Besides being quite thin and uniformly covering all surfaces, a suitable coating should resist noticeable colour changes in the denture base. The present study aimed to apply hybrid coatings on denture base and identify the main structural changes through scanning electron microscopy (SEM). The null hypothesis was that inorganic-organic hybrid coating would not influence the surface roughness, thickness and colour of PMMA used in the denture base.

Materials and Methods

Two sheets of resin plates were made of heat polymerized material (PMMA - SR Triplex Hot Acrylic Resin, Ivoclar Vivadent Inc; England) through a classical press-pack dough moulding technique of 2-mm thick wax-plate flaked based on the polymerization regime as suggested by the manufacturer. The flask was immersed in cold water, tempered up to 100°C, and maintained at that temperature for 60 minutes. The plates were all sectioned into 10×10-mm samples. Metallographic abrasive paper (MATADOR; Germany) at 600 and 800 mesh were sequentially used to polish the samples. Then, they were rinsed in ethanol and deionized water for 3 times (each time 3 minutes), and were stored until used.

For the hybrid coatings, 10.4g tetraethyl orthosilicate, 30g ethylene glycol diethyl ether, 5.85g deionized water, and 0.39g glacial acetic acid were stirred in a flask for 1.5 hours in water bath at 40°C. Then, 4.72g (2, 3-epoxypropoxy) propyltrimethoxysilane (all by Kimia-Gostar; Tehran, Iran) was added to continue the reaction for 6 hours at 60°C and, then, left for another 24 hours. The flask was supplemented with 4.26g glycidylmethacrylate, 2.16g acrylic acid, 9g methyl methacrylate, and 147g EGME (all by Kimia-Gostar; Tehran, Iran), and then placed in an oil bath. The flask was connected to a condenser and stirring apparatus. Stirring began after nitrogen was added to the flask. The nitrogen gas was infused for 15 minutes.

The oil bath was heated and stabilized at 70°C. Then, 0.10 g of azobisisobutyronitrile was dissolved in 3g ethylene glycol monomethyl ether and injected into the flask. The complex was allowed to progress for 10 hours and after it cooled down to the room temperature, the stirring and nitrogen gas influx were stopped. 2 -methylimidazole (Kimia-Gostar; Tehran, Iran) was then added at 10% of the molar mass of the epoxy group. The mixture was stirred at room temperature for 24 hours to obtain organic-inorganic hybrid coatings. The hybrid coating was applied over the surface of the resin plates, dried, placed in oven at 70°C for 1 hour, and polymerized at 90°C for 2 hours.

The prepared specimens were divided into an experimental (n=5) and a control group (n=5). The selected samples were subjected to SEM evaluation (Phenom ProX; Netherlands). SEM photomicrographs were taken at different magnifications for visual inspection. This system was also used to measure the surface roughness on 3 locations of each surface sample (Ra and Rz as profile roughness parameters). To calculate the Ra using an algorithm, we measured the average distance between the peaks and valleys, as well as the deviation from the mean line on the entire surface within the sampling length. To calculate the Rz, we also measured the vertical distance from the highest peak to the lowest valley within five sampling lengths; the distances were finally averaged.

The 3D Roughness Reconstruction software

helped the Phenom desktop SEM systems to generate three-dimensional images and submicrometer roughness measurements. The coating thickness was measured on the cross-section of the resin-coated samples. Meanwhile, the major discolourations were merely checked with naked eyes since the minor colour changes in the denture did not matter. The two groups were visually compared visually. The data related to changes from the baseline of wrinkles as well as the roughness features were analyzed using SPSS software version 18.0 (SPSS Inc., Chicago, IL, USA). Student's t test was performed and the significance level was set at $\alpha = 0.05$.

Results

The SEM inspection of the hybrid-coated acryl resin plates and control group revealed a coarser topography in the latter (Figure 1, a-d). However, the results of t test showed no statistically significant difference between the two groups (for Rz, $p = 0.053$ and for Ra $p = 0.110$) (Table 1). The cross-section view of the coated resin plates showed the thickness of the coating material (20μm) (Figure 2). Moreover, a perfect junction was observed between the acrylic resin and hybrid coating, i.e. it was quite uniform and had no gap. According to the SEM, the hybrid coating thoroughly covered the acryl surfaces. The hybrid coating was more homogeneous and compact than the acrylic resin plates. No dramatic discolouration was observed in the coated and control groups, as shown with naked eye (Figure 3).

Table 1: Surface roughness (Rz, Ra) of specimens in each group. Data are mean ±standard deviation (n=5)

group	Rz (μm)	Ra (nm)
Control	5.1 ± 0.15	518 ± 47
Experimental	4.48 ± 0.59	474 ± 27
p-value	0.053	0.110

The result was not significant at $p > 0.05$.

Discussion

So far, various options like fillers, plasticizers and coating material have been used to improve the properties of denture-base [17,18]. Such interventions could change the mechanical and antibacterial properties of the denture base. Denture coatings are often used as the antimicrobial agent [17,19-22]. Sato

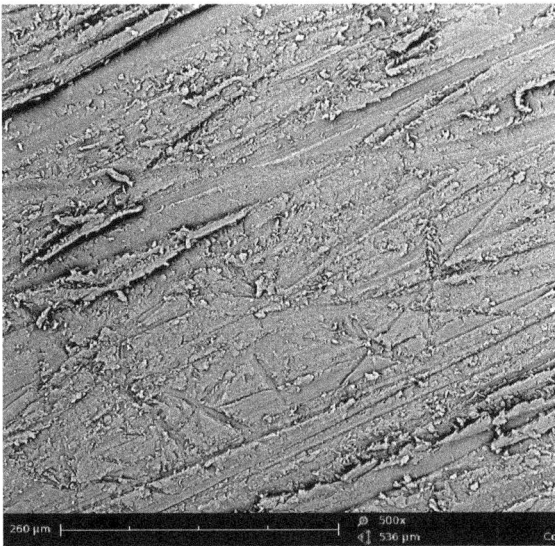

Figure 1-a: The surface roughness of a specimen in the control group at 500X

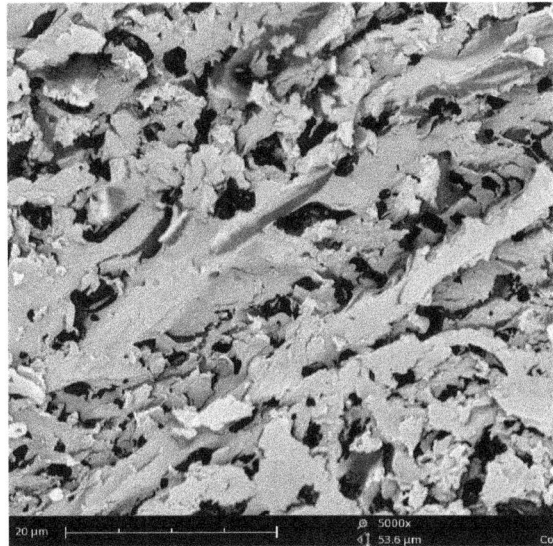

Figure 1-b: The surface roughness of a specimen in the control group at 5000X

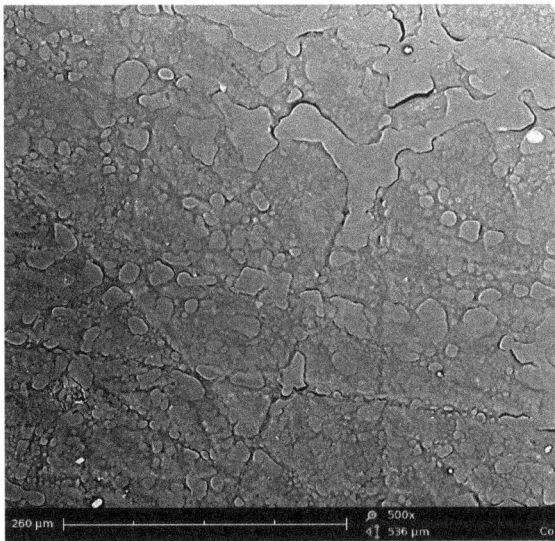

Figure 1-c: The surface roughness of a specimen in the coated group in 500X

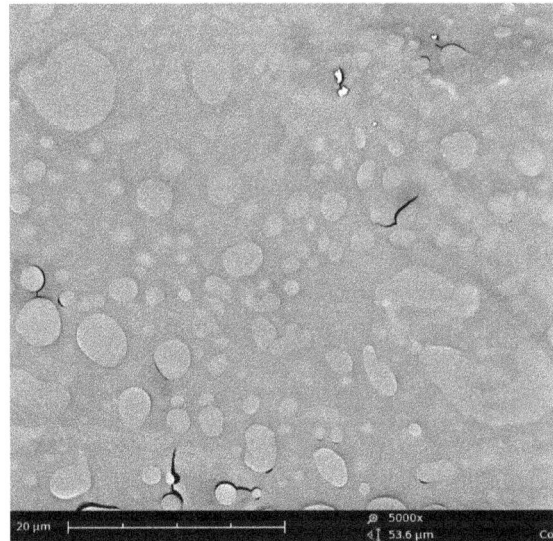

Figure 1-d: The surface roughness of a specimen in the coated group in 5000X

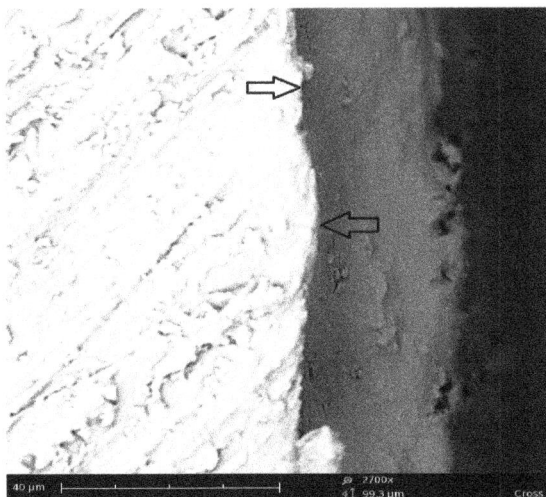

Figure 2: The cross-sectional view displaying the uniform junction. 20 μm thickness of coating (the coating is seen darker than the denture base).

et al. found that the use of mannan (the polysaccharide found in yeasts cell wall) coating on the denture base could prevent the adhesion of candida albicans [21]. Hybrid coating is also believed to improve the denture base properties [11,14,23]. It prevented water uptake into the base resin [11].

Zuo *et al.* noted that the hybrid coating effectively reduced the water uptake and solubility of the base resins and also improved the colour stability of the denture base. Moreover, they observed that this coating decreased the release of residual monomers and other particles of the resin, and prevented degradation of the denture base [11]. The network structure in hybrid coating is so dense that it decreases the adhesion and penetration of microorganisms like ceramic [23].

The denture roughness affects the adhesion

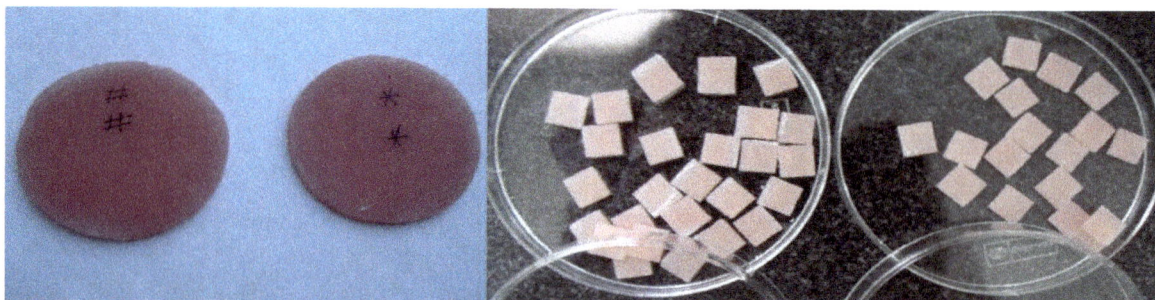

Figure 3: The control and coated groups. No significant discolouration was observable with naked eye. Visual comparison of the images confirms the absence of any significant difference in the discolouration between the two groups.

and retention of microorganisms, stain, plaque, and calculus [1]. Although the present study noted no statistically significant decrease in the surface roughness, more density and consistency was observed. This might be attributed to the reduced biofilm and plaque formation on the denture surface; however, it needs to be confirmed by more detailed studies. On the other hand, the wettability of the denture base is a determining factor in denture retention, especially in the maxilla [24]. It seems that the decreased surface roughness which is associated with lower surface contact results in lower wettability. This coating was hydrophilic, as Toselli et al. found that the hybrid coating improved the wettability since the coated acryl was more hydrophilic than pure acryl [23]. This coating can be used in nano science, as in coatings with nano-titania or nano-silver particles [17]. However, Wady et al. reported that the coating of silver nano-particles had no effect on candida albicans adherence [25].

The organic-inorganic hybrid used in the current study for coating of acryl resin disks provided a very thin coated layer of 20 μm thick (Figure 2). This feature can be an advantage for this coating as it does not interfere with the denture fit in denture users. Proper attachment of the hybrid layer to the resin is considerable because of chemical attachment. SEM evaluation showed continuous connection between the coating and the resin (Figure 2). Similarly, long-term coating should be insoluble.

The hybrid coatings are anti-scratch, as well [11,23]. The surface roughness promotes the denture base against candida adhesion, plaque accumulation, and stain. It was also reported by Toselli et al. and Mammeri et al. that the hybrid coating could resist the scratch and increase the surface hardness [10,23]. The employed hybrid layer formulation was transparent, so it did not alter the appearance and texture of the denture base [11]. Likewise, Toselli et

al. and Mammeri et al. visually compared the coating polymer films with control groups and found no colour change in the coating resin [10,23]. In those studies, the coating was so transparent that the writing on polymer films was readable after the coating.

Polymerization process of this coating layer was considered a repolymerization for the denture base and reduced the amount of residual monomer in denture base [2,11]. Likewise, Shim and Watts found that additional heat curing reduced the residual monomer in the resin [26]. Hybrid coating was found to have covered the microcracks and microporous, which can, in turn, make up for poor polymerizing or polishing, and improve the denture properties [10,11].

Conclusions

The hybrid coating employed in this study created a very delicate layer of 20μm thick with ideal junction on the acryl resin disks. Seemingly, this coating increases the quality and roughness of the denture base, and controls the microbial plaque formation. Yet, further studies are recommended to confirm the findings of the present study.

Conflict of Interest: None declared.

References

1. Farcaşiu AT, Antoniac IV, Antoniac A, et al. SEM Evaluation of Denture Base Materials Used in Clinical Practice. Key Engineering Materials. Trans Tech Pub. 2016;695:91-95.

2. Zarb GA, Hobkirk J, Eckert S, et al. Prosthodontic treatment for edentulous patients: complete dentures and implant-supported prostheses. 13th Edition. St. Louis, MO: Elsevier Mosby; 2013. p. 42-52.

3. Salerno C, Pascale M, Contaldo M, et al.

Candida-associated denture stomatitis. Med Oral Patol Oral Cir Bucal. 2011;16:139-143.

4. Papakonstantinou E, Raap U. Oral Cavity and Allergy: Meeting the Diagnostic and Therapeutic Challenge. Curr Oral Health Rep. 2016;3:347-355.

5. Zissis A, Yannikakis S, Polyzois G, et al. A long term study on residual monomer release from denture materials. Eur J Prosthodont Restor Dent. 2008;16:81-84.

6. Golbidi F, Jalali O. An evaluation of the Flexural Properties of Meliodent and Acropars Heat Polymerized Acrylic Resins. J Dent (Tehran) Univ Med Sci. 2007;4:68-71.

7. Jorge JH, Giampaolo ET, Vergani CE, et al. Effect of post-polymerization heat treatments on the cytotoxicity of two denture base acrylic resins. J Appl Oral Sci. 2006;14:203-207.

8. Bollenl CML, Lambrechts P, Quirynen M. Comparison of surface roughness of oral hard materials to the threshold surface roughness for bacterial plaque retention: A review of the literature. Dent Mater. 1997;13:258-269.

9. Jenkinson HF, Douglas LJ. Interactions between Candida species and bacteria in mixed infections. 1th Edition. ASM Press: Washington DC; 2002. p. 357-373.

10. Mammeri F, Rozes L, Sanchez C, et al. Mechanical Properties of SiO_2-PMMA Based Hybrid Organic-Inorganic Thin Films. J Sol-Gel Sci Technol. 2003;26:413-417.

11. Zuo W, Feng D, Song A, et al. Effects of organic-inorganic hybrid coating on the color stability of denture base resins. J Prosthet Dent. 2016;115:103-108.

12. Kickelbick G. Hybrid materials: synthesis, characterization, and applications. Available at: http://eu.wiley.com/WileyCDA/WileyTitle/productCd-3527312994.html

13. Huang ZH, Qiu KY. The effects of interactions on the properties of acrylic polymers/silica hybrid materials prepared by the in situ sol-gel process. Polymer. 1997;38:521-526.

14. Sassi Z, Bureau JC, Bakkali A. Structural characterization of the organic/inorganic networks in the hybrid material (TMOS–TMSM–MMA). Vib Spectrosc. 2002;28:251-262.

15. Drisko GL, Sanchez C. Hybridization in materials science–evolution, current state, and future aspirations. Eur J Inorg Chem. 2012;2012:5097-5105.

16. Kumar R, Münstedt H. Silver ion release from antimicrobial polyamide/silver composites. Biomaterials. 2005;26:2081-2088.

17. Song R, Jiao X, Lin L. Improvement of mechanical and antimicrobial properties of denture base resin by nano-titanium dioxide and nano-silicon dioxide particles. Pigm Resin Technol. 2011;40:393-398.

18. Tu M-G, Liang W-M, Wu T-C, et al. Improving the mechanical properties of fiber-reinforced acrylic denture-base resin. Mater Design. 2009;30:2468-2472.

19. Li X-l, Zuo W-w, Luo M, et al. Silver chloride loaded mesoporous silica particles and their application in the antibacterial coatings on denture base. Chem Res Chin Univ. 2013;29:1214-1218.

20. Marini M, De Niederhausern S, Iseppi R, et al. Antibacterial activity of plastics coated with silver-doped organic-inorganic hybrid coatings prepared by sol-gel processes. Biomacromolecules. 2007;8:1246-1254.

21. Sato M, Ohshima T, Maeda N, et al. Inhibitory effect of coated mannan against the adhesion of Candida biofilms to denture base resin. Dent Mater J. 2013;32:355-360.

22. Tsutsumi C, Takakuda K, Wakabayashi N. Reduction of Candida biofilm adhesion by incorporation of prereacted glass ionomer filler in denture base resin. J Dent. 2016;44:37-43.

23. Toselli M, Marini M, Fabbri P, et al. Sol–gel derived hybrid coatings for the improvement of scratch resistance of polyethylene. J Sol-Gel Sci Technol. 2007;43:73-83.

24. Kikuchi M, Ghani F, Watanabe M. Method for enhancing retention in complete denture bases. J Prosthet Dent. 1999;81:399-403.

25. Wady AF, Machado AL, Zucolotto V, et al. Evaluation of Candida albicans adhesion and biofilm formation on a denture base acrylic resin containing silver nanoparticles. J Appl Microbiol. 2012;112:1163-1172.

26. Shim JS, Watts D. Residual monomer concentrations in denture-base acrylic resin after an additional, soft-liner, heat-cure cycle. Dent Mater. 1999;15:296-300.

10

Microleakage Evaluation of Bulk-fill Composites Used with Different Adhesive Systems

Moosavi Hª; Moghaddas MJᵇ; Kordnoshahri Fᶜ; Zanjani Mᵈ*

ªAssociate Professor, Dental Materials Research Center, Department of Operative Dentistry, Mashhad Dental School, Mashhad University of Medical Sciences, Mashhad, Iran
ᵇAssociate Professor, Dental Materials Research Center, Department of Operative Dentistry, Mashhad Dental School, Mashhad University of Medical Sciences, Mashhad, Iran
ᶜGeneral Dentist, Mashhad Dental School, Mashhad University of Medical Sciences, Mashhad, Iran
ᵈPost graduate student, Department of Operative Dentistry, Mashhad Dental School, Mashhad University of Medical Sciences, Mashhad, Iran

ARTICLE INFO

Key words:
Bulk fill
Adhesive resin
Microleakage
Dye extraction

Corresponding Author:
Maryam Zanjani
Post graduate student,
Department of Operative
Dentistry, Mashhad Dental
School, Mashhad University of
Medical Sciences, Mashhad,
Iran
Email: Zanjanim941@mums.ac.ir

Abstract

Statement of Problem: The integrity of adhesive bond at the tooth/resin interface performs an essential role in the clinical success and survival of restorations.

Objectives: The purpose of this study was to compare microleakage of Class II cavities restored with total-etch or self-etch adhesives and different bulk-fill composites.

Materials and methods: Conventional class II cavities were prepared on forty sound human premolar teeth with approximately same size and shape. Half of the cavities restored with a sonic-resin placement system (SonicFill, Kerr), and the other half of the cavities with Tetric N-Ceram (TNC) composite with total-etch; Optibond Solo Plus or self-etch; Optibond XTR, adhesives. The samples stored in distilled water at 37 ° C for 24 hours, and then specimens were under 1000 thermal cycles. The teeth were covered with two layers of nail varnish except for one mm around gingival margins, and then were dipped in glass vials for 48 h at 37°C in a neutral-buffered 2% methy¬lene-blue solution. After removal from the dye, the teeth were rinsed and the varnish was removed, and stored individually in a glass vial containing 65% nitric acid. The vials were centrifuged, and 100 µl of the super¬natant from each was then analysed in a UV-Visible spectro¬photometer after a kinetic assay at 550 nm wavelength using concentrat¬ed nitric acid as the blank. So dye extraction was conducted to investigate the leakage test. Data were analysed by ANOVA test ($P<0.05$).

Results: The highest and lowest microleakage was related to self-etch/SonicFill and total-etch/Tetric N-Ceram groups respectively. The amount of microleakage was not significantly different among experimental groups ($P>0.05$).

Conclusions: Both of the bulk-fill composites with various adhesives had the same microleakage.

Introduction

In recent years, the composite resins are the first choice of restorative materials due to ever growing esthetic demand from the patients. Though the substantial improvements in esthetic, wear, and physical properties are achieved, the polymerization shrinkage is persisting as a major limitation [1]. The clinical consequences of the marginal gap include marginal leakage, postoperative sensitivity, secondary caries, discoloration, and cuspal strain [2]. The prevalence of proximal and cervical caries is on the rise due to large elder population and improved survival of teeth [3]. Several researchers have suggested the various techniques to reduce the polymerization shrinkage and consequently the better marginal integrity. The proposed methods are incremental placement, three sided light curing, centripetal build up, pulse cure, precured composite inserts, and intermediate layer; glass ionomer cement, auto polymerizing composites, and flowable composites [4-9]. Scientists have presented a new generation of composites and adhesives with less contraction property and also various techniques to reduce polymerization shrinkage and thus, better marginal integrity [5,10]. Few authors also suggested the bulk placement and curing to reduce the marginal gap and stress at the cavosurface margins [11]. The investigators have reported the reduced polymerization shrinkage with bulk curing methods [12]. Obtaining optimum seal between composites and tooth structure is critical for the clinical longevity of restoration and will contribute significantly toward the improved public oral health. SonicFill is a single-step composite system that doesn't require an additional capping layer. SonicFill system combines the advantages of a flowable composite with a universal composite. SonicFill system is comprised of a KaVo handpiece that enables sonic activation of a specially designed and conveniently delivered composite from Kerr. SonicFill's activation significantly reduces the composite viscosity to rapidly fill the cavity. However, this technique does not have cost benefit [6]. To overcome this disadvantage, a group of new products has been introduced known as bulk-fill composites that could be inserted in 4 mm bulk [7,8]. Using bulk-fill composites, clinical steps will be reduced by filling the cavity in single increment,

leading to less porosity and a uniform consistency [7]. Dental adhesive systems can be categorized based on the clinical procedure in "etch-and-rinse adhesives" and "self-etch adhesives". Other essential considerations concern the different anatomical characteristics of enamel and dentine which are involved in the bonding procedures that have also implications for the technique used as well as for the quality of the bond [13]. The restorative procedure with composites are very time-consuming and technically demanding, particularly concerning the application of the adhesive system. Therefore, together bulk-fill composites and self-etch adhesives could reduce operator error and chair side time. The microleakage under composite restoration is the topic of intense research for a long time. Hence, the purpose of this in vitro study was to compare the microleakage of class II bulk-fill composite restorations either with total-etch or self-etch adhesives.

Materials and Methods

This *in vitro* experimental study was conducted on forty intact human premolars of approximately the same size extracted within the past six months. The teeth were sound and had no carious lesions, cracks or fracture. The teeth were stored in Chloramine T 0/5 % solution at room temperature for disinfection. Conventional Class II cavities were prepared on one of the proximal surfaces of the teeth. Cavities were prepared with diamond bur (835/012‡) in a high-speed hand piece with water spray and the same size as much as possible, by one operator. It was used periodontal probes for measurement the depth and width with pulpal floor depth of 2 ± 0.5 mm, gingival width of 1.5 ± 0.5 mm, axial height of 2 ± 0.5 mm, and buccolingual width to 1/3 the distance between the tip of cusps. Therefore, the cervical margin of the cavity was extended about to the cementoenamel junction. The cavity had 90 cavosurface margins. The burs (Mani, INC. 8-3 Kiyohara Industrial Park, Utsunomiya, Tochigi, 321-3231, JAPAN) were replaced every five cavity preparations. The teeth were randomly divided into two groups (n=20). A transparent matrix was then placed on the tooth. Half of the cavities were restored with viscose bulk-fill composite resin (SonicFill, Kerr) with total-etch adhesives; Optibond Solo Plus (Kerr) or self-etch adhesive; Optibond XTR (Kerr) and the other half were restored with bulk-fill composite resin Tetric N-Ceram (Ivoclar Vivadent) with total-etch or self-etch technique, according to the manufacturer's instructions. For use Optibond Solo plus, the cavity was etched by 37% phosphoric acid on the enamel margins for five seconds and was then applied on dentin for 15 seconds, rinsed with air and water spray for 10 seconds and dried with cotton pellet. Optibond Solo Plus adhesive was then applied, air sprayed for 3-5 seconds from 1 cm distance and cured for 20 seconds. Using Optibond XTR adhesive, the initial Optibond XTR primer was applied on the enamel and dentin surfaces for 20 seconds and then was dried for 5 seconds with medium pressure air spray. To use Optibond XTR adhesive, it was primarily applied for 15 seconds on enamel and dentin and then dried out with air spray, light cured for 20 seconds using a Bluephase C8 (IvoclarVivadent, Schaan, Liechtenstein) light-curing unit with a light intensity of 800 mW/cm2. Cavities were then restored in one increment with the composite (SonicFill or Tetric N-Ceram) and cured with light for 20 seconds from occlusal, buccal and lingual sides. Restorative materials used in this study was shown in Table 1. After removing matrix, a scalpel and fine diamond burs were used to eliminate any excess material, especially at the gingival margin. A series of paper disks (Sof-Lex) were used to finish margins. Samples were stored in 37°C distilled water for 24 hours and thermocycled for 1000 cycles between 5 and 55 °C with a six minutes dwell time. 40 teeth were covered with 2 layers of nail varnish (VepaKozmetik, Istanbul, Turkey), except for one mm around gingival margin. The teeth were dipped in glass vials for 48 hours at 37°C in a neutral-buffered 2% methy¬lene-blue solution, under normal atmospheric pressure. After removing the dye, the teeth were rinsed under tap water for 30 min and the varnish was removed using a sharp scal¬pel, and then stored individually in a glass vial containing 600 μl of concentrated (65%) nitric acid for 3 days. The vials were centrifuged (LABNT, Spectrafuge 16M, USA) at 14000 rpm for 5 min, and 100 μl of the super-natant from each was then analysed in a UV-Visible spectro¬photometer (UNIC visible with scanner S2150,2100PC,USA) after a kinetic assay at 550 nm wavelength using concentrat¬ed nitric acid as the blank. In this manner, we recorded wavelength of diffused dye at tooth-restorative material interface. To check the normality of data distribution, Kolmogorov-Smirnov test was used. ANOVA test was conducted for evaluating of microleakage of experimental groups. The post-

Table 1: Materials, major components and manufacturers used in this study

Material	Major Components	Manufacturer
Optibond™ Solo Plus	Bis-GMA, HEMA, glycerol phosphate dimethacrylate (GPDM), sodium fluorosilicate, initiator, ethanol, water	Kerr, Orange, CA, USA
Optibond™ XTR	Primer : GPDM, hydrophilic co-monomers, water/ethanol, acetone Adhesive: resin monomers, inorganic fillers,ethanol	Kerr, Orange, CA, USA
SonicFill	Bis-GMA, TEGDMA, EBADMA, SiO2, glass, oxide, 83.5% filler	Kerr, Sybron Dental
Tetric N-Ceram	Bis-GMA, Bis-EMA, UDMA, barium aluminium silicate glass, Isofiller, ytterbium fluoride, spherical mixed oxide, camphorquinone plus an acyl phosphine oxide, dibenzoyl germanium derivative, 80% filler	IvoclarVivadent, Schaan, Liechtenstein

hoc multiple comparisons Tukey's test was used for pair wise comparisons. The statistical significance was set at p value less than 0.05. All statistical analyses were performed with Statistical Package for Social Sciences (SPSS) version 16 (SPSS Inc., Chicago, IL, USA).

Results

Table 2 illustrates the mean and standard deviation microleakage for all groups. ANOVA test was done to explore the difference in mean microleakage among studied groups. The analysis showed there was no difference among groups (P>0.05) and consequently, the type of adhesive and composite had no influence on the amount of microleakage (P= 0.13). All samples restored with SonicFill or Tetric N-Ceram composite and total-etch or self-etch adhesive showed the microleakage at the margins. The highest and lowest microleakage was related to self-etch/SonicFill (0.63) and total-etch/Tetric N-Ceram (0.43) groups respectively. However, this study showed that there was no difference between experimental groups in microleakage (P>0.05).

Table 2: Mean microleakage values and standard deviations for the experimental groups

groups	Number	Mean	Standard Deviation
Total-etch/SonicFill	10	0.58	0.04
Self-etch/SonicFill	10	0.63	0.01
Total-etch/TetricN-ceram	10	0.43	0.03
Self-etch/TetricN-ceram	10	0.45	0.01

Discussion

The present study was an effort to find the desirable material, which had least microleakage. This trial evaluated and compared the microleakage of two relatively new composite resins SonicFill and Tetric N-Ceram along with total-etch and self-etch adhesives in conventional class II cavities. In order to simulate oral cavity environment and clinical states, we used 1000 thermocycling test at 5-55° C according to 11450 ISO protocol. In our investigation, none of the tested adhesive systems eliminated microleakage in dentin margin of the cavity. This is in agreement with previ¬ous studies that evaluated microleakage of tooth-colour restorations at dentin interface [14-16]. In this study, selection of human permanent premolars of approximately the same size was based on maximum standardization and elimination of the possible effect of tooth anatomy on the results. It has been stated that etch-and-rinse adhesive systems generally perform better on enamel than self-etching systems which may be more appropriate for bonding to dentine. In order to escape a possible loss of the restoration, secondary caries or pulp damage due to bacteria penetration or due to cytotoxicity effects of eluted adhesive components, careful attention of several factors is essential in selecting the suitable bonding procedure and adhesive system for the individual patient situation [13]. Poggio et al. [17] evaluated microleakage of class II conventional and bulk-fill composite restorations with their gingival margin below the cementoenamel junction. All composite restorations showed some degrees of microleakage in their study but SonicFill composite showed minimum microleakage. However, in our study, Tetric N-Ceram bulk-fill with total-etch adhesive in comparison to SonicFill composite showed the best results, although the difference with other groups was not statistical significance. Moreover, it showed greater microleakage in dentin margin of conventional and bulk fill restorations, which was in accordance with our results and may be due to the lower thickness of enamel at the gingival margin, greater distance of light curing unit from the gingival margin and weaker bond to dentin compared to enamel [18]. A systematic review concluded that bulk-fill composites provide a bond to dentin as strong as that of conventional composites without the problems related to polymerization shrinkage of conventional composites and can be very useful particularly for deep cavities [19]. The microleakage test was designed taking into consideration; dye extraction, is the most frequent choices in test variables, as reported by prior studies [20,21]. Just like previous studies, in the present study, it was found that there was no statistical difference between SonicFill and Tetric N-Ceram composites in microleakage, as well two examined adhesives [22-24].Thus, our null hypothesis was verified. The highest average of microleakage was contributed to SonicFill group with self-etch adhesive, and the least average of microleakage was contributed to Tetric N-Ceram group with total-etch adhesive. This result is in agreement with earlier research [15,16]. It was found that the best marginal compatibility is contributed to Tetric N-Ceram composite which resembles our findings that indicate the least amount of microleakage is in this group [25]. Bulk-fill composites have been introduced to facilitate the placement of deep direct resin composite restorations. An ideal bulk-fill composite would be one that could be placed into a preparation having a high C-factor design and still exhibit very little polymerization shrinkage stress, while maintaining a high degree of cure throughout [26].

According to manufacturing claimed that Tetric N-Ceram bulk-fill enables posterior teeth to be restored with only one layer measuring up to four-millimetres in thickness, which considerably heightens efficiency. The patented light activator Ivocerin is responsible for ensuring the complete cure of the filling. Compared with conventional light initiators, the Ivocerin polymerisation booster is much more reactive. Therefore, polymerization is initiated even in very deep cavities and the material is fully cured. A specially conditioned shrinkage stress reliever keeps shrinkage and shrinkage stress during polymerization to a minimum. In addition, Tetric N-Ceram contains a mixture of bisphenol-A diglycidyldimethacrylate, urethane dimethacrylate, and ethoxylated bisphenol A dimethacrylate, all of which are high-molecular-weight monomers with high viscosity and low polymerization shrinkage [27]. Based on the most of studies done till now, an incremental layering technique has been the standard procedure in direct posterior composite restorations to diminish polymerization shrinkage stress and achieve sufficient curing [28,29]. SonicFill is a composite restoration where the viscosity of the composite is dramatically reduced up to 87%, due to the special rheological modifiers that react to sonic activation of the material delivered through the SonicFill hand piece during its placement, thus, increasing its flow and enabling rapid filling of the cavity. Precise adaptation to the cavity walls make the frequency and size of critical

voids located at the margin and along line angles of the cavity less pronounced compared to the conventional putty-like composites [30]. When the sonic energy is stopped, the composite returns to a more viscous, non-slumping state that is perfect for carving and contouring [31]. Generally, increasing the filler load in the resin matrix results in reduction of overall shrinkage of the composite due to the reduced availability of the monomer for the curing reaction. However, it may also result in increasing the viscosity of a material, thus posing difficulty in placement and more chances of gap formation and microleakage [29]. SonicFill consist of a special composite formulation that contains about 83.5% of fillers by weight, which is more higher when compared to the filler content of Tetric N-Ceram (80%wt) [30]. There was no significant difference in the microleakage between the two different bulk-fill materials used in this study, which might be attributed to the similarity in their filler loading. It has also been documented that an increase in filler volume content results in an increase in the stiffness of the material with high modulus of elasticity, thereby increasing the microleakage, which consents with the results of the current study [32]. Al-Harbi et al. [33] showed that SonicFill composite, with total-etch adhesive, had the best marginal integrity, though not statistically significant. Although the result of that research was different from our findings in composite type, it was in agreement with our study in adhesive type. This finding is similar to the study of Campos et al. that found no difference between bulk-fill and conventional composites [34]. Moreover, in our trial, there was no difference between total-etch adhesive and self-etch adhesive, similar to Delbons et al.[35]. The reason of this finding seems to be the presence of ethanol base solvent and the same adhesives that were employed. In another study, SonicFill composite with total-etch adhesives have shown the best marginal integrity [20]. Despite different method of analysis tests used, our study yielded the same results. Nevertheless, there were some unavoidable limitations in our study such as long-term storage of tooth hydration condition, absence of mastication forces, and patient dental habits, which might not necessarily be expected in actual practice.

It is obvious that dentists have always been looking

for a fast and reliable filling technique that allows reduction of layers, effort and time; therefore, the time-consuming incremental layering technique can be substituted with the bulk-fill technique using SonicFill as a bulk-fill material. Therefore, further research evaluating the properties of the materials with various adhesives and its clinical implications are recommended in future.

Conclusions

There was no difference between self-etch and total-etch adhesives with two bulk- fill composites, Tetric N-ceram and SonicFill resin composites, regarding their various placement methods, in term of cervical marginal microleakage.

Acknowledgments

Authors would like to thank for vice chancellor of research of Mashhad University of Medical Sciences for approve the grant for doing the research. The results presented in this study have been taken from a student thesis no: 2799, proposal code 931008.

Conflict of Interest: None declared.

References

1. Agrawal VS, Parekh VV, Shah NC. Comparative evaluation of microleakage of silorane-based composite and nanohybrid composite with or without polyethylene fiber inserts in class II restorations: An in vitro study. Oper Dent. 2012;37:E1-7.

2. Kaya S, Yigit Özer S, Adigüzel Ö, et al. Comparison of apical microleakage of dual-curing resin cements with fluid-filtration and dye extraction techniques. Med Sci Monit. 2015;21:937-44.

3. Somani R, Jaidka S, Arora S. Comparative evaluation of microleakage of newer generation dentin bonding agents: An in vitro study. Indian J Dent Res. 2016; 27:86-90.

4. Park J, Chang J, Ferracane J, et al. How should composite be layered to reduce shrinkage stress: incremental or bulk filling? Dent Mater. 2008;24:1501-5.

5. Lutz F, Krejci I, Luescher B,et al. Improved proximal margin adaptation of Class II composite resin restorations by use of light-reflecting wedges. Quintessence Int. 1986;17:659-64.

6. Eakle WS, Ito RK. Effect of insertion technique on microleakage in mesio-occlusodistal composite resin restorations. Quintessence Int. 1990;21:369-74.

7. Kanca J, Suh BI. Pulse activation: reducing resin-based composite contraction stresses at the enamel cavosurface margins. Am J Dent. 1999;12:107-12.

8. Hagge MS, Lindemuth JS, Mason JF, et al. Effect of four intermediate layer treatments on microleakage of Class II composite restorations. Gen Dent. 2001;49:489-95.

9. Majety KK, Pujar M. In vitro evaluation of microleakage of class II packable composite resin restorations using flowable composite and resin modified glass ionomers as intermediate layers. J Conserv Dent. 2011;14:414-7.

10. Giachetti L, Scaminaci Russo D, Bambi C, et al. A review of polymerization shrinkage stress: current techniques for posterior direct resin restorations. J Contemp Dent Pract. 2006;7:79-88.

11. Abbas G, Fleming GJ, Harrington E, et al. Cuspal movement and microleakage in premolar teeth restored with a packable composite cured in bulk or in increments. J Dent. 2003;31:437-44.

12. Belvedere PC. Contemporary posterior direct composites using state-of-the-art techniques. Dent Clin North Am. 2001;45:49-70.

13. Milia E, Cumbo E, Cardoso RJ, et al. Current dental adhesives systems. A narrative review. Curr Pharm Des. 2012;18:5542-52.

14. Sadeghi M. Influence of flowable materials on microleakage of nanofilled and hybrid Class II composite restorations with LED and QTH LCUs. Indian J Dent Res. 2009;20:159-63.

15. Osorio R, Toledano M, de Leonardi G, et al. Microleakage and interfacial morphology of self-etching adhesives in class V resin composite restorations. J Biomed Mater Res B Appl Biomater. 2003;66:399-409.

16. Koubi S, Raskin A, Dejou J, et al. Effect of dual cure composite as dentin substitute on the

marginal integrity of Class II open-sandwich restorations. Oper Dent. 2010; 34:150-6.

17. Poggio C, Chiesa M, Scribante A, *et al.* Microleakage in Class II composite restorations with margins below the CEJ: in vitro evaluation of different restorative techniques. Med Oral Patol Oral Cir Bucal. 2013;18:e793-8.

18. Juloski J, Carrabba M, Aragoneses JM, *et al.* Microleakage of Class II restorations and microtensile bond strength to dentin of low-shrinkage composites. Am J Dent. 2013;26:271-7.

19. Akah MM, Daifalla LE, Yousry MM. Bonding of bulk fill versus contemporary resin composites: A systematic review and meta-analysis. Indian J Sci Technol. 2016;9:1-13.

20. Asselin ME, Fortin D, Sitbon Y, *et al.* Marginal microleakage of a sealant applied to permanent enamel: evaluation of 3 application protocols. Pediatr Dent. 2008;30:29-33.

21. Cehreli ZC, Gungor HC. Quantitative microleakage evaluation of fissure sealants applied with or without a bonding agent: results after four-year water storage in vitro. J Adhes Dent. 2008;10:379-84.

22. Sivakumar JS, Prasad AS, Soundappan S, *et al.* A comparative evaluation of microleakage of restorations using silorane-based dental composite and methacrylate-based dental composites in Class II cavities: An in vitro study. J Pharm Bioallied Sci.2016;8:S81-S5.

23. Cantekin K, Gumus H. In vitro and clinical outcome of sandwich restorations with a bulk-fill flowable composite liner for pulpotomized primary teeth. J Clin Pediatr Dent.2014; 38:349-54.

24. Schwendicke F, Kern M, Dorfer C, *et al.* Influence of using different bonding systems and composites on the margin integrity and the mechanical properties of selectively excavated teeth in vitro. J Dent.2015; 43:327-34.

25. Agarwal RS, Hiremath H, Agarwal J, *et al.* Evaluation of cervical marginal and internal adaptation using newer bulk fill composites:

An in vitro study. J Conserv Dent. 2015; 18:56-61.

26. Tantbirojn D, Pfeifer CS, Braga RR, *et al.* Do low-shrink composites reduce polymerization shrinkage effects? J Dent Res. 2011; 90:596-601.

27. Gonçalves F, Kawano Y, Pfeifer C, *et al.* Influence of BisGMA, TEGDMA, and BisEMA contents on viscosity, conversion, and flexural strength of experimental resins and composites. Eur J Oral Sci. 2009 ;117:442-6.

28. Feilzer AJ, Gee AJD, Davidson CL. Setting stress in composite resin in relation to configuration of the restoration. J Dent Res. 1987;66:1636-39.

29. Jang JH, Park SH, Hwang IN. Polymerization shrinkage and depth of cure of bulk- fill resin composites and highly filled flowable resin. Oper Dent. 2015;40:172-80.

30. Hirata R, Pacheco RR, Caceres E, *et al.* Effect of Sonic Resin Composite Delivery on Void Formation Assessed by Micro-computed Tomography. Oper Dent. 2018;43:144-150.

31. Eunice C, Margarida A, João CL, *et al.* 99mTc in the evaluation of microleakage of composite resin restorations with SonicFillTM. An in vitro experimental model. Open J Stomatol. 2012;2:340-47.

32. Senawongse P, Pongprueksa P, Tagami J. The effect of the elastic modulus of low-viscosity resins on the microleakage of Class V resincomposite restorations under occlusal loading. Dent Mater J. 2010;29:324-9.

33. Al-Harbi F, Kaisarly D, Bader D, *et al.* Marginal Integrity of Bulk Versus Incremental Fill Class II Composite Restorations. Oper Dent. 2016; 41:146-56.

34. Campos EA, Ardu S, Lefever D,*et al.* Marginal adaptation of class II cavities restored with bulk-fill composites. J Dent. 2014;42:575-81.

35. Delbons FB, Perdigao J, Araujo E, *et al.* Randomized clinical trial of four adhesion strategies in posterior restorations-18-month results. J Esthet Restor Dent. 2015;27:107-17.

11

Development of a Method to Obtain more Accurate General and Oral Health Related Information Retrospectively

Golkari A[a,b]*****, **Sabokseir A**[a], **Blane D**[c], **Sheiham A**[b], **Watt RG**[b]

[a]Oral and Dental Disease Research Center and Department of Dental Public Health, School of Dentistry, Shiraz University of Medical Sciences, Shiraz, Iran
[b]Research Department of Epidemiology and Public Health, University College London, London, UK
[c]Department of Social Science and Medicine, Imperial College London, London, UK

ARTICLE INFO	Abstract
Key words: Data Collection Epidemiology Eetrospective Studies Early Childhood *Corresponding Author:* Ali Golkari Department of Dental Public Health, School of Dentistry, Shiraz University of Medical Sciences, Shiraz, Iran E-mail: golkaria@sums.ac.ir, aligolkari@yahoo.com	***Statement of Problem***: Early childhood is a crucial period of life as it affects one's future health. However, precise data on adverse events during this period is usually hard to access or collect, especially in developing countries. ***Objectives***: This paper first reviews the existing methods for retrospective data collection in health and social sciences, and then introduces a new method/tool for obtaining more accurate general and oral health related information from early childhood retrospectively. ***Materials and Methods***: The Early Childhood Events Life-Grid (ECEL) was developed to collect information on the type and time of health-related adverse events during the early years of life, by questioning the parents. The validity of ECEL and the accuracy of information obtained by this method were assessed in a pilot study and in a main study of 30 parents of 8 to 11 year old children from Shiraz (Iran). Responses obtained from parents using the final ECEL were compared with the recorded health insurance documents. ***Results***: There was an almost perfect agreement between the health insurance and ECEL data sets (Kappa value=0.95 and $p < 0.001$). Interviewees remembered the important events more accurately (100% exact timing match in case of hospitalization). ***Conclusions:*** The Early Childhood Events Life-Grid method proved to be highly accurate when compared with recorded medical documents.

Introduction

Life course epidemiology is a multidisciplinary approach to the study of health, its components, and its compromising factors. It attempts to integrate short- and long-term effects of different kinds of

physical and psychological factors that affect the development of diseases, and to study them longitudinally throughout the course of life of individuals, instead of looking at specific cross-sectional points of life [1]. The factors assessed include past health status, genetic differences, behaviours, and environmental exposures that may directly or indirectly affect the health of individuals or populations, starting from their gestational life or even previous generations [2]. Although life course epidemiology assembles a considerable amount of early childhood related data from cohort studies, especially birth cohorts, link registered methods and clinical assessments, the retrospective questionnaires remain vital for such studies [3]. Unfortunately, little research has been conducted to develop methods to collect accurate data from early life for life course studies.

Data Sources/ Data Collection for Use in Life Course Epidemiology

There are four main sources of life course data: cohort studies, linked-register method of collecting data, clinical assessments, and retrospective questionnaires. These methods are briefly reviewed here.

Birth cohort studies have been the main sources of data for life course epidemiologists, especially those with an interest in the role of early childhood. However, cohorts have their own disadvantages. That makes it impractical to exclusively rely on them. One disadvantage is that they are mainly done in more affluent countries because of their cost. Another problem is the long time needed to yield results [4]. For those reasons, the number of birth cohorts from which data can be used to assess influences of early childhood on later age is limited to those started in mid-20th century in northern countries and, therefore, cannot be extrapolated to less affluent countries. Cohorts are also vulnerable to the new questions that arise by advances in understanding of health components and risks [4].

Cohort studies, similar to other longitudinal studies, are affected by sample attrition over time. That is more common in birth cohorts where subjects frequently move from their residence. Last but not least is that although cohort studies are meant to be conducted as a contemporaneous observation, they are usually framed by several retrospective questionnaires asking subjects about events that occurred during short periods of their past, usually the period between the two questionnaires/interviews. This depends on remembering events of the past few months or years by them. Due to the disadvantages mentioned above, although the best type of life course epidemiology is still considered to be a cohort study from birth, many researchers have to use fully or partly retrospectively collected data.

Since the 1990s, linked-register methodologies have been used in a number of life course studies to assure the reliability of information obtained from the past. In this method, past life information obtained by a questionnaire is compared with documents kept by households, registered information from hospitals or clinics, and data gathered by other researchers [3]. This method is mainly used to obtain data from birth, as the most accessible registered data [5] and gestational life, as these are not included in most cohort studies [6,7]. Although most of the data obtained by this method are highly reliable, their application is limited by the limited amount of information that is recorded.

Clinical assessments such as clinical examination, anthropometric measurements, body activity tests, and most importantly, laboratory tests can also be used to obtain some data on the present and past health status and possible exposures to risk factors. The main disadvantage of these assessments is that they are restricted to physical measures. Non-organic past exposures cannot be readily assessed with this method. Moreover, this method would not provide much information, even on the past physical exposures, because they are masked by the affected tissues or healing of organs.

Retrospective questionnaires, although of questionable accuracy, is the only data collection option left to many epidemiologists. Nevertheless, it is vital to have a good questionnaire combined with a good method of interview to help people remember past events, especially to remember the precise timing of events. Designing such questionnaires so that an acceptable degree of accuracy is achieved, or development of methods to validate the previously obtained data, remains a challenge for many researchers.

Retrospective Data Collection

Retrospective data are mainly collected using either self-administered or interview-based questionnaires and by asking the subjects about themselves or their relatives' past experiences. Questionnaires rely on respondents answering questions correctly. Several factors may compromise the quality of the data obtained. However, the most important factors to improve the accuracy of data are: 1) convincing the respondents to participate and answer fully and honestly, and 2) to trigger their memory to remember events and their precise timings. The former is a matter of sample recruitment, design of questionnaire and attracting the subjects' interest and trust. These are usually tested and reported, for example, as the response rate and missing values or by comparing responses to parallel questions. The latter, however, has always been problematic, especially because it is difficult to measure the accuracy of people's memory.

The usual way to test the accuracy of the subject's answers is to compare them with the existing recorded documents. However, such documents covering the life course of subjects do not usually exist. If they do, there is no need to collect new data retrospectively. Even if such reports exist, no recorded document is perfectly accurate. Therefore, unknown level of accuracy of data can be considered as the main shortcoming applicable to many life course publications [3]. This is a further reason for developing better methods to improve the accuracy of people's recall and practical ways to validate them.

Several intuitive ways have been introduced (usually by psychologists) that claim to help people to remember their past events more accurately [8]. One method with the most promise is the life-grid method [4]. It has proved to make significant differences in reliability and accuracy of recalls, especially when precise time or age of events matters [9,10].

Life-grid method of collecting past life course data
Individuals differ in their capacity to remember. This is particularly true for autobiographical "extended special events" and "life time period" memories [11] which are the usual targets of life course epidemiology questionnaires. However, there are certain outstanding events that people remember better. Such events are personal landmarks such as birth, marriage, birth of children, death of close relatives, or important educational steps. Others are public landmarks that had impacts on the person's life. They include wars, natural disasters, and major political changes [4,12].

These outstanding events or "landmarks" can be used to improve the memory of other less important personal events. Even if the exact timings of some events are not remembered by respondents, they might still be able to recall the order of events by linking them to landmarks if each target event happened soon after or before a landmark event. Two or several landmark events with known timings can be used to help the subjects remember events that happened between landmarks, or to recall timing of an event. A method called bounded recall [12,13] was used to develop a technique called Event History Calendar (EHC). In EHC, the timings of a series of landmarks, either personal or public, are first discussed with the interviewee. Subjects will be prompted by the interviewer, first to trigger their memory and later to anchor their memory and place events with unknown timings in the time period between two landmarks [14].

The EHC was further developed into a well-designed life-grid method of collecting retrospective data. In the original method, introduced by Blane [4], the questionnaire is accompanied with a grid-like table with four major columns; the first 4 columns of the current study's early childhood events life-grid. The first column is called external line and contains time and important events outside the family known as public landmark events. All subjects or at least those who live in one area share the external line. The second column is called personal lifeline. Information regarding important events inside the family, such as births, deaths, marriages and divorces, are put in this column. The third column called residential line, contains data about type, size, facilities and addresses of all houses that the target person has lived in. The last column is occupational line and is about changes in a person's work status and certain conditions of jobs. The information related to each column is gathered and checked in relation to other columns and corrections made as the interviewee remembers more details.

Studies by Blane showed that people were happy with the method as they remembered precise details of their life with this method and reported reasonable proportions of precise data collection when results of the life-grid were compared with documents. The proportion dramatically increased from 41% -100% to 83% - 100%, when small mistakes were ignored [4, 10].

There is a controversy about letting the respondent see the grid while it is getting completed, as that will help the process of remembering events. Showing people the results of their pervious answers may give them more ideas about the events related to them, but at the same time it omits the triggering effects of an event being prompted by the interviewer. Moreover, the way the life-grid was used in recent studies looks complicated and might cause confusion or loss of orientation. On the other hand, having some illustrative material may be a simple timeline showing two ends of the period of time being discussed in the interview and locating events between them. That has proved to significantly increase the accuracy of answers [8,15,16]. A semi-structured method of questioning, which includes free recalls inside each column, also improves the quality of data obtained by giving time for the respondent to think and choose from those events that they remember first [16,17].

Since its introduction, the life-grid method has been extensively used worldwide and has shown to be very good at obtaining accurate timing of the past events in both qualitative and quantitative studies [8-10,16,18-22]. In most of these studies the life-grids were slightly changed and adapted to gain desirable information based on the objectives of each study.

Despite the extensive use of the life-grid and the event history calendar (EHC) methods by epidemiologists during the last decade, only two studies have used a rigorous approach to test the concurrent validity of these methods by comparing their findings with the recorded documents or previously collected data. Berney [10] compared the family and household data of 26 subjects obtained by the life-grid method after 50 years with recorded documents when exact timing of events was not one of objectives. He reported a kappa value between 0.41 and 1.0 for the agreement between the two data sets. The levels of agreement increased markedly when "$\pm$ unit" was added to the exact matches (0.83 < k < 1.0)[10].

Belli *et al.* [23] interviewed more than 600 randomly selected subjects on social and economic events occurring in the past 2-3 years by either the conventional question-list method or an event history calendar (EHC) method. They compared the results of both groups with the previously collected data as "gold standards". The agreement between data collected by EHC with the gold standards was substantial for 7 categorical variables (0.63 < k <0.79) and significantly higher than the conventional method for 2 of them. They also found significantly higher correlations between the EHC method and gold standard than the conventional method for 6 out of 9 continuous variables. Again timing of events was not an objective [23].

All published papers using the life-grid or EHC methods have reported high levels of satisfaction and accuracy either tested by qualitative methods or based on the researchers' experience. The method has been used as the best available method in collecting the past life course data in two well-known studies, the national English Longitudinal Study of Aging (ELSA, 2008) and an international Survey of Health, Aging and Retirement in Europe (SHARE) [8,24]. Computerised versions of the life grid method were used in SHARE study. Through computer based grids, a wide range of information on landmarks is provided for both interviewee and interviewer and, therefore, more accurate data are collected in relatively short interviews [8].

Shortcomings in Methods for Early Childhood Data Collection and Validation

The significance of the early years of childhood is the frequency and variation of important developmental milestones and occurrence of affective life events [25]. As subjects would not have much idea about

these events, parents/caregivers should be asked about them. However, there is a tendency for parents to remember dates, duration, and severity of only a few adverse events in their children's early life, especially when they occur close to each other. Parents may not be aware of children's important life events if the child had other caregivers, or parent may mix up the events that occurred to their children if they had two or more children born shortly after each other. In addition to the unreliable memory of parents, partially and inaccurately recorded medical and dental documents, if any, make it difficult to assess the health-related risk factors occurring in this crucial period of life [26].

Despite the emphasis on the outcomes of the early childhood events, life course epidemiology has made few efforts to develop methods to collect accurate data from early life. Looking at the broad span of life, most life course approaches use long periods of time, years and decades, as their index. So, even when the early childhood events are considered in their data collection, several events occur in one period, and are, therefore, not accurately recorded.

The life-grid and the event history calendar methods were originally developed for adults, especially the aging groups. Childhood data collected in some studies using these methods, whilst being the best method used in life course retrospective data collection, are too inaccurate [4,21,27]. This led the authors to consider developing better life-grid methods for accurate collection of early childhood data. The best method would be a special life-grid designed for early childhood containing developmental milestones and shorter periods of time for the earlier years, filled in by questioning parents or caregivers. The objectives of the current study were to develop a life-grid method to collect data on events in early childhood and test its content and concurrent validity.

Materials and Methods

A life-grid was developed to collect data on events in early childhood events. Ethical permission to collect data based on the development of a life-grid was obtained from Shiraz University of Medical Sciences. The life-grid was used with a simple life line from birth to the present age of the child. Relevant questions entered into each grid. A pilot study was conducted on 12 children followed by a main one on 30 children aged 8-11 years of age. Their parents were contacted and interviewed after explaining the objective. Content validity and relevance of the columns of the life-grid was assessed in the pilot study. Accuracy and concurrent validity of the life-grid was tested in the main study.

The Early Childhood Events Life-grid
The early childhood events life-grid is a table with 22 rows and 11 columns (Table 1). The first row is for headings. The other 21 rows contain age periods from "immediately after birth" to "7-8 years" and events happening during them. The first age periods are shorter as they are more important in physical and mental development and contain more changes in the

Age(and External line)	Personal life line	Residential status	Occupational line	Child activity line	Height	Weight	Illnesses	Medication	Hospitalization	Accidents/falls
Table 1: The early childhood events life-grid										
Immediately after birth										
Up to 1 month										
months 1-2										
months 2-3										
months 3-4										
months 4-5										
months 5-6										
months 6-9										
months 9-12										
months 12-15										
months 15-18										
months 18-21										
months 21-24										
years 2-2.5										
years 2.5-3										
years 3-3.5										
years 3.5-4										
years 4-5										
years 5-6										
years 6-7										
years 7-8										

child's life and activity.

The first column is the external life line and contains age periods and codes of some national and local events which are easy to remember and easy to relate to the past life. The second column is personal life line. Events such as birth of younger brother(s) and sister(s), death of a close relative, divorce and new marriage of parents and the time at which older brother(s) or sister(s) went to school/nursery are recorded in this column. The third column is for information regarding residential status of the family. Changes of address, changes to the shape or plan of the house, and owning a car, landline telephone or mobile phone numbers would be written in this column based on questions on Card 2. The fourth column of the life-grid belongs to the occupational status of parents/caregivers. This information is obtained based on questions on Card 3. The fifth column records the child's activities including infant feeding practices. Questions regarding the child's activities are shown in Card 4. Columns 6 and 7 show the height and weight of the child obtained from the child's growth chart and inserted into appropriate cells. Columns 8 to 11 were marked by codes based on questions about illnesses, medicine used, hospitalization, and accidents and falls in Card 5.

Life Line

As the life-grid was rather complicated, a simple line was shown to parents during the interview. The line started with the child's birth and ended at the current time. While the questions are answered by the parents, each event is marked on the line based on the approximate time given. As the interview proceeds, more events are marked and some previous markings are corrected based on the new answers.

Cards as illustrative materials

Five cards were used:

- Card 1-4: Contain questions relating to the second to fifth columns of the life-grid (personal life line, residential status, occupation of parents/guardians, and child activity line).
- Card 5: Contains questions on illnesses, medication and hospitalization and a list of important diseases.

Calibration of Interviewers

The main examiner (AG) was trained and calibrated to conduct life-grid interviews by two international experts in this method and gained experience of doing so by interviewing several parents of school-aged children. The main examiner (AG) then acted as the "gold standard" interviewer to train and calibrate the 4 others, all being professional health workers. At the end of the calibration process, one person (ASa) was chosen based on having the highest intra-examiner reproducibility and highest inter-examiner agreement with the gold standard examiner.

Explaining the Study and Gaining Consent

Upon arrival at the clinic and before conducting any investigation, the purpose and stages of the study were explained to the parents in detail and their consent was requested. Ethical permissions were shown with the request, and the researchers' contact details were recorded in case they were interested in the results of the study.

Interview

Each interview with parents/caregivers was conducted by two of the three calibrated interviewers. First, personal data were double checked with the interviewee. Then, questions regarding the child's birth conditions were asked. In the next step, the interviewees were asked questions regarding family life, residential status, and occupation of the parents/caregivers, child's activities, illnesses, medication, hospitalization, accidents and falls in a life-grid method and based on cards 1 to 5.

As the interviewee did not need to read the questionnaire, it was not translated into Farsi. However, two tools were used to facilitate the interview: 1) a list was shown to the interviewee to remind him/her of some important and common childhood diseases, and 2) a single line showing the child's birth and present age at the two ends was used. Each event remembered by the interviewee was marked on the line in relation with other events to obtain the correct time and order of the events.

It was possible to enter each life event as a code in the appropriate cell of the life-grid. However, in practice it was confusing for the interviewers and could increase the possibility of making mistakes. Thus, it was decided to write the name of each illness, as mentioned by the parent, into the appropriate cell. Medication, if used, was marked in its own columns of the life-grid. If the child had been hospitalized, that was marked in the appropriate cell. For boys, circumcision status and the date it was done was one of the questions.

Height and weight of the child from birth to the current date was entered from the child's growth chart into the respective column of the life-grid. The whole interview was tape recorded for further investigations by using a digital voice recorder if the interviewee agreed.

The pilot study

A convenient sample of twelve 8 to 10-year-old children was selected from the patients attending a clinic in Shiraz. They were usually accompanied by their mother or grandmother. The Relevance of Columns in the Life-grid was tested in two ways. First, the impact of the questions/answers of each column on the correctness of the answers given was observed. Then, after each interview, the interviewee's opinion was obtained about the importance of each category of questions (columns), helping them to remember the past events.

Main study

A multi-stage random sample of 110 children aged between 8 to 11 years was chosen from primary schools of Shiraz city. Their parents were asked to bring the children's health documents, such as birth card, growth charts, immunization card, and medical insurance records, to the interview. Parents were entered into the study only if 1) the documents covered their child's whole life and were fully filled in, 2) the parent/caregiver was in charge of caring for the child from birth to the present time, and 3) they gave consent for interview and access to the child's health documents.

The exact age of the occurrence of any change of address, any hospitalization, any accidents/falls, and those illnesses reported by the interviewee were extracted from the health documents. This information was assumed as "gold standard". Validity of the life-grid was assessed against this gold standard by using Kappa agreement coefficient. SPSS statistical software version 18.0 (SPSS Inc., Chicago, IL, USA) was used for statistical analysis.

Results

The average time for interviews was 50-60 minutes. The life-grid collected all desired factors that were considered when designing the life-grid such as strong psychological events, change of address, feeding pattern, and milestones in child activities, viral and non-viral illnesses, medication, hospitalization, falls and accidents.

All 12 interviewees participating in the pilot study agreed that the life-grid method was very useful to help them remember events and to correct the times of events. Most columns of the life-grid had a great impact on the correction of timing recorded in the other columns (Table 2). The child's activity line

Table 2: Number of cases that each column of the life-grid helped to correct the timing of events in other columns (N = 12).

Column	External Line	Personal life line	Residential status	Occupational line	Child activity line	Illnesses	Hospital-ization	Accidents /falls
Number of cases that corrected other columns events by using this column	0	2	5	3	10	3	3	1

had the greatest impact on the correction of the other columns. Different child's activities also helped the interviewees to correct the timing of other activities in the same column. The external line had the least impact. During the pilot study, it was shown that the number of older and younger brothers and sisters, and also the mother's age at the time of the child's birth were important information to be asked about and recorded.

Among the 110 parents who were asked to bring their children's health documents, 94 replied. Only 30 had the desired criteria to be included in the study. Fifty five of them did not have all the documents we needed. Three parents indicated that their children were raised by their grandparents up to a specific period and, therefore, they were unaware of some of their children's early childhood events. And six more did not want to participate in the study after the aim and process of the interview was explained to them. There was no significant difference in age (*p*-value = 0.723), sex (*p*-value = 0.899), or area of living (*p*-value = 0.095) between parents who included and those who were excluded from the study.

Table 3 shows the agreement between the findings of the life-grid and recorded events in the health documents (the gold standard) in relation to the four main variables. All events reported by the life-grid were found in the health records. Less exact matches were found for less important health related events such as change of address, and more exact matches were found for the more important ones, such as hospitalization. The Kappa agreement value was 0.95 when only exact time matches were assumed as agreement.

In the next step, if an event reported by the parents was in the adjacent grid to that found in the health document (just one grid difference between the time reported in ECEL and found in the documents), it was

Table 3: Agreements and disagreements between the findings of the life-grid method and the recorded health documents (N=30).

Event	Exact time Match	One grid Disagreement	Two or more grids disagreement	Not reported in life-grid but recorded in health documents	Total	Agreement level (k) of exact matches
Change of address	32(82.1%)	1(2.5%)	0(0%)	6(15.4%)	39(100%)	0.90
Illness	68(95.8%)	3(4.2%)	0(0%)	-	71(100%)	0.98
Accidents/falls	17(89.5%)	0(0%)	0(0%)	2(10.5%)	19(100%)	0.94
Hospitalization	12(100%)	0(0%)	0(0%)	0(0%)	12(100%)	1.0
Total	129(91.5%)	4(2.8%)	0(0%)	8(5.7%)	141(100%)	0.95

assumed to be an agreement. In that way, the Kappa agreement was increased to 0.97. These values show that there was an almost perfect agreement between the life-grid and the data recorded in health documents [28], and thereby high concurrent validity was found for the ECEL method. The agreement level between the two data sets for each variable is shown in Table 3.

Discussion

The life-grid method collected the past childhood life events accurately in terms of the number, nature, and exact timing of events. The agreement level (k = 0.95) between the findings of the life-grid method and recorded health documents was almost perfect. Less than 10 percent of events recorded in the health documents were not reported by the respondents or were reported a few months sooner or later than the time recorded in documents. There was no event that was only reported by the life-grid and not in the records.

In cases of disagreement, there was no way to find out which one was correct as the health record may have been wrong. It was a usual practice for Iranian doctors not to fully complete the health forms [29]. However, it was very unlikely that any agreement between the life-grid and health documents was wrong or achieved by chance [10]. A false agreement needs the respondent to give an inaccurate answer that exactly matches the wrong answer recorded in the health documents. Neither the respondent nor the interviewee was aware of any accidental mistake in the health document.

Accuracy of data obtained by the ECEL ($0.90 < k < 1.0$) was significantly ($p < 0.001$) higher than those

of the only comparable studies which reported $0.41 < k < 1.0$ (10) or $0.63 < k < 0.79$ [23]. Of course, the difference between the results of this study and those of Barney and Blane [10] was not significant after + one unit and + one grid were added to exact matches. This was due to the limited space for improvement in Kappa values related to the early childhood events life-grid, as it was already very high, compared to the other study.

Both interviewers and parents considered that the life histories of children were well displayed on paper as evidenced by the friendly interaction between interviewers and respondents. The method of prompting by the interviewer using previous answers triggered the respondent's memory. A short silence showed that they were thinking again, and then a correct answer was given with more confidence.

Participation in the interview, despite being a long procedure, was pleasant and encouraging for the respondents. Even the least interested respondents, who started the interview with doubts about the study, were, by the end of the session, excitedly participating in correcting the answers. The process of interview with a life-grid with several lines and words looks at the first glance to be a hard task for interviewers. In practice, however, the interviewers found the whole process easy.

The external line had the least impact, as interviewees mostly could not relate the events of this line with those of other lines. This was consistent with the findings of [30], indicating that the respondents were not able to correlate the external landmarks as well as personal landmarks to their life events. The value of this line is also consistent with the other studies in which crucial external events (like a war or an earthquake) were used in broader time periods such as years or decades [10,16]. The SHARELIFE project, a European study collecting data on past life events of people aged 50 or more, tested a solution to this problem. Their interviews are computer-based. A long list of important public events is preprogrammed. The respondents had the chance to choose the events that they remember better and the computer finds the exact date of them [8]. This method is used in Europe and might be difficult to employ in developing countries, where a computer might not be available in all interviews, or interviewees might be familiar with such computer aided and rather complicated process.

A limitation of this study was the unavailability of health documents that forced the researchers to exclude about half of the the invited samples. The response rate (27%) was low for that reason. Of course, this low rate cannot undermine the fact that the ECEL methods showed high content and concurrent validity, especially because there was no significant demographic difference between the included and excluded samples. The poor state of record keeping in Iran [29,31] was another important issue. Less than half of the invited children had relatively complete medical insurance records. In some cases, parents had thrown their older records away. The possibility of accidental or intended 'mistakes' in health documents forced the author not to include "illnesses recorded in documents but not reported in the life-grid" in the life-grid method's validation study. For the same reason, it was not possible to say which one, the record or the life-grid, was correct in the case of disagreement between them.

Conclusions

The Early Childhood Events Life-Grid method proved to be highly accurate when compared with recorded medical documents. However, the accuracy can be further improved if any available recorded document is first accessed. The findings from such documents can be used by interviewers as landmarks; solid events with known dates. Further work may reveal how external line (public events) can be used in early childhood events life-grid. Furthermore, the method's reliability needs to be tested.

Conflict of Interest: None declared.

References

1. Kuh D, Ben-Shlomo Y, Lynch J, *et al.* Life course epidemiology. J Epidemiol Community Health. 2003;57:778-783.

2. Ben-Shlomo Y, Kuh D. A life course approach to chronic disease epidemiology: conceptual models, empirical challenges and interdisciplinary perspectives. Int J Epidemiol. 2002;31:285-293.

3. Blane D, Netuveli G, Stone J. The development of life course epidemiology. Rev Epidemiol Sante Publique. 2007;55:31-38.

4. Blane D. Collecting retrospective data: development of a reliable method and a pilot study of its use. Soc Sci Med. 1996;42:751-757.

5. Koupilová I, Leon DA, Vågerö D. Can confounding by sociodemographic and behavioural factors explain the association between size at birth and blood pressure at age 50 in Sweden? J Epidemiol Community Health. 1997;51:14-18.

6. Leon DA, Johansson M, Rasmussen F. Gestational age and growth rate of fetal mass are inversely associated with systolic blood pressure in young adults: an epidemiologic study of 165,136 Swedish men aged 18 years. Am J Epidemiol. 2000;152:597-604.

7. Leon DA, Koupil I, Mann V, *et al.* Fetal, developmental, and parental influences on childhood systolic blood pressure in 600 sib pairs: the Uppsala Family study. Circulation. 2005;112:3478-3485.

8. Schröder M, Börsch-Supan A. Retrospective data collection in Europe. Available at: http://www.mea.mpisoc.mpg.de/uploads/user_mea_discussionpapers/pszm6txdgq331udz_komplett%20neu.pdf.

9. Bell AJ. "Oh yes I remember it well!" Reflections on using the life-grid in qualitative interviews with couples. Qual Sociol Rev. 2005;1:51-67.

10. Berney LR, Blane DB. Collecting retrospective data: accuracy of recall after 50 years judged against historical records. Soc Sci Med. 1997;45:1519-1525.

11. Woll S. How we represent, organize, and retrieve autobiographical memories? Everyday thinking : memory, reasoning, and judgment in the real world. 1th Edition. Mahwah, N.J.: London, Lawrence Erlbaum; 2002. p. 220-261.

12. Loftus EF, Marburger W. Since the eruption of Mt. St. Helens, has anyone beaten you up? Improving the accuracy of retrospective reports with landmark events. Mem Cognit. 1983;11:114-120.

13. Neter J, Waksberg J. A study of response errors in expenditures data from household interviews.

J Am Stat Assoc. 1964;59:18-55.

14. Freedman D, Thornton A, Camburn D, *et al*. The life history calendar: a technique for collecting retrospective data. Sociol Methodol. 1988;18:37-68.

15. Vinson DC, Reidinger C, Wilcosky T. Factors affecting the validity of a Timeline Follow-Back interview. J Stud Alcohol. 2003;64:733-740.

16. Wilson S, Cunningham-Burley S, Bancroft A, *et al*. Young people, biographical narratives and the life-grid: young people's accounts of parental substance use. Qual Res. 2007;7:135-151.

17. Jobe JB, White AA, Kelley CL, *et al*. Recall strategies and memory for health-care visits. Milbank Q. 1990;68:171-189.

18. Dawson J, Thorogood M, Marks SA, *et al*. The prevalence of foot problems in older women: a cause for concern. J Public Health Med. 2002;24:77-84.

19. Dawson J, Juszczak E, Thorogood M, *et al*. An investigation of risk factors for symptomatic osteoarthritis of the knee in women using a life course approach. J Epidemiol Community Health. 2003;57:823-830.

20. De Souza V, MacFarlane A, Murphy AW, *et al*. A qualitative study of factors influencing anti-microbial prescribing by non-consultant hospital doctors. J Antimicrob Chemother. 2006;58:840-843.

21. Edwards R, Pless-Mulloli T, Howel D, *et al*. Does living near heavy industry cause lung cancer in women? A case-control study using life grid interviews. Thorax. 2006;61:1076-1082.

22. Holland P, Berney L, Blane D, *et al*. Life course accumulation of disadvantage: childhood health and hazard exposure during adulthood. Soc Sci Med. 2000;50:1285-1295.

23. Belli RF, Shay WL, Stafford FP. Event history calendars and question list surveys: a direct comparison of interviewing methods. Public Opin Q. 2001;65:45-74.

24. ELSA. Health and lifestyle of people aged 50 and over: ELSA wave 4 interviewer project instruction. Availabl at: https://www.elsa-project. ac.uk/uploads/elsa/docs_w3/lh_interviewer.pdf

25. Slentz K, Krogh S. Early childhood development and its variations. Available at: https://www.am-azon.com/Early-Childhood-Development-Varia-tions-Education/dp/0805828842

26. Suckling GW, Herbison GP, Brown RH. Etiological factors influencing the prevalence of developmental defects of dental enamel in nine-year-old New Zealand children participating in a health and development study. J Dent Res. 1987;66:1466-1469.

27. Wainwright NW, Surtees PG. Childhood adversity, gender and depression over the life-course. J Affect Disord. 2002;72:33-44.

28. Landis JR, Koch GG. The measurement of observer agreement for categorical data. Biometrics. 1977;33:159-174.

29. Pourasghar F, Malekafzali H, Kazemi A, *et al*. What they fill in today, may not be useful tomorrow: lessons learned from studying Medical Records at the Women hospital in Tabriz, Iran. BMC Public Health. 2008;8:139.

30. Gaskell GD, Wright DB, O'Muircheartaigh CA. Telescoping of landmark events: implications for survey research. Public Opin Q. 2000;64:77-89.

31. Pourasghar F, Malekafzali H, Koch S, *et al*. Factors influencing the quality of medical documentation when a paper-based medical records system is replaced with an electronic medical records system: an Iranian case study. Int J Technol Assess Health Care. 2008;24:445-451.

12

Hertzian Load-bearing Capacity of Hybrid and Nano-hybrid Resin Composites Stored Dry and Wet

Farmani S[a], Orandi S[b], Sookhakiyan M[a], Mese A[c]

[a]Student Research Committee, Shiraz Dental School, Shiraz University of Medical Sciences, Shiraz, Iran
[b]Postgraduate Student , Department of Prosthodontics, School of Dentistry, Shiraz University of Medical Sciences, Shiraz, Iran
[c]Department of Prosthodontics, School of Dentistry, Dicle University, Diyarbakir, Turkey

ARTICLE INFO	Abstract

Key words:
Hertzian Indentation
Load-bearing Capacity
Resin Composites

Corresponding Author:
Ayse Mese,
Department of Prosthodontics,
School of Dentistry,
DicleUniversity,
Diyarbakir, Turkey

Email: amese@dicle.edu.tr

Statement of Problem: Hertzian indentation test has been proven to be an efficient and reliable alternative upon Vickers hardness test. This method has been used to test dental ceramics, amalgams, glass ionomers and luting cements.There is limited published information about the load-bearing capacity of resin composites using Hertizian indentation test.

Objectives: To investigate the load-bearing capacity of hybrid and nano-hybrid resin composites stored dry or wet up to 30 days, using Hertzian indentation test.

Materials and Methods: Three resin composites were used: two nano-hybrids (Filtek Supreme, and Luna) and one hybrid, (Rok). A total of 108 disc-shaped specimens (1mm thick x 10 mm diameter) were prepared using polyethylene mould. The specimens of each material were randomly divided into 6 groups of 6 (n=6) and stored at 37⁰C either in distilled water or dry for 1, 7 and 30 days. The specimens were tested using Hertzian jig aligned in the universal testing machine. The specimen was placed on the top of a disc-shaped substrate. The load was applied at the center of each specimen and the load at the first crack was recorded. Data were analyzed by ANOVA, Tukey'sand student's t-test using SPSS version 18.0.

Results: Three-way ANOVA showed a significant interaction between all the factors ($p = .0001$). The load bearing capacity of almost all materials reduced significantly in the wet condition in comparison with the dry condition ($p = .0001$). After seven days of immersion in distilled water, Filtek Supreme had significantly lower values than those of Rok and Luna, there was no significant differences between materials in the dry condition.

Conclusions:In contrast to dry condition, the load-bearing capacity of specimens stored in distilled water decreased significantly over the 30 days of immersion. The load bearing capacity of nano-hybrid composites tested in this study was shown to be comparable with that of the hybrid composite.

Introduction

Increasing demands for cosmetic dentistry and new developments in resin composites and adhesives have guided many dentists to use these materials, instead of amalgam, to restore posterior teeth. Over the last two decades, much research has been conducted to enhance the aesthetics and strength of resin composites.

Dental composites are composed of a polymeric matrix, reinforcing fillers, silane coupling agent for binding the filler to the matrix, and chemicals that stimulate or control the polymerization reaction [1,2]. Since their introduction, filler particle sizes incorporated in the resin matrix have reduced from the traditional to the nano particles to improve the mechanical properties of resin composites [3]. Today resin composites are mostly classified as hybrid, micro-hybrid, nano-hybrid, and nanoFill [3]. The particle sizes are 0.04-5 μm in hybrid, 0.04-1 μm in micro-hybrid, 5 - 75 nm in nano-hybrid, and 0.6 μm to 1.4 μm in nanofill composites [4].

It is believed that there are no factual differences between particle sizes of micro-hybrid and nano-hybrid composites. The logic behind this claim is that adding more commercialised nanoparticles and nanoclusters bounded in the resin matrix of micro-hybrid composites results in an optimized nano-hybrid with possible pre-polymerized resin fillers [5]. Therefore, these two types of composites should have the same load bearing capacity under the Hertzian indentation test.

Immersion of resin composites in the solution in laboratory over the period of time simulates the oral environment and is known to be responsible for the degradation of the materials, leading to loss of their mechanical properties [6-8]. Some studies reported that water storage led to a decrease in the elastic modulus [9], flexure strength [10], tensile strength [11], and fracture toughness of composites [12]. On the other hand, some others have shown no change or an increase in flexure strength [13] and fracture toughness [14] after aging in distilled water.

The Hertzian indentation in which a spherical indenter is used to apply a load to a flat surface has been proven to be a simple and clinically-relevant test method [15]. This method has been employed to test the dental ceramics [16], dental amalgams [17,18], glass ionomer restoratives [19] and resin-based luting cements [20].

Aging in distilled water leads to a significant change of material's strength as water is an existing element in the matrix and also the media of reaction [21]. It has been shown that aging in artificial saliva produces a consistent degradation by means of sorption and solubility of more leachable ions [22]. On the other hand, it is reported that although exposure to the air begins the loss of water, thus shrinking and generating cracks, load bearing capacity is not greatly affected [22]. Wang et al. in their study of measuring load-bearing capacity of ceramic-reinforced glass ionomer cement kept wet and dry found that the failure load was relatively stable for air-stored specimens but it showed a significant decrease for wet-stored specimens [22]. Chenglin et al. also showed that load-bearing capacity of all-ceramic crowns was reduced due to cement aging in distilled water [23].

Based on limited information about the load-bearing capacity of resin composites stored wet and dry using Hertzian indentation test, the aim of the current study was to investigate the load-bearing capacity of hybrid and nano-hybrid resin composites stored dry or wet up to 30 days, using Hertzian indentation test.

Materials and Methods

Specimen preparation

Three resin composites were tested (Table 1) in two conditions (wet and dry) and three time intervals (1,7 and 30 days). A total of 108 disc-shaped specimens of 1mm $\pm$ 0.1 mm thick and 10 mm in diameter were prepared using polyethylene mould. Resin composite was placed in the mould using a plastic instrument, packed gently with hand pressure and pressed between two plastic matrix strips and glass slabs to extrude the excess material. The top glass slab was removed and the resin composite was cured according to the manufacturer's recommended exposure times using an LED curing light at a wavelength range of 440–480 nm and output of 1500 mW/cm2 (Radii plus; SDI, Melbourne, Vic., Australia). The excess material around the mould was removed by wet grinding both sides of the specimen with 600-grit silicon carbide paper. Then, the specimen was removed from the mould and the thickness of each specimen was adjusted to 1 ($\pm$ 0.1) mm using a digital caliper (Mitutoyo Company, Japan). The specimens of each material were randomly divided into 6 groups of 6 (n = 6) and stored at 37∘C either in distilled water or dry for 1,7 and 30 days. After each time interval, the specimens were tested as explained below.

Specimen testing

The test set-up and conditions have been previously described by Wang *et al.* [17]. The specimen was

test were employed for sub-group analysis comparing the materials, times and conditions individually. $p < 0.05$ was considered statistically significant.

Results

Three way ANOVA showed a significant interaction

Table 1: Materials used in the present study

Name	Manufacturer	Type	Matrix/Filler (type, size and vol%)	Lot no./shade
Filtek Supreme XTE	3M /ESPE, St Paul, MN, USA	Nano-hybri resin composite	Resin: Bis-GMA,UDMA ,TEGDMA, PEGDMA, Bis-EMA Filler: combination of nonaggregated 20 nm sillica filler,non aggregated 4-11 nm zirconia filler & aggregated zirconia cluster filler(0.6-10 μm);59 vol%	N564759/A2
Luna	SDI, Vic, Australia	Nano-hybri resin composite	Resin: UDMA, Bis-EMA, TEGDMA Filler :SAS,AS 0.02-2 μm ,200-400nm ;61 vol%	130951T/A2
Rok	SDI, Vic, Australia	Hybrid resin composite	Resin: UDMA, TEGDMA, Bis-EMA Filler: SAS, AS, (0.04 -2.5 μm); 67.7 vol%	140454Z/A3

Bis-GMA=bisphenol a glycidyldimethacrylate,TEGDMA=triethylene glycol dimethacrylate, PEGDMA=Poly(ethylene glycol) dimethacrylate, UDMA = urethane dimethacrylate ,SAS= Strontium alumino silicate, AS= amorphous silica, Bis-EMA= bisphenol a Ethylmethacrylate,

placed on the top of a disc-shaped substrate, 5-mm thick ×10-mm diameter (nylon 6,6 [30 % glass fiber-reinforced polyamide]), with an elastic modulus of 10 GPa, (Good Fellow Cambridge, Huntingdon, UK). The jig was aligned to the loading axis of the universal testing machine (Zwick/Roll Z020; Zwick GmbH, Ulm, Germany). The load was applied at the center of each specimen at a cross-head speed of 1 mm/min. It was recorded at the first audible detection of a crack.

Statistical Analysis

Data were analyzed using SPSS version 18.0 (SPSS Inc., Chicago, IL, USA). Three –way ANOVA was used to assess the interaction effects between the three factors. One-way ANOVA, Tukey's and student's t

between the following factors; material ×time, material ×condition, and condition × time ($p = .0001$). Results of one-way ANOVA and pair comparison are shown in Table 2. The effect of time on materials was condition dependent. Over the time, wet condition significantly decreased the load bearing capacity of almost all materials in comparison with dry condition ($p = .0001$) except for Luna after 1 day of immersion in dry condition that showed slightly lower values than wet condition. At one day of wet condition, Luna (199 ± 15.6) showed significantly ($p = .011$) greater values than those of Rok (147.3 ± 37.4), while in the dry condition, there was no significant difference between the three materials.

After 7 days of wet condition, Filtek Supreme (115.1 ± 22.1) had significantly lower values than

Table 2: Means and standard deviations (±) of Hertzian load capacity for all tested materials, times and conditions (n = 6)

Material \ Condition	Wet			Dry		
	1D	7D	30D	1D	7D	30D
Rok	[A]147.3 ± 37.4	[A]141.± 16.1	[AB]115 ± 2.3	[A]171.9 ± 13.9	[A]212 ± 18.8	[A]221 ± 54.9
Filtek.supreme	[AB]162.6 ± 11.5	[B]115.1 ± 22.1	[A]95.4 ± 31.1	[A]193.6 ± 20.3	[A]214.5 ± 5.4	[B]155.3 ± 2.1
Luna	[B]199 ± 15.6	[A]167 ± 8.5	[B]169.3 ± 5.3	[A]186.5 ± 6.5	[A]207.2 ± 11.1	[A]215 ± 7.3

Different upper case shows significant differences in each column.

D=Day

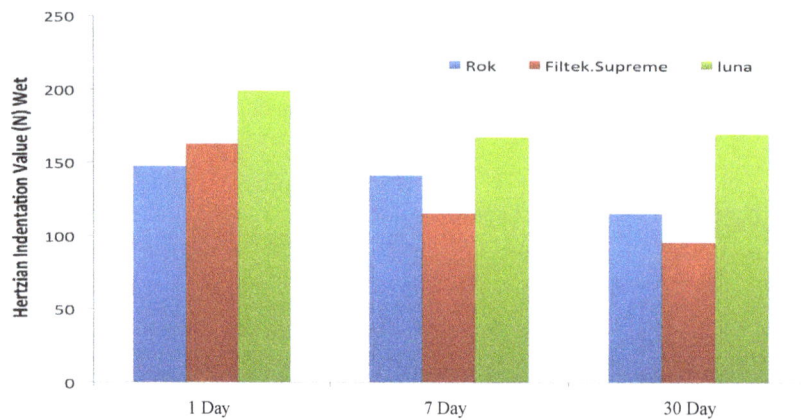

Figure 1: Load-bearing capacity values for specimens stored in wet condition up to 30 day

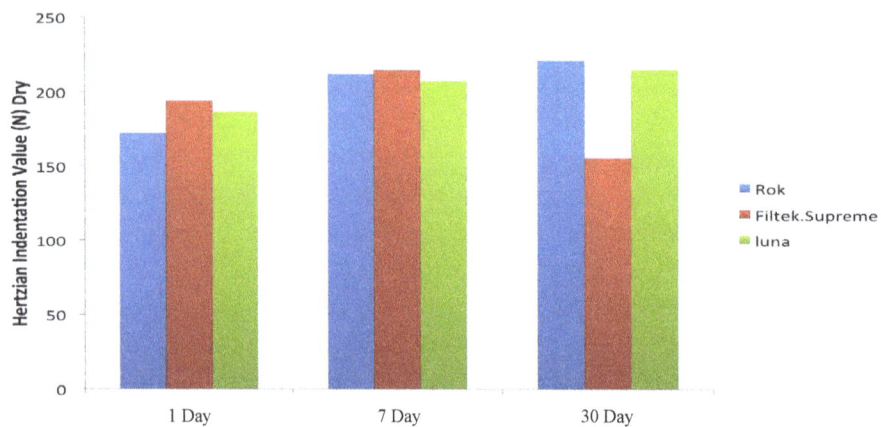

Figure 2: Load-bearing capacity values for specimens stored dry up to 30 day

those of Rok (212 ± 18.8; p =.037) and Luna (167 ± 8.5; p =.0001), but there was no significant difference between materials in dry condition. At 30 days of wet condition, Luna (169.3 ± 5.3) revealed significantly greater values than those of Filtek Supreme (95.4 ± 31.1; p =.0001), and in dry condition Filtek Supreme (155.3 ± 2.1) showed significantly lower values than those of Rok (221 ± 54.9; p =.002) and Luna (215 ± 7.3; p =.002). The differences between times in each condition are graphically shown in Figure 1 and 2.

Discussion

Results of this study showed that the load bearing capacity of nano-hybrid composites is comparable with or even higher than that of hybrid composite depending on the aging and storage condition. Wet condition significantly decreased the load bearing capacity of almost all materials in comparison with dry condition (p =.0001). A possible explanation for these results would be related to water sorption of the materials in the wet environment. Due to water uptake by the polymer, the interface between the resin matrix and the filler may collapse. In addition, water uptake causes a softening effect on the polymer matrix by swelling the network and reducing the frictional forces between the polymer chains [24,25] and reduces the strength of the material.

The load bearing capacity of all materials reduced consistently over the period of time up to 30 days which could be due to plasticization and that the further water uptake may cause cracking or degradation of either the resin matrix or filler/matrix interface [26-28]. Rok, as a hybrid resin composite, showed a lower baseline strength (171.9 ±13.9) compared to nano-hybrid materials but increased significantly after 30 days of being stored dry (221 ± 54.9). In contrast, the wet stored specimens showed a consistent decrease up to 30 days. Long-term water sorption has been shown to be lower for UDMA than for Bis-GMA and TEGDMA due to the presence of hydrophilic ether linkages in TEGDMA [7]. These observations might contribute to the very consistent behavior of Rok during storage.

In this study, two tested nano-hybrid resin composites, Luna and Filtek Supreme, performed differently with the highest values of load bearing capacity for Luna. This performance could be affected by the material's composition such as filler volume percentages, filler type and sizes, prepolymerized resin fillers, type of resin matrix, and the ratio of high molecular monomer (Bis-GMA) to the low molecular ones (UDMA, TEGDMA, Bis-EMA) [26,29-31]. Some studies showed that with increasing urethane content, the solubility values of resin composites decreased; this may imply that the degree of conversion and rate of cure are higher for Urethane based composites compared to BisGMA-based ones [32,33]. This may support the lower load bearing capacity of Filtek Supreme (BisGMA-based composite) than Luna (low molecular-based monomers). It has also been reported that decrease in the filler volume results in greater water sorption [34,35] which may be another reason for lower load bearing capacity of Filltek Supreme (59 vol%) in wet condition compared to Luna (61 vol%). In addition, based on the manufacturer's claim, Filtek Supreme has PEGDMA [Poly (ethylene glycol) dimethacrylate] as part of its resin matrix; this was used to replace a part of the TEGDMA component to moderate the shrinkage in Filtek Supreme XTE restorative.

Hertzian indentation test has been considered an effective simulator of oral loadings with two variables: contact load and indenter radius [15]. A spherical indenter is used to apply the load to a flat surface [17]. Two advantages of Hertzian indentation test upon Vickers hardness test are its ball shape indenter compared to the indenter tip in Vickers hardness and the substrate is used under the specimens [17]. The ball shape indenter prevents the contact stress field produced by the indenter tip, and the substrate acts as the elasticity of the dentin under the restoration to absorb the main forces applied to the specimen [17].

Conclusions

Within the limitations of this study, the following conclusions are drawn. Nano-hybrid composites tested in this study were shown to have comparable or even higher load bearing capacity than that of hybrid composite. In comparison with dry condition, specimens stored in distilled water showed significantly lower load bearing capacity. Time was found to be an effective factor. Further long-term studies are needed to compare the effect of aging on the load bearing capacity of resin composites more objectively.

Acknowledgements

The authors thank the Vice-Chancellor of Shiraz University of Medical Sciences for supporting this research (Grant# 9617).The authors thank Dr. Mehrdad Vossoughi Statistician in Shiraz Dental School for his help with the statistical analysis, and SDI and 3M/ESPE for providing the materials used in this study. The authors also thank Mrs. Marjan Bagheri for her valuable help throughout the experiment.

References

1. Klapdohr S, Moszner N. New inorganic components for dental filling composites. Monatshefte für Chemie. 2005;136:21-45.
2. Wassell R, Walls A, McCabe J. Direct composite inlays versus conventional composite restorations: 5-year follow-up. J Dent. 2000;28:375-382.
3. Wilson N, Wilson M, Wastell D, et al. A clinical trial of a visible light cured posterior composite resin restorative material: five-year results. Quintessence Int. 1988;19:675.
4. Sensi LG, Strassler HE, Webley W, et al. Direct composite resins. Inside Dentistry. 2007;3:76.
5. Ilie N, Hickel R. Investigations on mechanical behaviour of dental composites. Clin Oral Investig. 2009;13:427-438.
6. Ferracane J, Marker V. Solvent degradation and reduced fracture toughness in aged composites. J Dent Res. 1992;71:13-19.
7. Shin MA, Drummond JL. Evaluation of chemical and mechanical properties of dental composites. J Biomed Mate Res. 1999;48:540-545.
8. Soderholm K-J, Roberts M. Influence of water exposure on the tensile strength of composites. J Den Res. 1990;69:1812-1816.
9. Ferracane JL, Hopkin JK, Condon JR. Properties of heat-treated composites after aging in water. Dent Mater. 1995;11:354-3588.
10. Drummond J, Miescke K. Weibull models for the statistical analysis of dental composite data: aged in physiologic media and cyclic-fatigued. Dent Mater. 1991;7:25-29.
11. Fujishima A. Evaluation of environmental durability in water of light cure composite resins by the direct tensile test. Jpn J Dent Mater. 1988;7:44-61.
12. Mair L, Vowles R. The effect of thermal cycling on the fracture toughness of seven composite restorative materials. Dent Mater. 1989;5:23-26.
13. Drummond J, Savers E. In vitro aging of a heat/pressure-cured composite. Dent Mater. 1993;9:214-216.
14. Pilliar R, Vowles R, Williams D. The effect of environmental aging on the fracture toughness of dental composites. J Dent Res. 1987;66:722-726.
15. Lawn BR, Deng Y, Thompson VP. Use of contact testing in the characterization and design of all-ceramic crownlike layer structures: a review. J Prosthet Dent. 2001;86:495-510.
16. Deng Y, Lawn BR, Lloyd IK. Characterization of damage modes in dental ceramic bilayer structures. J Biomed Mater Res. 2002;63:137-145.
17. Wang Y, Darvell B. Failure mode of dental restorative materials under Hertzian indentation. Dent Mater. 2007;23:1236-1244.
18. Darvell B. Development of strength in dental silver amalgam. Dent Mater. 2012;28:e207-e217.
19. Wang Y, Darvell B. Failure behavior of glass ionomer cement under Hertzian indentation. Dent Mater. 2008;24:1223-1229.
20. Bagheri R, Vojdani M, Mogharabi S, et al. Effect of home bleaching on the mechanical properties of resin luting cements using Hertzian indentation test. J Investig Clin Dent. 2015;6:234-239.
21. Crisp S, Lewis B, Wilson A. Characterization of glass-ionomer cements 1. Long term hardness and compressive strength. J Dent. 1976;4:162-166.
22. Wang Y, Darvell B. Hertzian load-bearing capacity of a ceramic-reinforced glass ionomer cement stored wet and dry. Dent Mater. 2009;25:952-955.
23. Lu C, Wang R, Mao S, et al. Reduction of load-bearing capacity of all-ceramic crowns due to cement aging. J Mech Behav Biomed Mater. 2013;17:56-65.
24. Ferracane J, Berge H, Condon J. In vitro aging of dental composites in water—effect of degree of conversion, filler volume, and filler/matrix coupling. J Biomed Mater Res. 1998;42:465-472.
25. Ferracane J, Condon J. Degradation of composites caused by accelerated aging. J Dent Res. 1991;70:480.

26. Bagheri R, Tyas MJ, Burrow MF. Comparison of the effect of storage media on hardness and shear punch strength of tooth-coloured restorative materials. Am J Dent. 2007;20:329.

27. Asmussen E. Softening of BISGMA-based polymers by ethanol and by organic acids of plaque. Scand J Dent Res. 1984;92:257-261.

28. Wassell R, McCabe J, Walls A. Subsurface deformation associated with hardness measurements of composites. Dent Mater. 1992;8:218-223.

29. Bagheri R, Fani M, Ghasrodashti AB, et al. Effect of a home bleaching agent on the fracture toughness of resin composites, using short rod design. J Dent. 2014;15:74.

30. Ferooz MG, Azadeh N, Berahman N, et al. The role of home bleaching agent on the fracture toughness of resin composites using four-point bending test. J Dent Biomater. 2014;1:9-15.

31. Taha NA, Ghanim A, Tavangar MS. A comparison evaluation of mechanical properties of resin modified glass ionomer with resin composite restoratives. J Dent Biomater. 2015;2:47-53.

32. Schmidt C, Ilie N. The effect of aging on the mechanical properties of nanohybrid composites based on new monomer formulations. Clin Oral Investig. 2013;17:251-257.

33. Deepa C, Krishnan VK. Effect of resin matrix ratio, storage medium, and time upon the physical properties of a radiopaque dental composite. J Biomater Appl. 2000;14:296-315.

34. Kim K-H, Ong JL, Okuno O. The effect of filler loading and morphology on the mechanical properties of contemporary composites. J Prosthet Dent. 2002;87:642-649.

35. Kim K, Park J, Imai Y, et al. Microf racture Mechanisms of Dental Resin Composites Containing Spherically-shaped Filler Particles. J Dent Res. 1994;73:499-504.

13

Laboratory Comparison of the Anti-Bacterial Effects of Spearmint Extract and Hypochlorite Sodium on Enterococcus Faecalis Bacteria

Hajimaghsoodi S[a], Zandi H[b], Bahrami M[c*], Hakimian R[d]

[a]Department of Oral Medicine, Shahid Sadoughi University of Medical Sciences, Yazd, Iran
[b]Department of Microbiology, Shahid Sadoughi University of Medical Sciences, Yazd, Iran
[c]Shahid Sadoughi University of Medical Sciences, Yazd, Iran
[d]Department of Endodontics, School of Dentistry, Shahid Sadoughi University of Medical Sciences, Yazd, Iran

---

ARTICLE INFO

Key words:
Hypochlorite Sodium
Spearmint Extract
Root Canal Irrigation
Enterococcus faecalis

Corresponding Author:
Mohsen Bahrami
Shahid Sadoughi University
of Medical Sciences, Yazd,
Iran
E-mail: shmaghsoodi@
yahoo.com

Abstract

Statement of Problem: It is necessary to use irrigation solutions during cleaning and shaping of root canals to efficiently reduce the number of micro organisms. Sodium hypochlorite is used as an effective antibacterial endodontic irrigants. However, the extract of pennyroyal plant has also shown anti-bacterial characteristics comparable with antibacterial drugs.

Objectives: To compare the anti-bacterial effect of spearmint extract on Enterococcus faecalis bacteria with that of sodium hypochlorite 5.25%.

Materials and Methods: In this experimental study, Muller Hinton medium, including 5% sheep blood was prepared. The two solutions used including sodium hypochlorite 5.25% and spearmint extracts were put adjacent to Enterococcus faecalis bacteria after preparing. Two groups, each containing 10 samples, with the total of 20 samples were used. The disks, including each solution were placed 2 cm apart on a plate containing Muller Hinton medium and the bacteria. The plate was subsequently incubated at 37°C for 48 hours. After incubation, the mean diameter of the halo around each disk, which represents the lack of bacterial growth, was measured and compared using a ruler. Penicillin disk was used for positive control and a sterile blank disk containing physiologic serum was utilized as the negative control. This process was repeated 10 times for each solution. Data were analyzed in SPSS 17 statistical software using t-test.

Results: The results showed that the mean diameter of halo in the spearmint extract group was zero and in the sodium hypochlorite group it was 23.7 ± 1.49 mm. There was a significant difference between the mean diameter of the lack of growth halo of the spearmint extract and that of hypochlorite sodium 5.25% on Enterococcus faecalis bacteria ($p \leq 0.001$).

Conclusions: Considering the limitations of an experimental study, it seems that spearmint extract does not have any anti-bacterial effect against Enterococcus faecalis bacteria, in contrast to hypochlorite sodium 5.25%.

Introduction

The role of bacteria and their products has been confirmed as a major factor in the pulp and periapical diseases. As a result, removing these bacterial products is the main purpose of root canal treatment [1]. Mechanical preparation and irrigation of the canal, using an irrigating solution which is compatible with oral and periapical tissue, is a necessary task. The solution should be able to remove the bacteria and neutralize the bacterial products without damaging the host tissue. Therefore, the most suitable irrigating solution is the one that has a high anti-bacterial effect, causing the least damage to the host tissue [2]. Sodium Hypochlorite is used as an effective antibacterial irrigation material in root canal treatment procedures. It was observed that sodium hypochlorite solution can remove organic components of the dentin, without solving inorganic components that could cause dentin friability. Since in high concentrations, it causes removal of healthy tissues in addition to necrotic ones, transferring this solution from the root apex to the periapical area can cause severe complications in this area. We can also point to the unpleasant odor, causing sensitivity to the patient's eye, corrosion and instruments' colour change, as the other shortcomings of sodium hypochlorite [3].

Going back to the nature and using drugs with plants' origin has been done in the present era, where the modern human is faced with the side effects of the chemical drugs despite all the advertisements [4]. Medical properties of the pennyroyal plants have been proved [5]. Menthe pulegium is one of the twenty mint species known as pennyroyal. In medical sciences, the anti-bacterial effects of this plant on gram positive and gram negative bacteria have been proved. It has been shown that pennyroyal has anti-bacterial effect on Helicobacter Pylori, Salmonella, E. coli, Candida albicans and Staphylococcus aureus, compared to other drugs [6]. Entrococcus faecalis exhibits a high level of resistance to a wide range of antimicrobial agents [7] and it is among the few facultative bacteria associated with persistent apical periodontitis [8].

Since the extract of pennyroyal plant has shown anti-bacterial effect, this study aimed to determine whether spearmint extract impact on Entrococcus *faecalis* is comparable with that of sodium hypochlorite or not. The null hypothesis was that there is no difference between the anti-bacterial effects of those two solutions.

Materials and Methods

In this experimental study, two groups, each containing 10 samples, with the total of 20 samples were used, considering significance level of 5% and test power of 80%, based on s = 0.4 standard deviation of halo diameter, representing the lack of bacterial growth [9]. Based on the standards, Entrococcus faecalis bacteria with ATCC code of 29212 were cultured in rich blood agar medium, containing 5% sheep blood and incubated at 37°C for 24 hours. After the incubation and appearance of the bacterial colonies on the medium, one colony of bacteria was introduced to Tryptic Soy Broth (TSB) medium in the test tube to create bacterial suspension with 5% turbidity, tube of McFarland. To test the antibacterial effect of the solutions, a sample was prepared from bacterial suspension using soap and it was cultured in Muller Hinton medium including 5% sheep blood.

The method of spearmint extract preparation is in this way: after grinding the dried plant, it is kept in 80% ethanol for 48 hours. After filtering, ethanol is removed from the solution by rotary devices, so a pure extract is obtained which can be evaluated. In this study, the extract was prepared by Zarband company. Grouping of all the 20 disks was done between the two groups. The two solutions, sodium hypochlorite 5.25% and Spearmint extract (Zarband Company, Tehran, Iran), were applied on two separate disks. These disks were placed 2cm apart on a plate containing Muller Hinton Medium with 5% sheep blood and the bacteria. The plate was incubated in 37°C for 48 hours. After incubation, the mean diameter of the halo around each disk, which represents the lack of growth, was measured and compared using a ruler. To increase the accuracy, this process was repeated 10 times for each solution and the findings were calculated and compared (Figures 1 & 2).

Penicillin disk was used for positive control and a blank sterile disk with physiologic serum was used for negative control. In the process of preparing the disks, the blank sterile disk was prepared by pouring 0.01 milliliter of solution using a sampler. The disk was used after the solution was absorbed and dehydrated. This procedure was performed for each solution. Data were analyzed in SPSS 17 software. Mann-Whitney U test was used to compare the diameter of halo between the groups. The significance level was considered as alpha = 0.05.

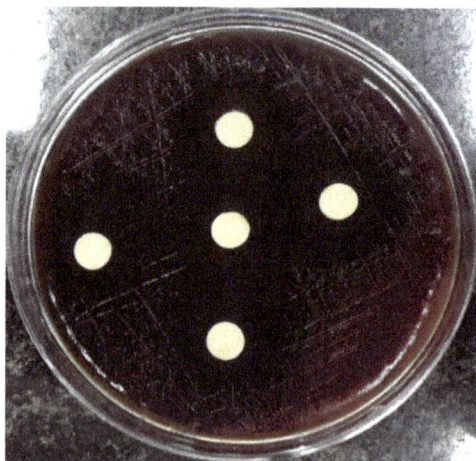

Figure 1: Bacterial growth in the hypochlorite sodium group

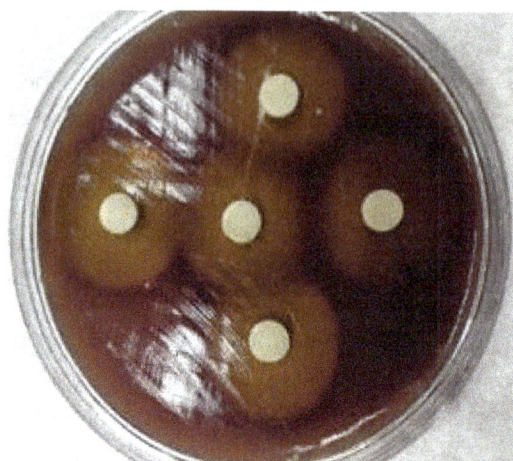

Figure 2: Bacterial growth in the spearmint extract group

Results

The results showed that the mean diameter of the halo in the Spearmint extract group was zero and in the sodium hypochlorite group it was 23.7 ± 1.49 mm. A significant statistical difference was observed in the comparison of the mean diameter of the halo in the two study groups based on Mann-Whitney U test ($p < 0.001$) (Table 1).

Table 1: Mean value and standard deviation of halo diameter of lack of microbial growth, (mm) in the two studied groups

Group	Number	Mean	SD	p-value
Hypochlorite sodium	10	23.70	1.49	
Spearmint extract	10	0	0	0.001>

SD: Standard Deviation

Discussion

The purpose of the present study was to investigate the anti-bacterial effect of the spearmint extract in comparison with that of sodium hypochlorite on E. faecalis bacteria which is the main anaerobic gram positive bacteria existing in the root canal with the ability of growth in agar medium [7]. The results showed that the mean diameter of the halo in the Spearmint extract group was zero, and in contrast to sodium hypochlorite, it did not have any effect on E. faecalis bacteria.

Sodium hypochlorite is one of the most common irrigating solutions of root canal during the treatment with the ability of removing biofilms and bacteria [10,11]. In the present study, 5.25% Sodium hypochlorite was selected because based on previous studies this concentration has a high efficacy against E. faecalis [12-15]. Thus, this concentration was used in this study and its antibacterial effect was compared with that of Spearmint extract.

Janzani, et al. reported that Spearmint extract has antibacterial properties due to the presence of Polgoon, Menton, and Neomenton groups in this plant that can cause the destruction of different polysaccharides, fatty acids, and phospholipids of bacteria membrane and subsequently, change the permeability of the bacterial cell membrane and destroy the bacterial wall [9]. Results of the study of Bonyadian and Moshtaghi [16] showed that Spearmint extract has antibacterial property against microorganisms such as Salmonella typhimurium, Listeria monocytogenes, Yersinia enterocolitica, Bacillus cereus, Clostridium perfringens, Staphylococcus aureus, Helicobacter pylori, Pseudomonas aeruginosa and Klebsiella pneumonia with the highest anti-bacterial effect against Salmonella typhimurium.

Indeed, we should notice that the antibacterial effect of the Spearmint extract for irrigating the root canal was tested in this study in laboratory conditions and these effects may be different in clinical conditions. Differences between PH of the saline and medium used in laboratory, mouth temperature and incubator temperature and also the presence of blood in the medium and oxidation power and survival in different areas of oral cavity could influence the results [13]. Therefore, compared to laboratory condition, the antimicrobial efficacy of irrigants is decreased in the tooth model. Also, the antimicrobial effects of different solutions are also affected by experimental methods, biological indices and the time duration when the bacteria are subjected to the solutions [17].

In the present study Agar diffusion method was used. One of the Agar diffusion test shortcomings is inability to distinguish between bacteriostatic or bactericidal properties of the studied materials. In addition, due to the need to sufficient time for efficient diffusions of the materials in the agar medium, we cannot distinguish its immediate effects. Also, it is not possible to study long-term effects of materials because they dry after 1 to 2 days.

It is important to notice that in plates including medium, antibacterial solutions were in contact with microbe permanently, but in the oral cavity materials are removed after a few seconds and the factors existing in the mouth neutralize their effect. Therefore, compared to laboratory condition, the antimicrobial efficacy of irrigants is decreased in the tooth model.

Because of the importance of the role of remaining bacteria in the failed root canal treatments and by considering the fact that using medicinal plants is one of the sources of new medicaments, further studies on other medicinal plants are recommended.

Conclusions

The results showed that the mean diameter of the halo of lack of growth in the Spearmint extract group was zero and in contrast to sodium hypochlorite, it did not have any effect on E.faecalis bacteria. Based on the results of this study and considering the constraints of a laboratorial study, it seems that spearmint extract does not have any anti-bacterial effect against Enterococcus faecalis bacteria, in contrast to hypochlorite sodium 5.25%.

Acknowledgements

We would like to thank the Vice-chancellor of Research and Technology, Shahid Sadoughi University of Medical Sciences, who approved this study.

Conflict of Interest: None declared

References

1. Zhang C, Hou BX, Zhao HY, *et al*. Microbial diversity in failed endodontic root-filled teeth. Chin Med J (Engl). 2012;125:1163-1168.

2. Yaghooti-Khorasani M, Assar S, RezaHoseini O. Comparison of Antimicrobial Effects of Persica and Chlorhexidine with Sodium Hypochlorite on Enterococcus Fecalis and Candida Albicans: An In vitro study. J Mash Dent Sch. 2010;34:153-160.

3. Mohammadi Z, Shalavi S. Antimicrobial activity of sodium hypochlorite in endodontics. J Mass Dent Soc. 2013;62:28-31.

4. Rashidi Sh, Farajee H, Jahanbin D, *et al*. Evaluation of Knowledge, Belief and Operation of Yasouj People Towards Pharmaceutical Plants. J Med Plants. 2012;11:177-184.

5. Chami N, Chami F, Bennis S, *et al*. Antifungal treatment with carvacrol and eugenol of oral candidiasis in immunosuppressed rats. Braz J Infect Dis. 2004;8:217-226.

6. Lindsay WP, Lamb CJ, Dixon RA. Microbial recognition and activation of plant defense systems. Trends Microbiol. 1993;1:181-187.

7. Heath CH, Blackmore TK, Gordon DL. Emerging resistance in Enterococcus spp. Med J Aust. 1996;164:116-120.

8. Haapasalo M, Ranta H, Ranta KT. Facultative gram-negative enteric rods in persistent periapical infections. Acta Odontol Scand. 1983;41:19-22.

9. Jazani NH, Ghasemnejad-Berenji H, Sadeqpoor S. Antibacterial effects of Iranian Mentha pulegium essential oil on isolates of Klebsiella sp. Pak J Biol Sci. 2009;12:183-185.

10. Clegg MS, Vertucci FJ, Walker C, *et al*. The effect of exposure to irrigant solutions on apical dentin biofilms in vitro. J Endod. 2006;32:434-437.

11. Heling I, Rotstein I, Dinur T, *et al*. Bactericidal and cytotoxic effects of sodium hypochlorite and sodium dichloroisocyanurate solutions in vitro. J Endod. 2001;27:278-280.

12. Berber VB, Gomes BP, Sena NT, *et al*. Efficacy of various concentrations of NaOCl and instrumentation techniques in reducing Enterococcus faecalis within root canals and dentinal tubules. Int Endod J. 2006;39:10-17.

13. Kangarloo-Haghighi A, Tashfam B, Nasseri M, *et al*. In-vitro comparison of antibacterial efficacy of a new irrigation solution containing nanosilver with sodium hypochlorite and chlorhexidine. J Dent Sch. 2013;30:261-267.

14. Retamozo B, Shabahang S, Johnson N, *et al*. Minimum contact time and concentration of sodium hypochlorite required to eliminate Enterococcus faecalis. J Endod. 2010;36:520-523.

15. Tirali RE, Turan Y, Akal N, *et al.* In vitro antimicrobial activity of several concentrations of NaOCl and Octenisept in elimination of endodontic pathogens. Oral Surg Oral Med Oral Pathol Oral Radiol Endod. 2009;108:117-120.

16. Bonyadian M, Moshtaghi H. Bacteriocidal Activity of Some Plants Essential Oils Against Bacilhis cereus, Salmonella typhimurium, Listeria monocytogenes and Yersinia enterocoliûca. Res J Microbiol. 2008;3:648-653.

17. Estrela C, Ribeiro RG, Estrela CR, *et al.* Antimicrobial effect of 2% sodium hypochlorite and 2% chlorhexidine tested by different methods. Braz Dent J. 2003;14:58-62.

14

Effect of Three Common Desensitizers in Reduction of the Dentin Hypersensitivity after Periodontal Surgery

Salahi S[a], Ghanbari M[b], Moosaali F[a]

[a]Oral and Dental Diseases Research Center AND Kerman Social Determinants on Oral Health Research Center AND Department of Periodontics, School of Dentistry, Kerman University of Medical Sciences, Kerman, Iran
[b]General practitioner, Faculty of Dentistry, Kerman University of Medical Sciences, Kerman, Iran.

ARTICLE INFO	Abstract

Key words:
Dentin Hypersensitivity
Dentin Sensitivity
Sensikin Gel
Sodium Fluoride Gel
Varnish Fluoride

Corresponding Author:
Fereshteh Moosaali,
Department of Periodontics,
Faculty of Dentistry, Kerman
University of Medical
Sciences, Kerman, Iran.

Email: moosaaly@kmu.ac.ir

Statement of Problem: Dentin hypersensitivity is one of the most common complaints of patients after periodontal treatments which occur after tissue shrinkage.

Objectives: The aim of this study was to determine and compare the effectiveness of sensikin gel (10% potassium nitrate and 0.22% sodium fluoride) with sodium fluoride gel (2.7%) and fluoride varnish (5%) in reducing the dentin hypersensitivity after periodontal surgery.

Materials and Methods: Twenty-two patients who, after full mouth periodontal surgery, had a complaint of dentin hypersensitivity (DH) in at least three quadrants were selected. Then a specific treatment was randomly selected for each quadrant which was applied once a day for one week and then stopped. A visual analog scale (VAS) was used to assess the subjects' responses to air blast and periodontal probe stimuli at baseline at one week, and one, three and 6 months after treatment. To analyze the data, repeated measures ANOVA test, Tukey test and variance analysis test were used.

Results: At all given intervals, almost both sodium fluoride and sensikin gel significantly reduced the dental sensitivity caused by stimulants. There were no significant differences between sensikin gel and other two desensitizers in reducing the dentin hypersensitivity after 1 week, 1 month, 3 months, and 6 months with respect to air blast stimuli. Sensikin gel was more efficient than Fluoride varnish in reducing the sensitivity caused by periodontal probe after 1 month.

Conclusions: Sensikin gel, sodium fluoride gel and fluoride varnish can all be prescribed to reduce dental sensitivity in patients who have undergone periodontal treatments. In the case of severe sensitivity to mechanical stimulations, a treatment with a long-run effectiveness such as sensikin and/or sodium fluoride gel is preferred.

Introduction

Dentin hypersensitivity (DH) is a common oral health problem which can be developed due to pulpal inflammation and/or tissue shrinkage subsequent to periodontal surgery. It can also be developed by some common factors like removal of the enamel (as a result of attrition, abrasion and erosion), denudation of the root surface (by loss of the overlying cementum and periodontal tissues), or gingival recession (because of severe tooth brushing, pocket reduction surgery, excessive flossing or secondary to periodontal diseases).

It is associated with severe and persistent pain from the exposed dentin, in response to chemical (i.e. exogenous/endogenous non-bacterial acids, carbohydrate/hypertonic chemical substances), thermal (i.e. heat, cooling), evaporative, tactile (i.e. rubbing the sensitive area with a finger nail or toothbrush bristles) or osmotic stimuli which cannot be ascribed to any other form of dental defect or disease [1-6]. The most common form of the treatment of dentine hypersensitivity is the use of desensitizing agents; the tolerance of pain can vary substantially among different people, and even in the same person depending on time and circumstances, since the perception of pain depends on individual factors such as personality, psychological factors and educational level, so this may cause only partial pain relief in most cases [7-10].

Both the numbers of dentinal tubules per unit area and the tubule diameters in the hypersensitive teeth are significantly greater compared with non-sensitive teeth [11]. There are many studies in the literature related to dentin hypersensitivity. Plagmann et al. [12] in a study covering 8 weeks of product use by 115 subjects, by the use of tactile stimulus (Yeaple probe) and air blast test for quantifying the dentinal hypersensitivity with the aid of visual analogue scale (VAS) demonstrated that the use of 1400 ppm fluoride dentifrice, delivered either as amine fluoride or sodium fluoride, did not differ significantly with the placebo dentifrice.

Brahmbhatt et al. [5] assessed the pain response on a VAS, by using tactile, air blast and cold-water stimuli up to 3-month intervals. It was concluded that all treatment modalities were superior to placebo in reducing DH, as well as 2% NaF-iontophoresis and

HEMA-G were more effective than 2% NaF local application at all-time intervals. But at 3-months, 2% NaF-iontophoresis was more effective than HEMA-G, while placebo produced no significant effect in reduction of DH.

In a randomized clinical trial by Frechoso et al. [10], the immediate efficacy of two treatments was compared with bioadhesive gels with different concentrations of potassium nitrate (NK 5% versus NK 10%) on DH by the use of the evaporative stimulus (ES). The researchers indicated a greater reduction of DH after ES during 48 h of treatment when they compared the NK10% group with the NK 5% group and placebo group. This difference increased significantly at 96 h. They also supported the practicality of an NK 10% gel to reduce the DH after stimulation with a blast of air during the first 4 days of its appearance.

Wara-aswapat et al. [13] in a 12-week home study investigated the effect of new toothpaste (0.3% triclosan), a desensitizing agent (5% potassium nitrate) and an anticaries agent (0.76% sodium monofluorophosphate (SMFP)) on the gingival health, plaque formation and DH. They reported a significant difference between the three treatment groups for DH. The reductions in VAS sensitivity scores, for the test group and the control group for both the tactile and air stimuli were significantly greater than the benchmark group. The sensitivity score for air stimulus from baseline to week 4 in the test group decreased more rapidly while no overall differences were found between the test and the control groups.

Camilotti et al. [14] in 2012 differentiated the effectiveness of different desensitizing agents in the treatment of painful symptoms caused by cervical dentin hypersensitivity (CDH) using modified U.S. Public Health Service criteria. 252 teeth of 42 patients presenting with dentin sensitivity to thermal changes in the oral environment were distributed among seven groups: G1 – placebo; G2, G3, G4 and G6 – fluoride varnishes (FV); G5 – sodium fluoride (SF); and G7 – potassium oxalate. It was found out that after the second week, there were statistically significant differences for all materials compared with the baseline, while after 30 days a significant gradual reduction was seen in Group G7 along with all the evaluated time intervals. They concluded that all the materials can reduce DH, with the exception of the G1 and G5 group.

As there is no specific study on the impact of materials used in this study on reducing DH after periodontal surgery, the aim of this study was to determine and compare the effectiveness of sensikin gel with sodium fluoride gel and fluoride varnish in reducing the dentin hypersensitivity after periodontal surgery.

Materials and Methods

This study was a randomized, split-mouth, single-blind clinical trial, involving 22 patients of both sexes (15 female and 7 male, aged between 23 to 66 years with a mean age of 48.2 years) with the complaint of dentin hypersensitivity in at least three quadrants after full mouth periodontal surgery. The number of patients was selected according to related literature [5,15-18]. The study was approved by the Ethics Committee of Kerman University of Medical Sciences (IR.KMU.REC.1394.252). Convenience sampling was performed for enrolling the patients in the study. After describing the study protocol (the characteristics and the conditions of the research) to all participating subjects, an informed consent was taken from the patients and all the patients' information was kept confidential. All of the patients were allowed to leave the study at any time they decided. The inclusion criteria were as follows:

Signing the informed consent, patients of either gender over 18 years of age, tooth brushing with Bass technique, and having at least 3 teeth (either canines or premolars) with an exposed root surface from which a painful response could be elicited by both a dental explorer and air blast [6,10].

The exclusion criteria were as follows:

The use of analgesic medications or desensitizing materials during the previous 6 weeks; any smoking habits; pregnancy or lactation; a history of long-term use of analgesic medications, antibiotic, antimicrobial, antidepressant, antiepileptic, or anti-inflammatory drugs as well as antihypertensive agents; specific oral allergy to any of the desensitizing materials to be evaluated; eating disorders; chronic systemic diseases; the use of orthodontic appliances within the last 3 months [10,13,19]; previous history of hypersensitivity reactions; the presence of large

or defective restorations, cracked enamel, caries, or occlusal overload on the hypersensitive tooth [4,5,6].

At the first visit, demonstration of proper brushing using Bass technique was given to each subject with the help of clinician. Afterwards, they were given a common soft-bristled toothbrush (Oral-B, 3 effects, soft, P&G south African trading) and toothpaste (Crest-complete, Procter & Gamble Gmbh, Gross Gerau, Germany). All the patients received non-surgical therapy for pocket elimination with the slurry of a mildly abrasive prophylaxis paste (Golchay, Iran). Afterwards, before the initiation of the study, all subjects have had identical or nearly identical primary clinical conditions such as mouth hygiene, gingival health and etcetera.

The mechanical examination is done by blasting air from a dental instrument at a distance of approximately 2 mm for 3 seconds onto the sensitive area, or gentle scratching (vertically and laterally over the exposed surface) with a dental probe (Yeaple probe) and measured using Visual Analogue Scale (VAS) to determine the most sensitive tooth in each quadrant [4,15,19]. If this provokes a positive pain response and other pathologies can be excluded, DHS therapy should be initiated. In any case, when the discomfort became intolerable, the stimulus was immediately removed. The test stimuli were applied in the same order during the study, with 10-minute interval between the applications of different stimuli. During the test, all the other teeth were isolated by cotton rolls and the desired tooth dried by air. We used two scales (one for air, another for periodontal probe) for every tooth examined at each visit.

A VAS is a horizontal line, 100 mm in length, anchored by word descriptors at each end, as illustrated in Figure 1. The patients specified their perception of pain by drawing a point on the VAS. The distance from this point to the left hand end of the line was VAS score [1,19].Then three quadrants were selected randomly and the specific treatment regime was considered for each of them.

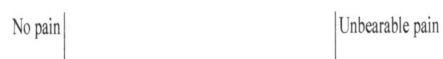

No pain   Unbearable pain

Figure 1: Visual analogue scale

In this stage, the patients who demonstrated at

Table 1: Comparison of VAS scores recorded for 2 different stimuli for all the three groups (SG, SF, and FV)

| | Air blast | | | | Periodontal probe | | | |
| | SG | SF | FV | p value | SG | SF | FV | p value |
	$\bar{x} \pm$ SD	$\bar{x} \pm$ SD	$\bar{x} \pm$ SD		$\bar{x} \pm$ SD	$\bar{x} \pm$ SD	$\bar{x} \pm$ SD	
Baseline	6.90 ± 2.87	6.45 ± 2.50	6.95 ± 2.49	0.78	4.31 ± 3.38	3.77 ± 2.99	3.86 ± 2.79	0.82
1 week	4.20 ± 2.74	5.90 ± 2.57	4.55 ± 2.52	0.10	2.45 ± 2.92	2.00 ± 2.69	1.55 ± 1.87	0.53
1 month	3.38 ± 2.72	2.71 ± 2.72	3.25 ± 2.95	0.71	2.09 ± 2.64	1.90 ± 2.23	0.47 ± 0.98	0.028*
3 month	3.78 ± 3.08	4.0 ± 2.82	5.15 ± 2.69	0.29	1.68 ± 1.85	2.88 ± 3.28	1.00 ± 2.05	0.72
6 month	3.88 ± 2.08	3.12 ± 3.11	5.68 ± 2.62	0.017*	1.00 ± 1.79	1.21 ± 1.96	0.63 ± 1.38	0.58

least 3 hypersensitive teeth in each quadrant were included and treated every day for a period of one week by the clinician. The treatment protocol was carried out with the three substances: material No.1 (sodium fluoride gel 2.7%, pascal, USA), material No.2 (sensikin gel, 10% potassium nitrate and 0.22% sodium fluoride, laboratorieskin, Spain), and material No.3 (fluoride varnish 5%, Pascal, USA).

Each one of the three studied materials was randomly used for the treatment of the hypersensitive teeth in one quadrant according to the lottery method. The materials were randomly numbered 1 to 3 and each quadrant of the patient (A-up and right, B-up and left, C-down and right and D-down and left) was assigned a unique label. Each label was placed in a bowl and mixed thoroughly. Then three of the labeled tags were picked from the bowl by a blindfolded person. All the quadrants bearing the labels picked

by the researcher were investigated. Afterwards, the treatment was done as follows: The first selected quadrant by the material No.1, the secondary selected quadrant by the material No.2 and the 3rd selected quadrant by the material No.3. Eating and drinking

was prohibited immediately after the treatment to half an hour post-treatment.

After 1 week, 1 month, 3 months, and 6 months, the patients were called again and the rate of sensitivity of the treated teeth was re-measured and recorded. To analyze the data, repeated measures ANOVA test, Tukey test and variance analysis test were used.

Results

The statistical analysis revealed no significant differences between the pretreatment groups (Table 1-2).

Table 2: The p value in the 3 groups at different time intervals versus baseline

| | Air blast | | | Periodontal probe | | |
	FV	SF	SG	FV	SF	SG
1 week	0	0	0.06	0.01	0.06	0
1 month	0.03	0.01	0.04	0.76	0.03	0
3 month	0.46	0	0.09	0.14	0.01	0.02
6 month	0.02	0.01	0.05	0.3	0.01	0

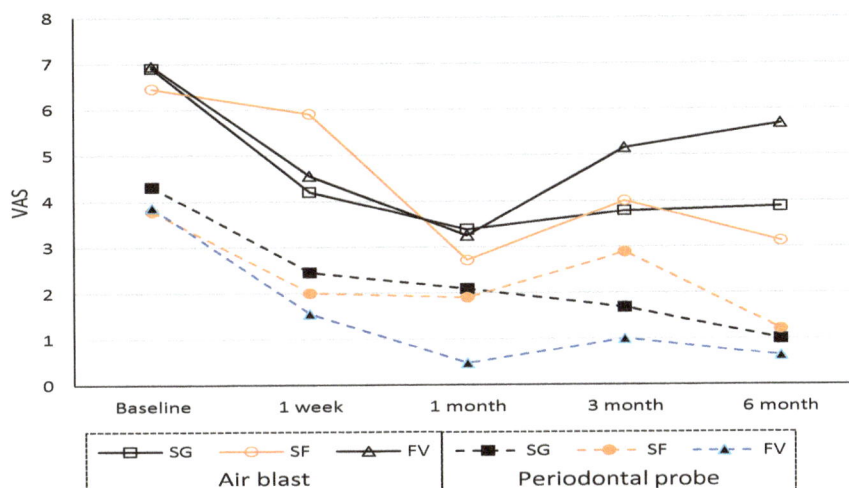

Figure 2: Comparison of VAS scores at baseline, 1st week, 1st month and 3rd and 6th months with two types of stimulus

Sensikin gel after 1 and 6 months and FV at the 1st week, 1st month and 6th month compared to pretreatment significantly reduced the amount of tooth sensitivity to stimulation caused by air blast while the reduction was almost significant at the ($p \leq 0.05$) level at 1 week and at 3 months ($p = 0.06$ and $p = 0.09$, respectively). Moreover, it reduced the dentin hypersensitivity to periodontal probe stimuli ($p < 0.05$) at all-time intervals compared to the baseline (Figure 2). Regardless of the 1st week after periodontal probe stimuli, SF significantly reduced the dentin hypersensitivity to various stimuli ($p < 0.05$) at all-time intervals compared to the baseline.

As shown in Table 3, SF with respect to air blast and SG with respect to the periodontal probe exhibited a greater reduction in DH than FV at 6 months and 1 month, respectively. However, SG was almost significantly more effective than FV in this time period. At all other time intervals, no significant difference was seen between the three groups in all testing parameters ($p > 0.05$). Mean VAS scores in the SF group always were lower for the air stimulus than for the probe stimulus, but it was the opposite for the SG group (Table 1).

Among the patients with complaint of dentin hypersensitivity to a variety of stimuli such as thermal, evaporative, tactile, osmotic, or chemical, the patients' chief complaint (18.2%) was sensitivity to cold and biting pain. The most hypersensitivity was related to the mandibular right lateral (10.6%),

Table 3: The significance of pairwise comparative efficacy of the materials used for treatment of dentin hypersensitivity					
	Air blast			**Periodontal probe**		
	SF VS. FV	SG VS. FV	SG VS. SF	SF VS. FV	SG VS. FV	SG VS. SF
Baseline	0.80	0.99	0.83	0.99	0.87	0.82
1 week	0.24	0.90	0.10	0.84	0.50	0.84
1 month	0.81	0.98	0.72	0.074**	0.037*	0.95
3 month	0.43	0.31	0.97	0.06**	0.67	0.30
6 month	0.017*	0.10**	0.68	0.56	0.79	0.92

*p value < pp 0.05 is statistically significant.

**p value between 0.05 and 0.1 was considered statistically almost significant.

mandibular left canine (9.1%) and the mandibular right second premolar (7.6%), respectively.

Discussion

Dentin hypersensitivity is a common oral pain arising from the exposed dentine in response to an array of stimuli (i.e. mechanical, tactile, osmotic, or chemical), which cannot be ascribed to any other pathology like necrotizing ulcerative gingivitis, periodontitis, and traumatic tooth picking [16,20-21].

Of those complaining about hypersensitive teeth, 31.8 percent were male and 68.2 percent were female; this may indicate that DH is commonest in females. This finding is in agreement with previous reports published by others [4,10,22-24]. This may be because of bad tooth brushing habits such as using hard brushes, excessive forces and scrubbing at the cervical areas in the females.

Abed *et al.* [15] clinically evaluated the efficacy of Neodymium-Doped Yttrium Aluminum Garnet (Nd: YAG) Laser Therapy and Sensikin gel in treatment of DH. They used VAS to quantify sensitivity by the cold air syringe. They found that in Sensikin gel treated group, the amount of VAS index significantly reduced at 1 week, 1, 3 and 6 months after application compared with the baseline. Table 2 shows that this finding is almost in line with our findings. Potassium nitrate and sodium fluoride are some active ingredients of Sensikin gel, individual efficacy of which has been shown in the study of Ritter *et al.* In the SG group, 1 week and 3 months after the application of VAS index, when tested with air blast and periodontal probe, it almost differed significantly but it differed significantly from the baseline, respectively. Unlike SF, Sensikin gel was not exactly significantly different at all-time intervals when tested with air blast.

Ritter AV. *et al.* found that the teeth desensitized with the FV had significantly lower mean VAS scores when tested with air blast at 8 and 24 weeks post-treatment in comparison with baseline scores [17]. In this study, we found that in the FV treated group, the amount of VAS index significantly reduced when tested with air blast at 1 week, 1 and 6 months while it only significantly reduced when tested with periodontal probe at 1 week after application

compared with the baseline.

Fluoride varnishes are theoretically ideal desensitizing agents for several reasons. Importantly, they are inexpensive, convenient to use in the office, as well as quick and easy in application. The varnish is reported to set on the teeth in the presence of the saliva, so it is unnecessary although advisable to thoroughly dry all tooth surfaces prior to treatment, the varnish stays on the teeth for hours and in some instances for days that causes immediate relief and is the primari cause of the high levels of fluoride uptake [18].

Within the limitations of this study, such as lack of control group, the 3 groups presented improvements in DH as expressed by the comparison between the initial and final means obtained during and after the treatment. When groups FV, SG and SF were compared at 1 month, SG was significantly more effective than FV and SF was almost significantly more effective than FV for the probe stimulus while at 6 months SF was significantly superior to FV and SG was almost significantly superior to FV for the air stimulus. At other time intervals, there were no statistically significant differences between the 3 groups. This made it possible to establish which of the materials were clinically effective. These outcomes are in line with those of other studies that reported a similar action for different fluoridated products used in the treatment of DH after a few weeks of application [1,17].

Conclusions

There was no significant difference between sensikin gel, sodium fluoride gel and fluoride varnish in reducing dentin hypersensitivity after 1 week, 1 month and 3 months with respect to air stimuli. Sensikin gel was more efficient than fluoride varnish in reducing sensitivity caused by periodontal probe after 1 month. Sensikin gel, sodium fluoride gel and fluoride varnish can all be prescribed to reduce dental sensitivity in patients who undergo periodontal treatments. In the case of severe sensitivity to mechanical stimulations for immediate treatment, fluoride varnish is recommended and if the pain persists, a treatment with a long-run effectiveness such as sensikin and/or sodium fluoride gel is suggested.

References

1. Aranha ACC, Pimental LAF, Marchi GM. Clinical evaluation of desensitizing treatments for cervical dentin hypersensitivity. Braz Oral Res. 2009;23:333-339.

2. Aparna S, Setty S, Thakur S. Comparative efficacy of two treatment modalities for dentinal hypersensitivity: a clinical trial. Indian J Dent Res. 2010;21:544-548.

3. Pamir T, Dalgar H, Onal B. Clinical evaluation of three desensitizing agents in relieving dentin hypersensitivity. Oper Dent. 2007;32:544-548.

4. Bahsi E, Dalli M, Uzgur R, et al. An analysis of the aetiology, prevalence and clinical features of dentin hypersensitivity in a general dental population. Eur Rev Med Pharmacol Sci. 2012;16:1107-1116.

5. Brahmbhatt N, Bhavsar N, Sahayata V. et al. A double blind controlled trial comparing three treatment modalities for dentin hypersensitivity. Med Oral Patol Oral Cir Bucal. 2012;17:483-490.

6. Pretha MS, Setty S, Ravindra S. Dentinal hypersensitivity? Can this agent be the solution?Indian J Dent Res. 2006;17:178-184.

7. Dababneh RH, Khouri AT, Addy M. Dentine hypersensitivity - an enigma? A review of terminology, mechanisms, aetiology and management. Br Dent J. 1999;187:606-611.

8. Walters PA. Dentinal hypersensitivity: a review. J Contemp Dent Pract. 2005;6:107-117.

9. Addy M, Urquhart E. Dentine hypersensitivity: its prevalence, aetiology and clinical management. Dent Update. 1992;19:407-408,410-412.

10. Frechoso SC, Menendez M, Guisasola C, et al. Evaluation of the efficacy of two potassium nitrate bioadhesive gels (5% and 10%) in the treatment of dentin hypersensitivity.a randomized clinical trial. J Clin Periodontol. 2003;30:315-320.

11. Absi EG, Addy M, Adams D. Dentine hypersensitivity. A study of the patency of dentinal tubules in sensitive and non-sensitive cervical dentine. J Clin Periodontol. 1987;14:280–284.

12. Plagmann HC, Konig J, Bernimoulin JP, et al. A clinical study comparing two high-fluride dentifrices for the treatment of dentinal hypersensitivity. Quintessence Int. 1997;28:403-408.

13. Wara-aswapati N, Krongnawakul D, Jiraviboon D, et al. The effect of a new toothpastecontaining potassium nitrate and triclosan on gingival health, plaque formation and dentin hypersensitivity. J Clin Periodontol. 2005;32:53-58.

14. Camilotti V, Zilly J, Busato PMR, et al. Desensitizing treatments for dentin hypersensitivity: a randomized, split-mouth clinical trial. Braz Oral Res. 2012;26:263-268.

15. Abed AM, Naghsh N, Birang R. et al. Clinical Evaluation of the Efficacy of Neodymium-Doped Yttrium Aluminium Garnet (Nd: YAG) Laser Therapy and Sensikin in Treatment of Dentine Hypersensitivity. J Lasers Med Sci. 2012;3:61-66.

16. Parveen N, Lal V, Hafeez S, et al. Clinical effectiveness of tooth mousse in dentinal hypersensitivity dentine or pulp. Pakistan Oral Dent J. 2014;34:344-347.

17. Ritter AV, de L Dias W, Miguez P, et al. Treating cervical dentin hypersensitivity with fluoride varnish. J Am Dent Assoc. 2006;137:1013-1020.

18. Clark DC, Hanley JA, Geoghegan S, et al. The effectiveness of a fluoride varnish and a desensitizing toothpaste in treating dentinal hypersensitivity. J Periodontal Res. 1985;20:212-219.

19. Ide M, Wilson RF, Ashley FP. The reproductibility of methods of assessment for cervical dentine hypersensitivity. J Clin Peridontol. 2001;28:16-22.

20. West NX. Dentine hypersensitivity: preventive and therapeutic approaches to treatment. Periodontol. 2000;48:31–41.

21. Canadian Advisory Board on Dentin Hypersensitivity. Consensus-based recommendations for the diagnosis and management of dentin hypersensitivity. J Can Dent Assoc. 2003;69:221–226.

22. Miglani S, Aggarwal V, Ahuja B. Dentin hypersensitivity: Recent trends in management. J Conserv Dent. 2010;13:218-224.

23. Azodo CC, Amayo AC. Dentinal sensitivity among a selected group of young adults in Nigeria. Niger Med J. 2011;52:189–192.

24. Udoye CI. Pattern and distribution of cervical dentine hypersensitivity in a Nigerian tertiary hospital. Odontostomatol Trop. 2006;29:19–22.

15

Influence of Incorporating Fluoroapatite Nanobioceramic on the Compressive Strength and Bioactivity of Glass Ionomer Cement

Khaghani M[a], Alizadeh S[a], Doostmohammadi A[b]

[a]Young Researchers and Elite Club, Najafabad Branch, Islamic Azad University, Najafabad, Iran
[b]Materials Department, Engineering faculty, Shahrekord University, Shahrekord, Iran

ARTICLE INFO

Key words:
Fluoroapatite
Nanoparticle
Glass Ionomer Cement
Simulated Body Fluid

Corresponding Author:
Sara Alizadeh
Young Researchers and Elite
Club, Najafabad Branch,
Islamic Azad University,
Najafabad, Iran
Email: sarah.alizadeh@smt.
iaun.ac.ir

Abstract

Statement of Problem: In order to increase the performance of glass ionomer cement, it is reinforced with metal powders, short fibers, bioceramics and other materials. Fluoroapatite ($Ca_{10}(PO_4)_6F_2$) is found in dental enamel and is usually used in dental materials due to its good chemical and physical properties.

Objectives: In this study, the effects of the addition of synthesized fluoroapatite nanoceramic on the compressive strength and bioactivity of glass ionomer cement were investigated.

Materials and Methods: The synthesized fluoroapatite nanoceramic particles (~ 70 nm) were incorporated into as-prepared glass ionomer powder and were characterized using X-ray diffraction (XRD), Fourier transform infrared spectroscopy (FTIR) and scanning electron microscopy (SEM). Moreover, the compressive strength values of the modified glass ionomer cements with 0, 1, 3 and 5 wt% of fluoroapatite were evaluated.

Results: Results showed that glass ionomer cement containing 3 wt% fluoroapatite nanoparticles exhibited the highest compressive strength (102.6 ± 4) compared to the other groups, including control group. Furthermore, FTIR and SEM investigations indicated that after soaking the glass ionomer cement- 3 wt% fluoroapatite composite in the simulated body fluid solution, the intensity of O-H, P-O and C-O absorption bands increased as a result of the formation of apatite layer on the surface of the sample, and the rather flat and homogeneous surface of the cement became more porous and inhomogeneous.

Conclusions: Addition of synthesized nano-fluoroapatite to as-prepared glass ionomer cement enhanced the compressive strength as well as nucleation of the calcium phosphate layer on the surface of the composite. This makes it a good candidate for dentistry and orthopedic applications.

Introduction

This study is a continuation of our previous studies: synthesis of flouroapatite [1] and glass ionomer powders [2]. In recent years, apatites [$Ca_{10}(PO_4)_6(OH, F, Cl)_2$] have attracted considerable interest in a broad range of applications such as biomedical uses [3], drug delivery carriers [4], catalysts carriers [5] and adsorbents [6].

Among the apatite group, fluoroapatite (FA) is considered as a biomedical material due to its low solubility, excellent chemical durability, excellent biocompatibility and the moderate resistance to radiation-induced amorphization [7,8]. Although FA is structurally very similar to hydroxyapatite (HA), it has higher thermal stability, more acid solubility tolerance and greater mechanical strength than HA [9,10]. The performance of FA in biological applications is affected by the nano-scale morphology and crystallinity [7]. Hence, owing to the importance of techniques for the preparation of FA with a controlled structure, they have been widely investigated through several methods, such as precipitation [11], sol-gel [12], hydrolysis [13], hydrothermal [14], sonochemical [15] and mechanochemical [10] synthesis.

Glass ionomer cements (GICs) have recently attracted increasing interest in clinical dentistry because of their excellent properties such as biocompatibility, low cytotoxicity, ability of the material for regeneration of hard tissues, low coefficient of thermal expansion, good adhesion to moist tooth structure and anticariogenic properties due to the fluoride ion release [16-18]. Remarkable improvements have been achieved since the invention of GICs to increase their performance which include reinforcement with metal powders [19], modification with resin [20] and incorporation with short fibers [21,22], bioceramics [12,17,23] and other materials.

Moshaverinia et al. [12] synthesized nano-fluoroapatite via an ethanol based sol-gel technique using $(NH_4)_2HPO_4, Ca(NO_3)_2.4H_2O$ and NH_4F as the starting materials. They indicated that the addition of nano-HA and FA to Fuji II commercial GIC enhanced the mechanical properties of the resulting cements and their bond strengths to dentin.

As reported by some researchers, fluoride release is the main factor involved in the antibacterial activity of GIs [24]. In the current study, the effects of the addition of FA nanoceramic on properties of the synthesized glass ionomer cement were evaluated.

Materials and Methods

Synthesis of nanofluoroapatite
For the preparation of fluoroapatite nanoparticles

via sol-gel method, 0.192 g of phosphorus pentoxide (P_2O_5, GR, Merck, Darmstadt, Germany) was dissolved in 20 cc of absolute ethanol (GR, Merck, Darmstadt, Germany) to a concentration of 0.5 M. Simultaneously, 7 g of calcium nitrate tetrahydrate ($Ca(NO_3)_2.4H_2O$, GR, Merck, Darmstadt, Germany) was dissolved in absolute ethanol (20 cc) to form 0.5 M solution to be the Ca precursor. Subsequently, suitable amounts (1.140 cc) of hexafluorophosphoric acid (HPF_6, GR, Sigma-Aldrich, St. Louis, MO, USA) were added to the P precursor and afterwards the Ca/P ratio was adjusted to 1.67 by the slow and drop-wise addition of Ca precursor in order to obtain the starting solution. The mixture was stirred on a magnetic stirrer at room temperature (r.t.) for 24 h, and the gel was aged for at least 24 h at r.t. The as-prepared FA gel was dried at 120 °C for the next 24 h. The obtained solids were grounded and finally calcined at 600 °C for 1 h (heating rate = 3 °C/min) [1].

Preparation of GI powder
The ceramic part of glass ionomer cement was synthesized by the melting method as described in the previous study [2]. In brief, having mixed a defined weight percentage of the starting materials, including aluminum oxide (Al_2O_3, Merck, Darmstadt, Germany), silicon oxide (SiO_2, Merck, Darmstadt, Germany), fluoride strontium (SrF, Merck, Darmstadt, Germany), aluminumphosphate ($AlPO_4$, Merck, Darmstadt, Germany), and calciumfluoride (CaF_2, Merck, Darmstadt, Germany), in a ball mill, the researchers placed the powder in an electric melting furnace and heated it for three hours with the rate of 5 °C/min, to reach the temperature of 1400 °C. Melted glass, resulted from melting the mentioned crystalline materials at 1400 °C, was cooled at ambient temperature and undergone shattering process for 5 hours in a ball mill. At this stage, the obtained powder was passed through a 200 mesh sieve. The obtained powder was the ceramic part of glass ionomer cement and in the next stage, it was mixed with a polymer liquid (polyacrylicacid, Sigma-Aldrich, St. Louis, MO, USA).

Glass ionomer-fluoroapatitenanocomposite
In order to prepare glass ionomer-fluoroapatite nanocomposite, 0, 1, 3 and 5 wt% of nano-FA (~70 nm) were added to the synthesized glass ionomer powders and mixed in amalgamator for 30 s, separately. Then,

GI-FA powders were mixed with polyacrylic acid for 30 s, where the powder/liquid (P/L) ratio was set at 2.7/1. After that, cement mixes were poured into the aluminum moulds (4 mm in diameter and 6 mm in height). The moulds were covered with glass slides, flattened and gently pressed by hand to remove air bubbles from the cements. Finally, after 1 h, the specimens were carefully removed.

The phase composition of samples was carried out by the Philips X-ray diffractometer (XRD) with Cu Kα radiation (λ=0.154 nm) at 40 kV and 30 mA.

Compressive strength measurements
Compressive strength measurement (CS; MPa) was performed on a universal testing machine (Hounsfield, Model H25KS, England) with load cell of 25 kN at 0.5 mm/min. Cylindrical specimens with 4±0.1mm diameter and 6 ± 0.1mm height were prepared according to ASTM D695, and their compressive strength was calculated by the following equation:

$$CS=4P/\pi d^2 \qquad (1)$$

Where P is the load at fracture (N), and d is the diameter of the cylindrical specimen (mm). In each group, three samples were evaluated, and the mean values were compared.

In vitro bioactivity evaluation
In vitro bioactivity of the best performing glass ionomer-fluoroapatite nanocomposite was investigated by soaking in the simulated body fluid (SBF) prepared according to the standard procedure described by Kokubo and Takadama [25] at pH 7.4 for 28 days at 37 °C.

The apatite formation on the surface of the samples as a consequence of the dissolution and precipitation process of calcium phosphate was investigated by scanning electron microscopy (SEM, Seron Technology, AIS2100, Germany) and Fourier transform infrared spectroscopy (FTIR, 6300, JASCO, Japan) over a range of 4000 - 500 cm^{-1}at a resolution of 2.0 cm^{-1}.

Results

Characterization of glass ionomer-fluoroapatite nanocomposite
The XRD patterns of the as-prepared glass ionomer sample and FA-added GIC after being mixed with polyacrylic acid are shown in Figures 1a and b, respectively. The GIC sample (Figure 1a) does not show any sharp peaks in the XRD analysis, indicating that it is a predominantly amorphous material, whereas in the XRD pattern of the FA-added set GIC, peaks related to the crystalline apatite structure were observed between 20° and 35° (Figure1b).

Additionally, the SEM photomicrographs (Figure 2a and b) showed a good mixture of the particles in the matrix and a good bonding between the glass ionomer powder and polymer liquid. Moreover, the surface morphology of the GIC-FA composite exhibited a higher degree of integrity, smoother surface and fewer surface cracks in comparison to the GIC control group.

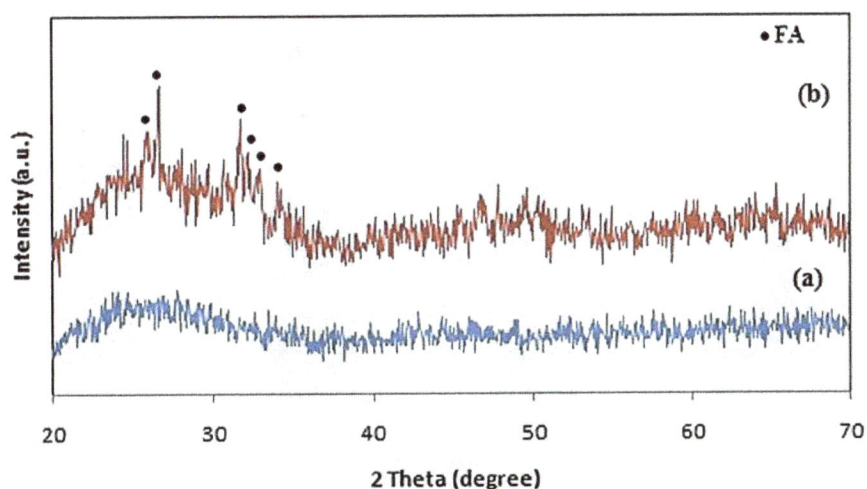

Figure1: XRD patterns of (a) as-prepared GIC and (b) FA-added GIC after mixing with polyacrylic acid.

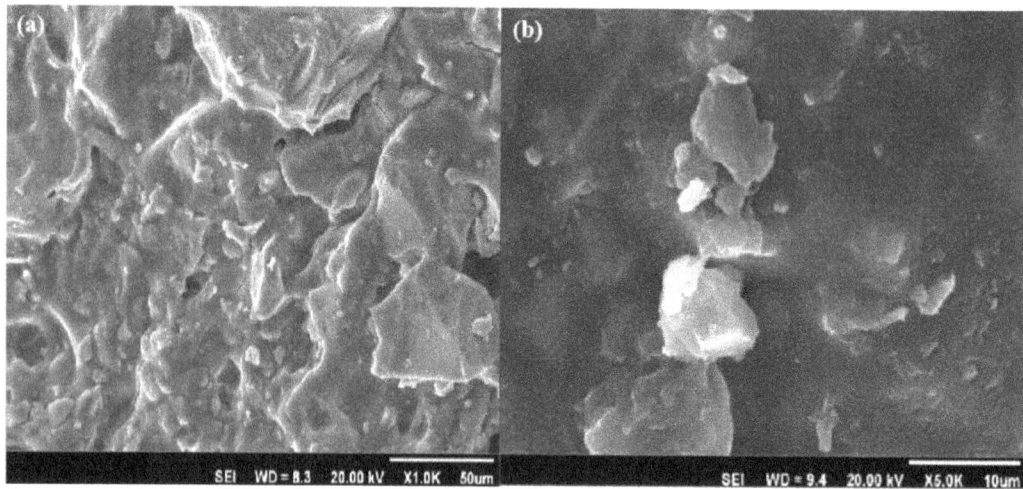

Figure 2: SEM images of FA-added GIC after mixing with polyacrylic acid at (a) X1.0K and (b) X5.0K magnifications.

Compressive strength testing

The mean values (standard deviation) of the measured compressive strength (CS) of at least three samples of each group are presented in Table 1 and graphically in Figure 3. In general, the compressive strength of

GIC increased when fluoroapatite nanoparticles were added to the matrix. Mechanical results also indicated that the compressive strength increased remarkably with increasing the concentration of fluoroapatite nanoparticles up to 3 wt%.

Table 1: Compressive strength values (mean ± standard deviation) of nano-FA-containing glass ionomer cement groups.

Group	Compressive strength (MPa)
GI-control	46.10 ± 3.39
GI-1% (w/w) FA	74.76 ± 5.60
GI-3% (w/w) FA	102.61 ± 4.00
GI-5% (w/w) FA	86.27 ± 4.51

In vitro bioactivity

The best performing GIC-FA nanocomposite as determined by mechanical testing, GIC-3% (w/w) FA, was chosen for the SBF trial. The qualitative investigation of precipitated apatite on the surface of GIC modified with 3 wt% fluoroapatite nanoparticles as a consequence of the dissolution and precipitation process of calciumphosphate was considered by SEM (Figure 4).

Furthermore, the results of evaluating the bioactivity of glass ionomer powder, carried out by Fourier transform infrared spectrometer, and

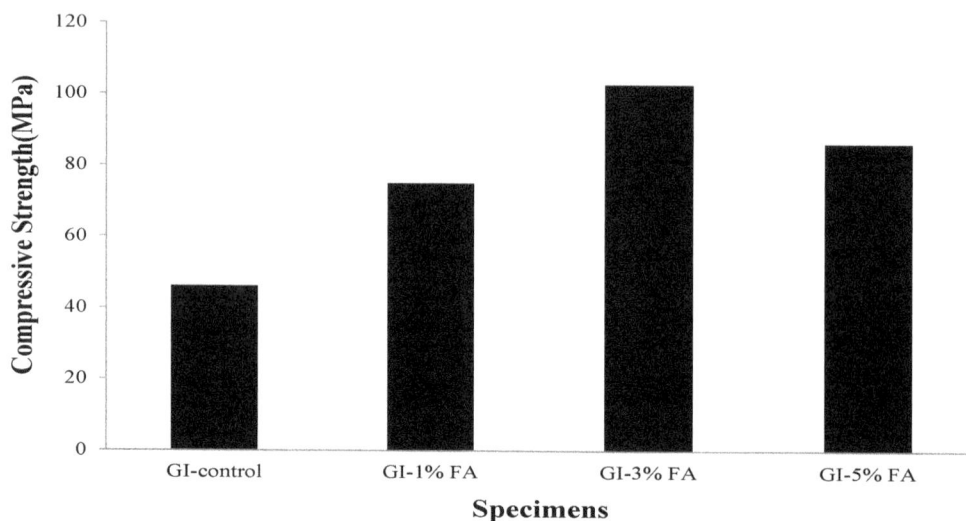

Figure 3: Compressive strength values of nano-FA-containing glass ionomer cement groups.

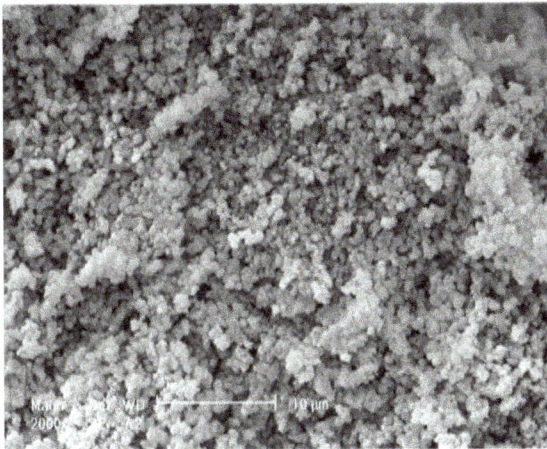

Figure 4: SEM micrograph of GIC-FA composite after keeping in SBF solution at 37 °C for 28 days.

comparing the powder sample before and after soaking in SBF for 28 days at the temperature of 37 °C, are shown in Figures 5a and b, respectively. According to the FTIR spectra of GIC and GIC-FA composite (Figures 5a and b), it is noticed that the intensity of O-H (3500 cm⁻¹), P-O (600-500 cm⁻¹ and 1100-950 cm⁻¹) and C-O (1440-1335 cm⁻¹) absorption bands [26] have increased after 28 days storage in SBF.

Discussion

In this study, FA particles were incorporated in the synthesized glass ionomer cement. As shown in Figure 1, after incorporating the FA particles into the glass ionomer cement, the intense peaks related to the apatite structure appeared in the amorphous matrix of GIC. This was in line with the findings reported previously by Moshavernia et al. [12].

Conventional glass-ionomer cements had low mechanical properties in comparison with other restorative materials, like composite resin or dental amalgam. In order to improve the strength of these materials, the researchers added dispersing agents, such as different powders and fibrous reinforcements, to the cement mixture. Many studies suggested that the mechanical properties were affected by the porosity of the cement, bonding between dispersing agents and the cement matrix, and the properties of particles dispersed through the matrix phase [27-30]. In the present study, mechanical test results indicated that all the GIC samples became stronger when they were incorporated with fluoroapatite nanoparticles; that is to say, nano-FA/ ionomer group exhibited higher compressive strength (with the mean values 74.7 ± 5.6, 102.6 ± 4 and 86.2 ± 4.5 for GIC containing 1, 3 and 5 wt% FA, respectively) in comparison with the control group (with the mean value 46.1 ± 3.4). The increase of compressive strength in the presence of fluoroapatite nanoparticles was due to the formation of crystal phases in the amorphous structure of glass

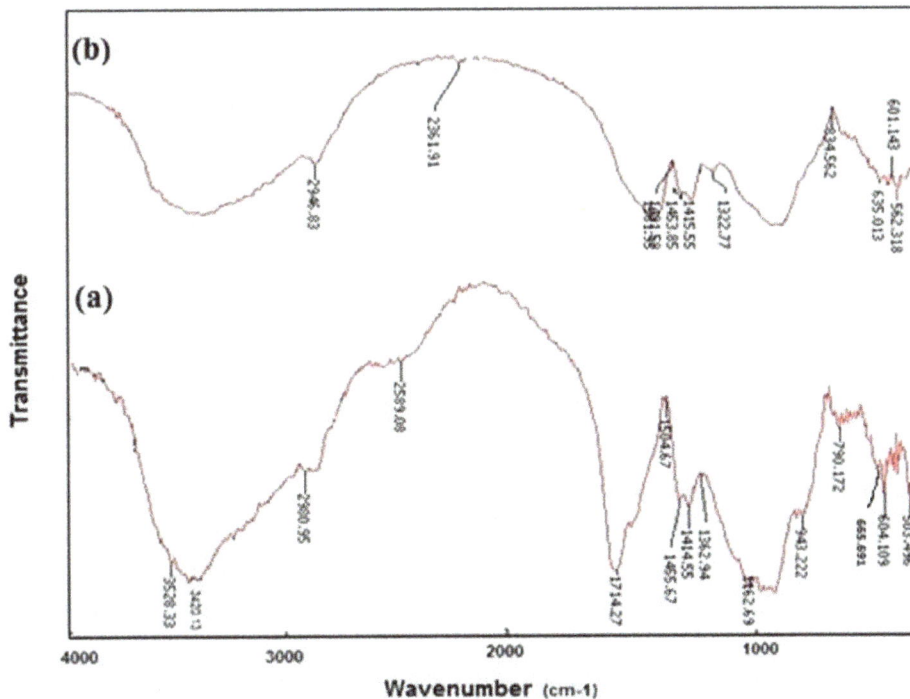

Figure 5: FTIR spectra of the GIC-FA composite: (a) before soaking in SBF, (b) after 28 days of soaking in SBF.

ionomer. Moreover, the combination of glass ionomer particles with larger particle size and FA particles with smaller one led to a wide distribution of particle size. This might cause a high packing density of the combined particles within the glass ionomer matrix, and therefore, a high mechanical strength [31].

Goenka *et al.* [32] examined the addition of synthesized nanocrystalline calcium deficient hydroxyapatite (nCDHA) by 5, 10 and 15 wt% to the commercial GIC. They concluded that ionic release percentage, weight loss and compressive strength of the nCDHA-GIC composite increased with nCDHA addition.

Li *et al.* [18] indicated that the mechanical strength of glass ionomer cement improved significantly when it was modified with niobium oxide (Nb_2O_5). In their study, the compressive strength obtained for Nb_2O_5-added GIC sample was about 142.25 MPa, which was about 50% higher than that of unmodified commercial GIC (94.81 MPa).

Strength reduction of the composites containing FA particles more than 3 wt% for CS is caused by the reduction of bond forces between ceramic and polymeric components of the GIC. In fact, the added fluoroapatite particles act as a barrier and prevent the complete bonding of the parts of glass ionomer cement [17,12,31]. On the other side, it should be noted that particles with a large specific surface area tend to form agglomerates. This effect can make nanoparticles more difficult to uniformly dispersed into polymer matrix, resulting in a strength reduction [33]. Similar results were also reported by Elsaka *et al.* [23] and Sayyedan *et al.* [17] for incorporating TiO_2 and forsterite nanoparticles into the glass ionomer cement, respectively.

The potential of apatite formation on the surfaces of cements in the presence of SBF was considered as a measure of their bioactivity behavior. At the first stage, cement samples were immersed in SBF for 28 days, and then their surfaces were analyzed by FTIR and SEM techniques.

After investigating the FTIR spectra of GIC-FA composite, before and after soaking in the SBF for 28 days at 37 °C and pH 7.4 (Figure 5a and b), we found that by immersing the GIC-FA composite in the SBF, the intensity of O-H, P-O and C-O absorption bands increased because of the formation of carbonate hydroxyapatite on the surface of the cement [34]. Formation of apatite layer after soaking

in SBF demonstrated the bioactivity behavior of this composite [2].

In addition, having qualitatively compared the scanning electron micrographs of GIC-FA cements presented in Figure 2 (before soaking in SBF) and Figure 4 (after 28 days soaking in SBF), we found that after soaking GIC-FA cements in the simulated body fluid, the rather flat and homogeneous surface of the cement transformed into a rather porous and inhomogeneous one. It is interesting to note that in Figure 4, the observable dispersed particles with the lighter colour are the apatite particles which are precipitated on the cement surface from the SBF [2]. The qualitative comparison made between Figure 4 in this study with Figure 4b and c (presented the surface of the GIC sample after 28 days of soaking in the SBF) in our previous study [2], shows that the rate of apatite's nucleation on the surface of GIC-FA nanocomposite is more than that on the surface of GIC [34].

Based on the results obtained from scanning electron micrographs and Fourier transform infrared spectra, it can be concluded the produced composite has an appropriate bioactive behavior.

Conclusions

The findings of this study revealed that the addition of synthesized nano-FA to the as-prepared GIC enhanced the compressive strength, especially by adding 3 wt% FA. However, adding more than 3 wt% FA may decrease the compressive strength due to the high tendency of nanoparicles to form agglomerates. Moreover, FTIR and SEM investigations indicated that calcium phosphate layer nucleated on the surface of the sample, and the rather flat and homogeneous surface of the cement has transformed into a rather porous and inhomogeneous one after soaking in SBF solution for a period of time. It can be concluded from the results that the addition of synthesized nano-fluoroapatite to the as-prepared glass ionomer cement makes it a good candidate for dentistry and orthopedic applications.

Conflict of Interest: None declared.

References

1. Khaghani M, Golniya Z, Monshi A, *et al.*

Preparation, characterization and bioactivity evaluation of fluor-hroxyapatite (FHA) nano-crystals. Adv Proc Mater. 2013;7:97-106.

2. Khaghani M, Doostmohammadi A, Golniya Z, et al. Preparation, physicochemical characterization, and bioactivity evaluation of strontium-containing glass ionomer cement. ISRN Ceram. 2013;2013:1-7.

3. Kannan S, Lemos AF, Ferreira JM. Synthesis and mechanical performance of biological-like hydroxyapatites. Chem Mater. 2006;18:2181-2186.

4. Komlev VS, Barinov SM, Koplik EV. A method to fabricate porous spherical hydroxyapatite granules intended for time-controlled drug release. Biomaterials. 2002;23:3449-3454.

5. Mori K, Yamaguchi K, Hara T, et al. Controlled synthesis of hydroxyapatite-supported palladium complexes as highly efficient heterogeneous catalysts. J Am Chem Soc. 2002;124:11572-11573.

6. Feng Y, Gong JL, Zeng GM, et al. Adsorption of Cd (II) and Zn (II) from aqueous solutions using magnetic hydroxyapatite nanoparticles as adsorbents. Chem Eng J. 2010;162:487-494.

7. Chen M, Jiang D, Li D, et al. Controllable synthesis of fluorapatite nanocrystals with various morphologies: Effects of pH value and chelating reagent. J Alloy Comp. 2009;485:396-401.

8. Chinthaka Silva GW, Ma L, Hemmers O, et al. Micro-structural characterization of precipitation-synthesized fluorapatite nano-material by transmission electron microscopy using different sample preparation techniques. Micron. 2008;39:269-274.

9. Wang H, Sun K, Li A, et al. Size-controlled synthesis and characterization of fluorapatite nanocrystals in the presence of gelatin. Powder Tech. 2011;209:9-14.

10. Ebrahimi-Kahrizsangi, R, Nasiri-Tabrizi B, Chami A. Characterization of single-crystal fluorapatite nanoparticles synthesized via mechanochemical method. Partic. 2011;9:537-544.

11. Chen Y, Miao X. Thermal and chemical stability of fluorohydroxyapatite ceramics with different fluorine contents. Biomaterials. 2005;26:1205-1210.

12. Moshaverinia A, Ansari S, Moshaverinia M, et al. Effects of incorporation of hydroxyapatite and fluoroapatite nanobioceramics into conventional glass ionomer cements (GIC). Acta Biomater. 2008;4:432-440.

13. Kurmaev EZ, Matsuya S, Shin S, et al. Observation of fluorapatite formation under hydrolysis of tetracalcium phosphate in the presence of KF by means of soft X-ray emission and absorption spectroscopy. J Mater Sci Mater Med. 2002;13:33-36.

14. Rodriguez-Lorenzo LM, Hart JN, Gross KA. Influence of fluorine in the synthesis of apatites. Synthesis of solid solutions of hydroxy-fluorapatite. Biomaterials. 2003;24:3777-3785.

15. Barandehfard F, Keyanpour-Rad M, Hosseinnia A, et al. Sonochemical synthesis of hydroxyapatite and fluoroapatite nanosized bioceramics. J Ceram Process Res. 2012;13:437-440.

16. Shiekh RA, Rahman IAb, Masudi SM, et al. Modification of glassionomercement by incorporating hydroxyapatite-silicanano-powder-composite: Sol–gel synthesis and characterization. Ceram Int. 2014;40:3165-3170.

17. Sayyedan FS, Fathi MH, Edris H, et al. Effect of forsterite nanoparticles on mechanical properties of glass ionomer cements. Ceram Int. 2014;40:10743-10748.

18. Li S, Su B, Ran J, et al. Effects of Niobium Oxide Addition on the Mechanical Properties of Glass Ionomer Cement. Mater Sci Forum. 2014;815:373-378.

19. Irie M, Nakai H. Mechanical properties of silver-added glass ionomers and their bond strength to human tooth. Dent Mater J. 1988;7:87-93.

20. Farrugia C, Camilleri J. Antimicrobial properties of conventionalrestorative filling materials and advances inantimicrobial properties of composite resins andglass ionomer cements-A literature review. Dent Mater. 2015;31:89-99.

21. Hammouda IM. Reinforcement of conventional glass-ionomer restorative material with short glass fibers. J Mech Behav Biomed Mater. 2009; 2:73-81.

22. Silva RM, Santos PH, Souza LB, et al. Effects of cellulose fibers on the physical and chemical properties of glass ionomer dental restorative materials. Mater Res Bull. 2013;48:118-126.

23. Elsaka SE, Hamouda IM, Swain MV. Titanium

dioxide nanoparticles addition to a conventional glass-ionomer restorative: Influence on physical and antibacterial properties. J Dent. 2011;39:589-598.

24. Loyola-Rodriguez JP, Garcia-Godoy F, Lindquist R. Growth inhibition of glass ionomer cements on mutans streptococci. Pediatr Dent. 1994;16:346-349.

25. Kokubo T, Takadama H. How useful is SBF in predicting in vivo bone bioactivity? Biomaterials. 2006;27:2907-2915.

26. Li Y, Wiliana T, Tam KC. Synthesis of amorphous calcium phosphate using various types of cyclodextrins. Mater Res Bull. 2007;42:820-827.

27. Moshaverinia A, Roohpour N, Chee WWL, et al. A review of powder modifications in conventional glass-ionomer dental cements. J Mater Chem. 2011;21:1319-1328.

28. Swift EJ, Dogan AU. Analysis of glass-ionomer cement with the use of electron microscopy. J Prothet Dent. 1990;64:167-174.

29. Miyata N. Dispersion toughening of ceramics. Bull Ceram Soc Japan. 1986;21:605-612.

30. Kon M, Kawano F, Tada Y, et al. Effect of crystallization on fracture strength of castable glass-ceramics containing two crystals. Dent Mater J. 1994;13:47-54.

31. Gu YW, Yap AU, Cheang P, et al. Effects of incorporation of HA/ZrO_2 into glass ionomer cement (GIC). Biomaterials. 2005;26:713-720.

32. Goenka S, Balu R, Sampath Kumar TS. Effects of nanocrystalline calcium deficient hydroxyapatite incorporation in glass ionomer cements. J Mech Behav Biomed Mater. 2012;7:69-76.

33. Zhao J, Xie D. Effect of nanoparticles on wear resistance and surface hardness of a dental glass-ionomer cement. J Compos Mater. 2009;43:2739-2752.

34. Sayyedan FS, Fathi MH, Edris H, et al. Fluoride release and bioactivity evaluation of glass ionomer: Forsterite nanocomposite. Dent Res J. 2013;10:452-459.

16

Computer-Based Oral Hygiene Instruction versus Verbal Method in Fixed Orthodontic Patients

Moshkelgosha V[a], Mehrvarz Sh[b], Saki M[c*], Golkari A[d]

[a]Orthodontic Research Center, Department of Orthodontics, School of Dentistry, Shiraz University of Medical Sciences, Shiraz, Iran

[b]Student Research Committee, School of Dentistry, Shiraz University of Medical Sciences, Shiraz, Iran

[c]Student Research Committee, Orthodontic Research Center and Department of Orthodontics, School of Dentistry, Shiraz University of Medical Sciences, Shiraz, Iran

[d]Department of Dental Public Health , School of Dentistry, Shiraz University of Medical Sciences, Shiraz, Iran

---

ARTICLE INFO

Key words:
Computer-Based
Fixed Orthodontic Appliances
Oral Hygiene

Corresponding Author:
Maryam Saki
Student Research Committee,
Orthodontic Research Center
and Department of Orthodontics,
School of Dentistry, Shiraz
University of Medical Sciences,
Shiraz, Iran
Email: mary_sa68@yahoo.com

Abstract

Statement of Problem: Fixed orthodontic appliances in the oral cavity make tooth cleaning procedures more complicated.

Objectives: This study aimed to compare the efficacy of computerized oral hygiene instruction with verbal technique among fixed orthodontic patients referred to the evening clinic of Orthodontics of Shiraz Dental School.

Materials and Methods: A single-blind study was performed in Orthodontic Department of Shiraz, Islamic Republic of Iran, from January to May 2015 following the demonstrated exclusion and inclusion criteria. The sample size was considered 60 patients with 30 subjects in each group. Bleeding on probing and plaque indices and dental knowledge were assessed in the subjects to determine pre-intervention status. A questionnaire was designed for dental knowledge evaluation. The patients were randomly assigned into the computerized and verbal groups. Three weeks after the oral hygiene instruction, indices of bleeding on probing and plaque index and the dental knowledge were evaluated to investigate post-intervention outcome. The two groups were compared by chi-square and student t tests. The pre- and post-intervention scores in each group were compared using paired t-test.

Results: In the computerized group, the mean score for plaque index and bleeding on probing index was significantly decreased while dental health knowledge was significantly increased after oral hygiene instruction, in contrast to the verbal group.

Conclusions: Within the limitations of the current study, computerized oral hygiene instruction is proposed to be more effective in providing optimal oral health status compared to the conventional method in fixed orthodontic patients.

Introduction

Presence of fixed orthodontic appliances disturbs the access of oral hygiene instruments to the teeth surfaces and leads to plaque buildup [1,2]. Plaque accumulation on the tooth surfaces is known to cause gingivitis, periodontal loss and enamel demineralization [3,4]. Development of white spot lesions is related to dental plaque around the orthodontic brackets [5,6]. The quality of life of patients with fixed orthodontic appliances will be altered because of the change in their oral health condition [7,8]. Therefore, such patients are normally counseled and treated by hygienists before being placed on the waiting list for receiving their fixed orthodontic treatment. Despite this pre-treatment screening, there is always a reduction in the effectiveness of oral hygiene when the orthodontic treatment phase starts [9].

Oral hygiene is a key factor for preservation of periodontal health as it decreases the microbial plaque that has been accumulated on the teeth and gingiva [10,11]. The effect of patient self-care procedures such as brushing and flossing on prevention of periodontal diseases has been clearly identified [12,13]. Some psychological models to behaviour management for oral hygiene-related behaviours have been demonstrated [14-18]. It is known that applying professional oral health advice on oral hygiene has a great influence on improving the level of oral hygiene of the patients [19,20].

Nowadays, as the technology improves, the use of computers extends, and computers are an inseparable component of an individual's life. A major advantage of computer-based training is its high degree of standardization, repeatability, and clarity. This is what has been called for in research into methods of oral hygiene instruction for a long time [21].

There is some controversy in the reported effects of the computerized oral hygiene instruction compared with conventional methods. In a study conducted on implant patients, a computerized oral health instruction program was compared with conventional oral health instructions. Lower plaque index, pocket depths and bleeding on probing were reported in the computerized group [22]. Another research compared the results of written, verbal and video tape methods of oral hygiene instructions for fixed orthodontic patients. It was declared that there was no significant difference between these methods and all methods had comparable results [23]. A study compared the effect of computer-based oral hygiene

instructions on modified Bass and Fones technique. The computerized oral hygiene instruction was proposed as the most standard technique in teaching both methods of brushing [21].

To the best of our knowledge, there is no research on comparing computerized oral hygiene instruction with other methods such as written or verbal for fixed orthodontic patients. On the other hand, we know that cultural differences can cause different results with each kind of instruction methods. This study aimed to compare the efficacy of computerized instruction with face-to-face verbal techniques among fixed orthodontic patients referring to Department of Orthodontics of Shiraz Dental School.

Materials and Methods

Study Design and Setting

A single-blind clinical trial was performed in the orthodontic specialist clinic of Shiraz Dental School, Shiraz University of Medical Sciences, Shiraz, Islamic Republic of Iran, from January to May 2015. They all underwent their routine orthodontic treatment based on their own orthodontist's recommendation. Their orthodontic treatment was not in any way affected by this study. The selected patients were then divided into two groups based on how they received the oral hygiene instruction.

Subjects, Sample size and Randomization

Fixed orthodontic patients who were admitted in the orthodontic specialist clinic of Shiraz University of Medical Sciences, with no history of previous orthodontic treatment selected using the convenient sampling method by one research assistant. The inclusion and exclusion criteria were: being literate, age range of 13-35, presence of at least 20 of their own teeth, 10 or more teeth showing plaque or bleeding, no study of dentistry, no smoking, no electrical tooth brushing, no dental treatment affecting gingival health or oral hygiene throughout the study, and no pregnancy or lactation during the study. Patients with diabetes, habit of smoking, and local factors predisposing them to plaque accumulation such as faulty restorations, calculus and unusual tooth crown morphology were also excluded. The sample size was considered 60 patients with 30 subjects in each group, based on consultation with a statistician. On the first session of banding and bonding of the lower arch, a self-designed questionnaire, consisting of patients' demographic information, chief complaint and 20 multiple-choice questions, was given to the subjects to assess their knowledge of dental health as a pre-intervention test score.

Validity and reliability of the questionnaire were assessed in a pilot study. First, two faculty members of Shiraz School of Dentistry, one from Department of Orthodontics and one from Department of Periodontics were asked to evaluate each question and the questionnaire as a whole. Revisions were made based on what these two experts found necessary to achieve the main objectives of this study. In the next step of the pilot study, a professional Farsi Language editor was asked to determine the readability of the questions, so that they would be suitable for the patients in this study, considering that the sample could contain teenagers and young adults with minimum literacy. The face validity of the questionnaire was assessed by seeking help from a professional designer. The final questionnaire was distributed among a convenient sample of 20 orthodontic patients. The internal validity was assessed using Cronbach's alpha ($\alpha = 0.73$). These 20 patients were asked to fill the questioner again after four weeks. The test-retest reliability of the questionnaire was assessed using kappa agreement test.

The questions covered knowledge of appliance care and diet and routine dental care during fixed orthodontic therapy. Each correct answer was given 1 score while an incorrect choice was given zero. Therefore, the total score of each patient was in the range of zero to 20. Afterwards, an outline form for recording the oral hygiene condition was filled out by one research assistant as a record of initial oral hygiene status before the intervention. The designed form consisted of patients' demographic information, plaque index and bleeding on probing index. The lower arches of the patients were banded and bonded by one trained technician. Similar brackets, bands [0.022 in, MBT prescription, Mini Master Series™ American Orthodontics™ metal brackets and bands (Sheboygan, WI, USA)], archwire [Nickel Titanium (NiTi) (3M Unitek, Monrovia, California, USA], primer (Ormco, Italy) and adhesive (light cure, Greenglue, Italy) with similar protocol of etching, bonding and curing, were applied in all patients. Brackets and band main tubes were placed on the middle of the tooth occlusogingivally and mesiodistally. Excess adhesive was checked and removed for each tooth. Patients who canceled their appointments, did not agree to participate or debonded their brackets were excluded from the study. After the

completion of pre-intervention form, the patients were randomly divided into two groups: computerized and verbal oral hygiene instruction. The randomization sequence was conducted using a computerized random number generator and the allocation was kept in sealed opaque consecutively numbered envelopes. This simple randomization scheme was independently prepared by a research assistant who was not involved in determining eligibility, providing the dental knowledge questionnaire and oral hygiene assessment form, or evaluating the outcome. After the randomized allocation, the two groups were checked regarding the matching of the probable confounding factors of age and gender.

Oral Hygiene Instruction

The oral hygiene instruction was performed at the end of the session of banding and bonding of the lower teeth. The oral care equipment specialized for orthodontic patients (Sunstar GUM, USA) were prescribed for all the subjects at the session of admission. The patients were asked to bring their equipment at the session of impression taking. Session of banding and bonding was not planned for the patients unless their equipment was checked. The content of the oral hygiene instruction of both groups was similar, consisting of five sections: brushing; flossing using interdental brush; oral rinse; fixed appliance care; and diet. Modified Bass brushing technique was instructed focusing on cleaning the gingival 3rd and the whole braces. Flossing using superfloss was demonstrated and prescribed once daily. Fluoridated oral rinse was introduced for daily use. The appliance care and diet excluding hard foods and sticky chocolates were also explained to the patients. The duration of instruction for both groups was set 10 minutes: 3 minutes for brushing, 1 minute for oral rinse, and 2 minutes for each section of flossing, interdental brush, and appliance care and diet. The prepared instruction was mainly derived from the website of Iranian Association of Orthodontists [24], the website of American Association of Orthodontists [25], the website of British Dental Health foundation [26], and the textbook of Carranza's clinical periodontology [27]. The validity of oral and computerized instruction was checked by two faculty members in each field of orthodontics and periodontics.

The patients in the verbal group received an instruction of oral hygiene procedures verbally by a trained dental student. All the instructions were shown on a dental model with braces. During the demonstration, the patients were not allowed to ask questions irrelevant to the content of the oral hygiene instruction. This was considered in order to minimize the different information the verbal group might got, compared with the computerized group.

The computerized group received the same information by software. The software was designed by an orthodontist who was a faculty member of Shiraz University of Medical Sciences ("Educational Dental Disc, Orthodontics", Jahan Pardaz Teb Company, Tehran, Iran). The software had the autorun ability and its window opened when the CD-ROM was inserted. The subjects were allowed to use the software only in the clinic. Each section had Farsi written and graphic demonstrations and ended with a training video clip. The narrator of the videos also spoke in Farsi. A section was opened by choosing it from the menu at the bottom of the software window.

After three weeks, the oral hygiene status was evaluated by another research assistant who was unaware of the study protocol to determine the post-intervention condition. The questionnaire of dental knowledge was filled out by the patients once again, the score of which was considered as the post-intervention grade. Patients who did not attend on the due date were excluded.

Outcome measures
The primary outcome was a change in the oral hygiene procedures both theoretically and practically which was determined by the post-intervention score of dental knowledge questionnaire and the illustrated plaque index. The lower arch (the arch to be banded and bonded) was assumed to be comprised of three segments: the segment distal to the right cuspid, that distal to the left cuspid, and that mesial to the right and left first bicuspids. Each segment was examined for debris or calculus. From each segment, one tooth with the greatest area covered by dental plaque was chosen for calculating the individual index, for that particular segment. Buccal and labial surface of each tooth was divided into nine segments using two imaginary horizontal and vertical lines that trisected the tooth surface occlusogingivally and mesiodistally, respectively [23]. The subjects were asked to chew one tablet of a disclosing agent (GUM Red Cote Disclosing Tablets 824 Sunstar Butler GUM, Chicago, USA) and swish around the mouth for 30 seconds without swallowing, expel, and rinse with water for one minute. Of the tooth surface, the gingival two third excluding the middle segment

of the total of nine which is the position of bracket placement or band tube was considered for plaque evaluation. One point would be attributed to each segment of a tooth which was covered with dental plaques. For the assessed individual tooth, the points were added together. The total score for the arch was also determined by adding up the individual scores of the three selected teeth. Therefore, the score range for each individual tooth and the lower arch were 0-5 and 0-15, respectively. The pre-intervention plaque index was measured before banding and bonding of the brackets.

The secondary outcome was presumed to be a change in periodontal health which was measured by the bleeding on probing (BOP) index. The buccal and labial surfaces of each selected tooth for plaque index assessment were also tested for BOP index. Using the same imaginary vertical lines, the BOP was evaluated in three mesial, middle and distal areas of the free gingiva. For each area, one point was considered if bleeding occurred between 30 seconds after gentle probing with a periodontal probe (Williams periodontal probe; Hu-Friedy, Chicago, USA). The sum of the points was regarded as the individual score of the selected teeth for BOP. These scores were added to comprise the total score of the arch. Conclusively, the range of BOP index of each tooth and the whole arch was 0-3 and 0-9, respectively. The pre-intervention BOP index was measured before banding and bonding of the brackets.

Ethical Consideration
Ethical approval was obtained from the Ethics Committee of Shiraz University of Medical Sciences (#94-01-37-9831). The study was in accordance with Helsinki Declaration of 1975 as revised in 2000 [28]. All participants were assured that their data would be kept confidential. All patients' parents signed a written informed consent about letting their data to be used in this study.

Statistical Analysis
The mean of the lower arch score of the plaque index and BOP index for the computerized and verbal groups was calculated. The mean of pre- and post-intervention score for the two groups was also determined. Data were analyzed through SPSS software (SPSS Software, Version 18.0; IBM, Chicago, IL). Matching of the age and gender among the two groups was checked using Student`s t and Chi-square test. The pre- and post-intervention score

Table 1: The descriptive statistics of the samples

Group	Female (%)	Male (%)	Age Range (Mean ± SD)	Aesthethic Chief Complaint	Functional Chief Complaint	P value
Verbal	24(80%)	6(20%)	13-31(23.7 ± 6.1)	26(86.7%)	4(13.3%)	
Computerized	25(83.3%)	5(16.7%)	13-31(21.6 ± 6.0)	24(80%)	6(20%)	>0.05
Total	49(81.67%)	11(18.33%)	13-31(22.7 ± 6.1)	50(83.3%)	10(16.7%)	

in each group was compared using Paired t-tests. The comparison between plaque and BOP index before and after the intervention in each group was also done using the same statistical test.

Results

Sixty subjects consisting of 49 females (81.67%) and 11 males (18.33%) were selected. After randomized allocation, 30 patients were allocated to each of the verbal and computerized groups. None of the subjects cancelled the second visit or debonded their brackets and the recruitment rate of both groups was 100%. The age and gender were matched between the two groups ($p > 0.05$). The descriptive data of the subjects in the verbal and computerized groups is shown in Table 1.

The mean score of plaque index, BOP index and dental health knowledge was not significantly different between the verbal and computerized groups before the oral hygiene instruction ($p = 0.85, 0.54, 0.71$) respectively.

After oral hygiene instruction, the mean score of plaque index, BOP index and dental health knowledge in the verbal group was slightly improved but not significantly different compared with the pre-intervention score ($p = 0.066, 0.161, 0.057$) respectively.

In the computerized group, the mean score for plaque index and BOP index was significantly decreased ($p = 0.037, 0.035$) respectively while dental health knowledge was significantly increased after the oral hygiene instruction ($p = 0.046$) (Figure 1).

Discussion

This study aimed to compare the efficacy of the verbal and computerized oral hygiene instruction among fixed orthodontic patients using plaque index, bleeding on probing index, and dental knowledge score. Oral hygiene can be considered as a behaviour which needs to be learned through oral hygiene instruction to improve the patients' oral health. Some psychological models to behaviour management for oral hygiene-related behaviours have been demonstrated [14-18]. When reviewing these models, some socio-psychological determinants of oral hygiene behaviour were proposed, most of which cannot be controlled. To put it simply, three domains of learning have been demonstrated in the process of behavioural change: cognitive, affective and behavioural [29]. The designed questionnaire for knowledge of dental health was used to evaluate the effect of oral hygiene instruction (OHI) on the cognitive domain. Plaque index was used as a

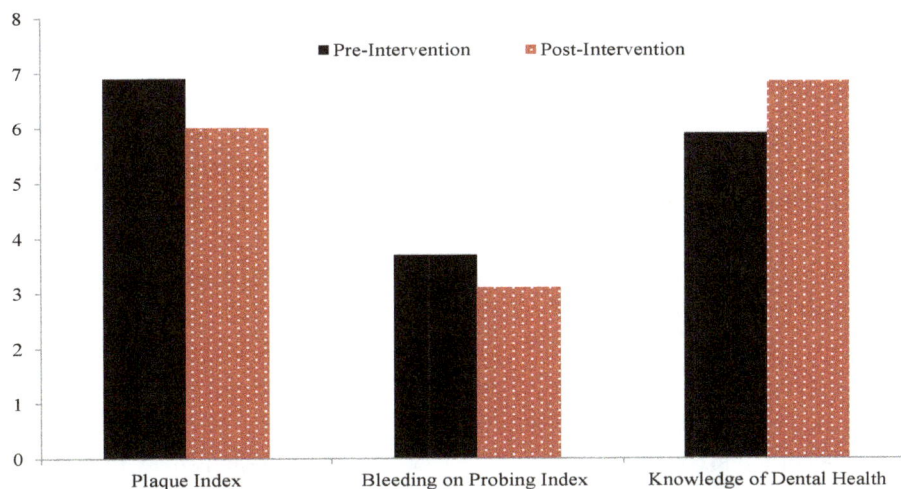

Figure 1: The mean score of plaque index, bleeding on probing index and dental health knowledge before and after computerized oral hygiene instruction

measure of the patient's oral hygiene status and identification of the effect of OHI on the behavioural domain. BOP index was used to assess the condition of the periodontal health which was considered to be the consequence of behavioural change.

The groups were examined to be matched regarding the primary plaque index, BOP index and dental health knowledge, in order to exclude the confounding effects on the result. The dental knowledge, status of oral hygiene and periodontal health were found not to be different between the participants of the two groups. As lifestyle, occupational status and gender are also confounding factors that can affect oral hygiene behaviour [30], they were also taken into consideration. The groups were matched considering the gender and age.

Three weeks after verbal oral hygiene instruction on the session of banding and bonding the lower arch, dental health knowledge and the status of oral hygiene and periodontal health did not change significantly. Regarding the two indices, it can be concluded that the verbal OHI was effective as the oral hygiene and periodontal health was expected to be worse if special oral hygiene procedures were not applied. Besides, considering the p values of the three parameters (p plaque index = 0.066, p BOP index = 0.161, p test = 0.057), it can be inferred that if the number of participants was higher in this group, the results would probably be statistically significant.

In the computerized OHI group, dental health knowledge and the condition of oral hygiene and periodontal health were improved significantly. Viewing the similar number of subjects in the verbal and computerized groups, it can be suggested that the computerized OHI is possibly more effective for fixed orthodontic patients within the age range of 13-31 years.

Since the orthodontic brackets and wire would disturb the cleansing procedures in the gingival two thirds, only these areas were evaluated for plaque index assessment, excluding the area of the bracket placement as in Less and Rock' study [23].

Sano and colleagues [22], comparing a computerized program with conventional oral hygiene instruction on implant patients, found that patients who used the computerized oral health instruction had lower plaque index, pocket depths and BOP; they concluded that the instruction program made it easier for the patients to understand their oral condition, and to learn and repeat appropriate self-care practices. The result of the plaque index and BOP index was in

agreement with the current study. In Sano's study, the oral hygiene index (OHI) was used rather than plaque index [22]. Oral hygiene index includes combined debris and calculus index. Confounding factors were not noted in sample selection or randomization, in contrast to our study in which they were mentioned as the exclusion criteria. The subjects were allowed to take the designed CD-ROM home. This might cause some interaction of the information in the CD-ROM between the two groups which may make the trial uncontrolled and the deductions cannot be relied on. There was control neither over the number of CD-ROM viewed by the subjects, nor the exchange of the CD-ROM between the verbal and the computerized groups. Besides, if the computerized OHI can be helpful only in the office, it will be of great value and will save money and time for the patients.

Less and Rock, comparing the results between written, verbal and video tape methods of oral hygiene instructions for fixed orthodontic patients, concluded that there was no significant difference between these methods and all methods had comparable results [23].This was in contrast to our results. The reason of this difference might be the fact that the patients participating in the study were banded and bonded during one to three previous months. It was not exactly stated when the patients were instructed how to clean their teeth and braces or if they were instructed with the same technique. This was probably a confounding factor in the study. If the subjects were not instructed in the first session of banding and bonding, it would be unethical.

Comparing the effect of computer-based oral hygiene instructions on modified bass and Fones technique on students, Harnake and co-workers concluded that computerized oral hygiene instruction is proposed as the most standard technique in teaching methods of brushing. Fones technique was concluded to be more advantageous than modified Bass technique [21]. Papillary bleeding index and Turesky modification of the plaque index of Quigley and Hein were assessed six, twelve, and twenty eight weeks after the visit of oral hygiene instruction. The subjects were students probably in similar age group of young adults; this was not stated clearly in the method or results of the research. In our study, the subjects were adolescents and young adults (13-31 years).

Our study had some limitations. In female subjects, the effect of menstrual cycle and hormonal changes could not be matched between the two groups. This might have confounded the result of the research. Moreover, the status of oral hygiene was evaluated only after three weeks and the maintenance of the oral hygiene behaviour was not assessed in further follow ups. Future studies with more follow ups and higher sample volume are suggested to be conducted.

Conclusions

Within the limitations of the current study, computerized oral hygiene instruction was suggested to be more effective in providing optimum oral health status compared to conventional method in fixed orthodontic patients.

Conflict of Interest: None declared.

References

1. Ousehal L, Lazrak L, Es-said R, *et al*. Evaluation of dental plaque control in patients wearing fixed orthodontic appliances: a clinical study. Int Orthod. 2011;9:140-155.

2. Klukowska M, Bader A, Erbe C, *et al*. Plaque levels of patients with fixed orthodontic appliances measured by digital plaque image analysis. Am J Orthod Dentofacial Orthop. 2011;139:463-470.

3. Axelsson P, Nyström B, Lindhe J. The long-term effect of a plaque control program on tooth mortality, caries and periodontal disease in adults. J Clin Periodontol. 2004;31:749-457.

4. Van Der Weijden F, Slot D. Oral hygiene in the prevention of periodontal diseases: the evidence. Periodontol 2000. 2011;55:104-123.

5. Tufekci E, Dixon J, Gunsolley J, *et al*. Prevalence of white spot lesions during orthodontic treatment with fixed appliances. Angle Orthod. 2011;81:206-210.

6. Enaia M, Bock N, Ruf S. White-spot lesions during multibracket appliance treatment: a challenge for clinical excellence. Am J Orthod Dentofacial Orthop. 2011;140:17-24.

7. Liu Z, McGrath C, Hägg U. Changes in oral health-related quality of life during fixed orthodontic appliance therapy: an 18-month prospective longitudinal study. Am J Orthod Dentofacial Orthop. 2011;139:214-219.

8. Chen M, Wang DW, Wu LP. Fixed orthodontic appliance therapy and its impact on oral health-related quality of life in Chinese patients. Angle Orthod. 2010; 80:49-53.

9. Atassi F, Awartani F. Oral hygiene status among orthodontic patients. J Contemp Dent Pract. 2010;11:25-32.

10. Turner Y, Ashley F, Wilson R. Effectiveness of oral hygiene with and without root planing in treating subjects with chronic periodontitis. Br Dent J. 1994;177: 367-371.

11. Stewart J, Strack S, Graves P. Development of oral hygiene self-efficacy and outcome expectancy questionnaires. Community Dent Oral Epidemiol. 1997;25:337-342.

12. van der Weijden GA, Slot DE. interdental oral hygiene: the evidence. In Bartold P, Jin L, editors. Multi-Disciplinary Management of Periodontal Disease. Hong Kong: Asian Pacific Society of Periodontology; 2012. p. 16-33.

13. Claydon NC. Current concepts in toothbrushing and interdental cleaning. Periodontol 2000. 2008;48:10-22.

14. Renz A, Ide M, Newton T, Robinson PG, Smith D. Psychological interventions to improve adherence to oral hygiene instructions in adults with periodontal diseases. Cochrane Database Syst Rev. 2007 Apr 18; (2):CD005097.

15. McCaul K, O'Neill K, Glasgow R. Predicting performance of dental hygiene behaviors: an examination of Fishbein and Ajzen Model and self-efficacy expectations. J Appl Soc Psychol. 1988; 18:114-128.

16. Tedesco L, Keffer M, Fleck-Kandath C. Self efficacy, reasoned action, and oral health behavior reports: a social cognitive approach to compliance. J Behav Med. 1991;14:341-355.

17. McCaul K, Sandgren A, O'Neill K, *et al*. The value of the theory of planned behavior, perceived behavior control, and self-efficacy expectations for predicting health-protective behaviors. Basic Appl Soc Psych. 1993;14:231-252.

18. Buunk-Werkhoven YA, Dijkstra A, van der Schans CP. Determinants of oral hygiene behavior: a study based on the theory of planned behavior. Community Dent Oral Epidemiol. 2011;39:250-259.

19. Ribeiro D, Pavarina A, Giampaolo E, *et al*. Effect of oral hygiene education and motivation on removable partial denture wearers: longitudinal study. Gerodontology. 2009; 26:150-156.

20. Jönsson B, Öhrn K, Oscarson N, *et al*. An individually tailored treatment programme for improved oral hygiene: introduction of a new

course of action in health education for patients with periodontitis. Int J Dent Hyg. 2009;7:166-175.

21. Harnacke D, Mitter S, Lehner M, *et al.* Improving oral hygiene skills by computer-based training: a randomized controlled comparison of the modified Bass and the Fones techniques. PLoS One. 2012;7:37072.

22. Sano T, Oishi K, Mizohata K, *et al.* Oral hygiene instruction program for implant patients Evaluation of clinical utility based on plaque control records and changes in prevalence of deep pocket probing depths and bleeding on probing. J Osaka Dent Univ. 2012;46:245-249.

23. Lees A, Rock W. A comparison between written, verbal, and videotape oral hygiene instruction for patients with fixed appliances. J Orthod. 2000;27:323-328.

24. "cares-orthodontics". Iao.ir. N.p., 2014. Web. 20 Dec. 2014. (http://iao.ir/cares-orthodontics.aspx).

25. "Instructional Videos | AAO Members". Aaoinfo. org. N.p., 2014. Web. 20 Dec. 2014. (https:// www.aaoinfo.org/node/3034)

26. "Oral Treatments And Dental Health › Orthodontics › Living With My Brace | The British Dental Health Foundation". Dentalhealth. org. N.p., 2014. Web. 20 Dec. 2014. (https:// www.dentalhealth.org/tell-me-about/topic/ orthodontics/living-with-my-brace)

27. Newman MG, Takei H, Klokkevold PR, Carranza FA. Carranza's clinical periodontology: 12th ed, Elsevier health sciences; 2015

28. "WMA Declaration Of Helsinki - Ethical Principles For Medical Research Involving Human Subjects". Wma.net. N.p., 2014. Web. 20 Dec. 2014. (http:// www.wma.net/en/30publications/10policies/b3/ index.html)

29. Daly B, Watt R, Batchelor P, *et al.* Essential Dental public health. 1st Edition. New York: Oxford University Press; 2002. p. 156.

30. Sakki T, Knuuttila ML, Anttila S. Lifestyle, gender and occupational status as determinants of dental health behavior. J Clin Periodontol. 1998;25:566-570.

17

The Effect of Bulk Depth and Irradiation Time on the Surface Hardness and Degree of Cure of Bulk-Fill Composites

Farahat F[a], Daneshkazemi AR[b], Hajiahmadi Z[c]

[a]Department of Operative Dentistry, School of Dentistry, Shahid Sadoughi University of Medical Sciences, Yazd, Iran
[b]Social Determinants on Oral Health Research Center and Department of Operative Dentistry, School of Dentistry, Shahid Sadoughi University of Medical Sciences, Yazd, Iran
[c]Yazd Dental School, Shahid Sadoughi University of Medical Sciences, Yazd, Iran

ARTICLE INFO	Abstract
Key words: Bulk-fill Composites Irradiation Time Microhardness Degree of Cure *Corresponding Author:* Zeynab Hajiahmadi Yazd Dental School, Shahid Sadoughi University of Medical Sciences, Yazd, Iran Email: Zeynab.dentist@yahoo.com	***Statement of Problem:*** For many years, application of the composite restoration with a thickness less than 2 mm for achieving the minimum polymerization contraction and stress has been accepted as a principle. But through the recent development in dental material a group of resin based composites (RBCs) called Bulk Fill is introduced whose producers claim the possibility of achieving a good restoration in bulks with depths of 4 or even 5 mm. ***Objectives:*** To evaluate the effect of irradiation times and bulk depths on the degree of cure (DC) of a bulk fill composite and compare it with the universal type. ***Materials and Methods:*** This study was conducted on two groups of dental RBCs including Tetric N Ceram Bulk Fill and Tetric N Ceram Universal. The composite samples were prepared in Teflon moulds with a diameter of 5 mm and height of 2, 4 and 6 mm. Then, half of the samples in each depth were cured from the upper side of the mould for 20s by LED light curing unit. The irradiation time for other specimens was 40s. After 24 hours of storage in distilled water, the microhardness of the top and bottom of the samples was measured using a Future Tech (Japan- Model FM 700) Vickers hardness testing machine. Data were analyzed statistically using the one and multi way ANOVA and Tukey's test ($p = 0.050$). ***Results:*** The DC of Tetric N Ceram Bulk Fill in defined irradiation time and bulk depth was significantly more than the universal type ($p < 0.001$). Also, the DC of both composites studied was significantly ($p < 0.001$) reduced by increasing the bulk depths. Increasing the curing time from 20 to 40 seconds had a marginally significant effect ($p \leq 0.040$) on the DC of both bulk fill and universal studied RBC samples. ***Conclusions:*** The DC of the investigated bulk fill composite was better than the universal type in all the irradiation times and bulk depths. The studied universal and bulk fill RBCs had an appropriate DC at the 2 and 4 mm bulk depths respectively and using the recommended curing time of 40s can led to the slightly better value of DC in both composites.

Introduction

To achieve a high level of aesthetics, physical and strength properties close to natural tooth structure has been among the factors to be considered for spread of resin based composites (RBCs) in restorative dentistry in recent years. Since emergence of composites, a lot of changes have been made in their chemical structure and filler to eliminate or improve the defects [1]. In addition to the numerous advantages of composites used in restorative dentistry, the presence of characteristics like low polymerization shrinkage and depth have always caused restrictions in the field of application of these materials [2].

For many years, the use of composites with a thicknesses of less than 2 mm in order to achieve a restoration with a high degree of cure (DC) and minimal shrinkage polymerization and stress has been proposed as a principle [3,4]. However, using this technique in restoration of deep cavities is time consuming and also there is probability of air bubbles confinement or contamination between layers of the composite [5]. Thus, search for strategies for rapid conduction of deep dental cavities caused tendency to develop and marketing new RBC materials with capability of increasing the depth of polymerization in recent years.

A new type of RBCs named bulk fill has recently been introduced to the market which contains lower amount of filler with larger size. Presence of large sized filler (up to 2μm) in the structure of this composite in general terms reduces the level of connectivity between matrix and filler and can improve the transmission of curing blue light into the deeper point of composite restoration [6]. Moreover, according to the manufacturers, bulk fill composites have capability of replacement in deep cavities with thicknesses of 4 to 5 mm in one layer without the need for longer curing process or more severe irradiation. Thus, restoration time will be shorter and treatment will be faster [7].

Surface hardness is one of the important mechanical properties of dental composites. Hardness of resin composites can be defined as resistance against permanent indentation or penetration on the surface of restoration. This specification affects the capability of polishing and resistance to scratches of the material [8].

Polymerization rate of composites also affects the mechanical properties, size stability and solubility, stability of colours and their biocompatibility [9]. Among various features, the ratio of bottom to top surface microhardness of RBCs in different irradiation times, called the degree of cure (DC), is widely used to evaluate the performance of dental RBCs in recent years [9]. Results of the references confirm the linear relationship between the surface and depth hardness of the composite restorations and their DC [7-10]. If the bottom to top surface microhardness of dental RBCs is more than 80 %, the DC of their restoration is acceptable [5,9].

In the studies conducted, different DCs have been reported for bulk fill and universal RBCs. For example, Czasch et al. showed that Venus Diamond and Surefil SDR composites have an acceptable DC if they are irradiated for 20 s to a depth of 4 mm [11]. The study by Tarle et al. showed that restorations with a depth of 4 mm with Quix Phil and X-TRA Fil composites have an acceptable DC if they are irradiated for at least 30 s, [6]. These researchers reported that by reducing the irradiation time to 10 s, especially for restorations with a depth of 4 mm, the microhardness of the bottom surface is greatly reduced, although in this case there is no significant change in the microhardness of top surface.

According to the above mentioned points, it can be concluded that the type of composites has a significant effect on the researches results. Most of the studies done by researchers in the field of dental materials have focused on different curing conditions or depth of restoration layers on the DC of the dental RBCs separately. For this reason in this study, the effect of curing time and material thickness on the DC of two groups of universal and bulk fill RBCs were considered. In addition, there was an attempt to investigate the validity of higher DC of bulk fill RBCs at thicker restoration layers and less curing time than the similar universal types as a part of the null hypothesis of the present work. Furthermore, investigation of acceptable DC of Tetric N Ceram bulk fill RBCs up to a depth of 4 mm, higher than universal type, based on their manufacturers' claim is another aim of this study.

Materials and Methods

The materials evaluated in this in vitro study were

Table 1: Properties of the composites studied

Composite type	Tetric N-Ceram	Tetric N Ceram bulk fill
Manufacturer	Ivoclar Vivadent - Italy	Ivoclar Vivadent - Italy
LOT #	T24404	T29061
Matrix	Dimethacrylate	Dimethacrylate
Filler	Barium Glass, Ytterbium Trifluoride, Mixed Oxide and Copolymer	Barium Glass, Ytterbium, Trifluoride, Prepolymer and Mixed Oxide
Filler (volume %)	55-57	53-55
Filler (weight %)	80-81	75-77

two nanohybrid resin based composites (RBCs) including universal (Tetric N Ceram) and bulk fill (Tetric N Ceram Bulk Fill) with shade A3 (Table 1). A total of 96 samples were prepared and then equally divided into 12 groups (n = 8) including the two types of investigated resin based composites (bulk fill and universal), the three various sample height (2,4 and 6 mm) and finally the two applied curing times (20 and 40 seconds) in the present work. In other words, each of 12 groups of samples consisting of 8 specimens were made from one of the two used composite types with a height of 2 or 4 or 6 mm and curing time of 20 or 40 seconds.

Sample preparation
Preparation of the specimens was performed in cylindrical Teflon moulds with a diameter of 5 mm and height of 2, 4 and 6 mm. The moulds were first mounted on the top of a glass slab with the dimensions of $1 \times 76 \times 76$ mm and a Mylar strip (PD, Switzerland) and then the mould was filled in bulk with one of the two investigated universal and bulk fill composites. The upper surface of the mould was covered with a second Mylar strip and glass slab. A load of 500 g was applied on the top of glass slab for 30 seconds to ensure consistent packing of the samples and elimination of the extra composite materials.

Afterwards, the load and top slab were removed and the samples were light cured only from the upper surface using LED Demi light curing unit

(Demi- Kerr- USA) with an output intensity of 1000 mW/cm² for 20 or 40 seconds. The tip (circular with a diameter of 10 mm) of light curing unit was kept centered and in direct contact with the top Mylar strip. It should be noted that the power density of the light curing unit was checked after curing every 5 specimens using a radiometer (Demetron, Kerr-USA). After removing the top Mylar strip, the samples were pushed out of the mould and unpolymerized extra composites material of the top surface edge was deleted with a bistoury blade. Then the surface of all composite samples was polished in the presence of water using red, orange, yellow and white Sof Lex (3M ESPE- USA) polishing discs for 5 seconds, respectively. The top surfaces of the samples were identified with an indelible mark. Finally, the samples were rinsed with water and kept in distilled water for 24 hours at 37 ° C in the light proof incubator (Memmert IPP55plus, Germany) chamber.

Measurement of microhardness and the degree of cure
After removing the samples from distilled water, the microhardness of top and bottom surfaces of them was measured by Future Tech (Japan-Model FM 700) Vickers hardness (VHN) tester. To perform the test, six selective indentations (3 on both the top and bottom surfaces) were made with 50 g load and dwell time of 15 seconds using a pyramid shaped diamond indenter head tip. The

location of indentation points on the surface and depth of composite samples were selected so that they had at least 2 mm distance from the sample edges and each other. Then with adjusting the electronic microscope index on the surface of sample, the diameter of the square indentation area was determined by tester. Finally, the surface and depth Vickers microhardness of specimens' calculations were made using computer processor of tester device based on Eq. 1 and final displayed results on the Vickers tester screen were recorded for further statistical consideration. The three measurement microhardness values on the top and bottom were averaged to obtain a single value for surface and depth Vickers microhardness of each specimen.

$$VHN = (1.8544P) / D^2 \qquad (1)$$

In which, VHN represents Vickers hardness of material (Kg/mm²), P is the predetermined load applied on the sample (Kg) and D is the average diagonal distance (mm) of the square resulting from indentation of the pyramid tip of Vickers hardness tester. After determining the amount of top and bottom microhardness, the degree of cure (DC) of each sample was calculated according to Eq. 2.

$$Degree\ of\ Cure\,(\%) = \frac{bottom\ Microhardness}{top\ Microhardness} \times 100 \qquad (2)$$

Statistical analysis
Statistical analysis was performed with IBM package for the social sciences (SPSS Inc., IBM Corporation- New York, USA) Statistics Version 18 for Windows. Three-way analysis of variance (ANOVA) was applied to investigate the effect of various studied restorative RBCs materials, thickness and irradiation times on mean surface and depth microhardness and the DC of samples. The post-hoc Tukey's HSD (Honestly Significant Difference) test was used for pair-wise comparison between the means when ANOVA test is significant.

Also, independent *t*-test had been applied to compare between two types of investigated bulk fill and universal composites and their depth and surface microhardness. In addition, one-way ANOVA have been used to evaluate the influence of sample height and irradiation time on the mean

surface and depth microhardness and DC followed by Tukey's test was used for pair wise comparison between the means when ANOVA test is significant. The significance level of statistical analysis was set $p \leq 0.05$.

Results

The mean values of surface and depth microhardness (VHN) of the tested points and the calculated degree of cure (DC) for are displayed in Table 2.

ANOVA showed the significant effect ($p = 0.001$) of the samples' thickness on depth microhardness of universal Tetric N Ceram RBCs; however, based on *Tukey*'s test output, this effect was not significant ($p = 0.389$) in the thicknesses of 4 (31.67 ± 3.74 VHN)and 6 mm (30.24 ± 3.28 VHN). On the other hand, it's obvious from the ANOVA results that the influence of irradiation time was noticeable ($p = 0.002$) on the depth microhardness of the universal Tetric N Ceram RBC samples.

Based on the ANOVA results, in the investigated Tetric N Ceram bulk fill composite change of samples thickness between 2 (92.77 ± 13.2 VHN), 4 (77.75 ± 7.27 VHN) and 6 mm (68.33 ± 7.83 VHN) had a significant ($p = 0.001$) effect on their depth microhardness. The results of *Tukey*'s test also confirms that change of sample thickness between 2, 4 and 6 mm have significant effect on the depth microhardness of investigated bulk fill RBCs at ($p \leq 0.003$). Also, ANOVA results indicate that different irradiation times did not have a significant effect ($p = 0.121$) on depth microhardness of bulk fill samples although the effect of this factor on depth microhardness of bulk fill was higher than the surface microhardness ($p = 0.147$). In addition, it was observed from the ANOVA results that increasing the thickness of the samples and irradiation time had no significant ($p \geq 0.05$) effect on the surface microhardness of both studied universal and bulk fill RBCs.

According to the three-way ANOVA results, surface microhardness of the investigated universal and bulk fill composites was not significantly affected by the type of composite material ($p = 0.388$) and any change of RBC samples thickness ($p = 0.592$) while the effect of different curing time on the surface hardness of bulk fill sample compared with universal type was slightly

Table 2: Results of surface and depth microhardness and degree of cure of the studied composites.

Resin composite	MT (mm)	IT (sec)	N	MTH (Kg/mm²)	SD	MBH (Kg/mm²)	SD	DC (%)	SD
Universal (Tetric N Ceram)	2	20	8	44.51	2.54	33.98	1.91	76.52	5.36
		40	8	45.72	2.69	35.38	1.43	77.68	6.51
		Total	16	45.12	2.60	34.68	1.79	77.10	5.80
	4	20	8	44.42	2.40	29.97	3.48	67.91	10.44
		40	8	45.31	2.21	33.36	3.35	73.82	8.70
		Total	16	44.87	2.28	31.67	3.74	70.87	9.78
	6	20	8	44.71	2.44	28.16	2.19	63.07	4.81
		40	8	46.63	3.10	32.31	2.89	69.65	8.58
		Total	16	45.67	2.87	30.24	3.28	66.36	7.53
bulk fill (Tetric N Ceram Bulk Fill)	2	20	8	44.88	3.10	40.74	3.74	90.95	8.06
		40	8	46.03	6.81	42.63	3.09	94.58	17.35
		Total	16	45.46	5.15	41.69	3.46	92.77	13.20
	4	20	8	44.97	2.98	34.64	2.19	77.42	8.16
		40	8	46.25	1.40	36.04	2.33	78.08	6.80
		Total	16	45.61	2.35	35.35	2.30	77.76	7.27
	6	20	8	45.20	3.10	29.68	2.43	65.93	7.03
		40	8	47.38	2.75	33.37	3.07	70.71	8.28
		Total	16	46.29	3.05	31.53	3.29	68.33	7.83

MT= Material thickness, IT= Irradiation time, N= Number of samples, MTH= Mean top surface microhardness, SD=- Standard deviation , MBH= Mean bottom surface microhardness and DC= Degree of cure

meaningful ($p = 0.032$). Further, the results of three-way ANOVA and *Tukey*'s test were showed that variation of all investigated factors including composite type, thickness of samples and curing times had a significant ($p \leq 0.001$) effect on the depth microhardness of studied resin composites.

Statistical analysis of the results related to the DC of composite samples using the three-way ANOVA method showed the significant superiority ($p = 0.001$) of DC value of bulk fill samples over the universal type in similar depth and irradiation time. Also, in both composite materials, by increase of samples height, the DC value of the samples decreased significantly ($p = 0.001$) and

the value of this parameter for curing time of 40 seconds was slightly ($p = 0.040$) longer than 20 s. In addition, according to the three-way ANOVA results, the effect of irradiation time on the DC of two composites studied in the same thickness did not show a considerable significance ($p = 0.676$). Further, it's clear from the three- way ANOVA results that the influence of variation of sample thickness on the DC of investigated composites with the same curing time is also considerable ($p = 0.010$) .

Discussion

Bulk fill RBCs are materials that, according to the

manufacturers' claim, can be cured in thicknesses of 4 or even 5 mm at one stage [9]. Validity of this claim was performed by investigating the effect of irradiation times and different thicknesses on the performance of Tetric N Ceram bulk fill RBCs based on the DC in this study. Furthermore, the results were compared with similar Tetric N Ceram universal RBC. On the other hand, comparison of the performance of the two composites under the study in similar depths and irradiation times showed the significant superiority of DC in bulk fill type over universal types in different thicknesses of 2, 4 and 6 mm.

The ratio microhardness of bottom to top surface as a common criterion for evaluating the DC of the dental RBC restoration [10,12,13] is used in this study. According to the possibility of increasing the DC of composite samples in a time interval after the curing process [14-18] as well as increasing their degree of polymerization by increasing the temperature of storage room [19], in this study all tests were performed 24 hours after curing the samples and keeping them in light proof incubator space at mouth temperature (37 °C).

The present results show that universal samples at 2 mm depth and bulk fill samples at 2 and 4 mm depths had an acceptable DC based on 80% microhardness drop-off hypothesis from top to bottom surface of specimens. This is in agreement with comparable studies [5,7,8,11] that showed different bulk fill materials had higher depth of cure than the common universal composites.

Many factors such as the size and composition of the filler, material translucency and intensity of LED, curing time, monomer composition and concentration of photo initiator can have considerable effects on the DC of dental RBCs [17]. Increase of filler content and also application of irregularly shaped filler in composites composition can lead to increased contact area of the resin and filler and reduce the amount of light transmittance through the RBCs [20]. Light transmission also reduces in composites with large sized filler (0.05-2μm) [18]. On the other hand, one of the best ways to enhance the DC of RBCs might be to increase the materials translucency by matching the refractive indices of fillers and matrix. Differences in the refractive indices of filler and the composite matrix may increase light scattering, which consequently

reduces the DC of the composite restorations [17].

The present study shows that the DC of Tetric N Ceram bulk fill RBC is more than universal Tetric N Ceram type. Considering the properties of studied RBCs (Table 1), it is clear that despite the similarity in shape and size of fillers, the higher translucency due to using different filler chemical composition [8] and lower filler content of bulk fill material (75-77 wt%, 53-55 vol%) compared with universal type (80-81 wt% , 55-57 vol%) can be some factors affecting present results. Several researches [3,7,21] such as Moszner et al. [20] and Bucuta et al. [8] have been done to evaluate the effects of amount and size of filler and the materials translucency on the DC of bulk fill and universal RBCs that their findings support the results of this work.

The chemical composition of the filler and matrix can have significant effects on the DC of RBCs. In the filler combination of Tetric N Ceram bulk fill composite prepolymerized fillers (PPF) containing barium glass and silica minerals is used. Based on other studies [7,8,11,21], due to the application of PPF, RBCs like Tetric N Ceram bulk fill are able to achieve a high filler load while maintaining a low specific surface between inorganic fillers and organic matrix, as a part of PPF is actually organic. Today, new types of photoinitiator such as Ivocerin and Benzoyl Germaniumare are used in the composition of PPF of bulk fill RBCs instead of the common type such as Camphorquinone (CQ) [22-24]. The higher capability of these materials in creation of free radicals per molecule unit can improve the light sensitivity of RBCs [25-28]. These changes have a positive effect on the light absorbance ability and DC of RBCs.

The manufacturers' instruction of placing the Tetric N Ceram bulk fill and Tetric N Ceram universal RBCs up to 4 mm and 2 mm bulks respectively and light curing for 10 s without a loss in acceptable DC seems to be of great interest for clinicians. Results of present study recommend an increase of the curing time from 20 to 40 s in clinical condition due to its marginally significant effects on the DC of both investigated RBCs. Also, present results indicate that in both investigated bulk fill and universal RBCs, the value of DC significantly decrease with any increasing of the sample thickness. Effects of material thickness and curing time on the performance of RBCs have been investigated in many research works [5,8,11,13,29-31]. Some others studied the effect of material thickness on the DC of various bulk fill RBCs for curing time of 20 s [5,8,30]. Their results show that in some types of bulk fill RBCs such as SDR the DC remains acceptable with increasing the material thickness only up to 4 mm in agreement with present results while some other bulk fill RBCs such as X-Tra, Venus and Tetric Evoceram can have reasonable depth of cure up to 6 or 8 mm in contrast to this study.

It seems that different results of many studies conducted on the microhardness of bulk fill and universal RBCs can be related to various factors such as material composition, time interval passing from samples preparation and performing tests, type of moulds, type and temperature of storage room and test design [32]. In general, evaluating the microhardness of the RBCs at 1 mm depth in addition to present investigated thickness of 2, 4 and 6 mm for different curing time of 10 and 30 s can provide a more comprehensive study.

Conclusions

Within the limitations of present in vitro study, it can be stated that the DC of Tetric N Ceram bulk fill RBCs is higher than similar universal type for all values of curing time and material thickness. Also, the producer recommended irradiation time of 20 s and appropriate curing depth up to 4 and 2 mm is sufficient for investigated bulk fill and universal RBCs, respectively. According to the marginally significant effect of the curing time on the DC of both Tetric N Ceram composite samples, increasing the irradiation time from 20 to 40 s in clinical condition is suggested.

Conflict of Interest: None declared.

References

1. Heymann HD, Swift EJ, Ritter AV. Sturtevant's art and science of operative dentistry. 6th Edition. St. Louis: Mosby:2013.
2. Furness A, Tadros MY, Looney SW, et al. Effect of bulk/incremental fill on internal gap formation of bulk-fill composites. J Dent. 2014;42:439-449.
3. Roggendorf MJ, Kramer N, Appelt A, et al. Marginal quality of flowable 4-mm base vs. conventionally layered resin composite. J Dent. 2011;39:643-647.
4. Ferracane JL. Resin composite-state of the art. Dent Mater. 2011;27:29-38.
5. Flury S, Hayoz S, Peutzfeldt A, et al. Depth of cure of resin composites: are the ISO 4049 method suitable for bulk fill materials. Dent Mater. 2012;28:521-528.
6. Tarle Z, Attin T, Marovic D, et al. Influence of irradiation time on subsurface degree of conversion and microhardness of high-viscosity bulk-fill composites. Clin Oral Investig. 2015;19:831-840.
7. Ilie N, Bucuta S, Draenert M. Bulk fill resin based composites: an in vitro assessment of their mechanical performance. Oper Dent. 2013;38:618-625.
8. Bucuta S, Ilie N. Light transmittance and micro-mechanical properties of bulk fill vs. conventional resin based composites. Clin Oral Investig. 2014;18:1991-2000.
9. Agrawal A, Manwar NU, Hegde S, et al. Comparative evaluation of surface hardness and depth of cure of silorane and methacrylate-based posterior composite resins: An in vitro study. J Conserv Dent. 2015;18:136-139.
10. Ilie N, Stark K. Effect of different curing protocols on the mechanical properties of low-viscosity bulk fill composites. Clin Oral Investig. 2015;19:271-279.
11. Czasch P, Ilie N. In vitro comparison of mechanical properties and degree of cure of bulk fill composites. Clin Oral Investig. 2013;17:227-235.
12. Bouschlicher MR, Rueggeberg FA, Wilson BM. Correlation of bottom to top surface microhardness and conversion ratios for a variety of resin composite compositions. Oper Dent. 2004;29:698-704.
13. Ilie N, Stark K. Curing behaviour of high-viscosity bulk-fill composites. J Dent. 2014;42: 977-985.
14. Truffier-Boutry D, Demoustier-Champagne S, Devaux J, et al. Physico-chemical explanation of the post-polymerization shrinkage in dental

resins. Dent Mater. 2006;22: 405-412.

15. Stansbury JW. Dimethacrylate network formation and polymer property evolution as determined by the selection of monomers and curing conditions. Dent Mater. 2012;28:13-22.

16. Skrtic D, Antonucci JM. Effect of chemical structure and composition of the resin phase on vinyl conversion of amorphous calcium phosphate-filled composites. Polym Int. 2007;56:497-505.

17. Johnston WM, Leung RL, Fan PL. A mathematical model for post-irradiation hardening of photo activated composite resins. Dent Mater. 1985;1:191-194.

18. Yearn JA. Factors affecting cure of visible light activated composites. Int Dent J. 1985;35: 218-225.

19. Price RB, Whalen JM, Price TB, et al. The effect of specimen temperature on the polymerization of a resin-composite. Dent Mater. 2011;27:983-989.

20. Moszner N, Fischer UK, Ganster B, et al. Benzoyl germanium derivatives as novel visible light photo initiators for dental materials. Dent Mater. 2008;24:901-907.

21. Arikawa H, Kanie T, Fujii K, et al. Effect of filler properties in composite resins on light transmittance characteristics and color. Dent Mater J. 2007;26:38-44.

22. Neshchadin D, Rosspeintner A, Griesser M, et al. Acylgermanes: photoinitiators and sources for Ge-centered radicals. Insights into their reactivity. J Am Chem Soc. 2013;135:17314-17321.

23. Neumann MG, Schmitt CC, Ferreira GC, et al. The initiating radical yields and the efficiency of polymerization for various dental photo initiators excited by different light curing units. Dent Mater. 2006;22:576-584.

24. Rueggeberg FA. State of the art: Dental photo curing - a review. Dent Mater. 2011;27:39-52.

25. Leloup G, Holvoet PE, Bebelman S, et al. Raman scattering determination of the depth of cure of light-activated composites: influence of different clinically relevant parameters. J Oral Rehabil. 2002;29:510-515.

26. Jakubiak J, Allonas X, Fouassier JP, et al. Camphorquinone amines photo initiating systems for the initiation of free radical polymerization. Polymer. 2003;44:5219-5226.

27. Leprince JG, Hadis M, Shortall AC, et al. Photoinitiator type and applicability of exposure reciprocity law in filled photoactive resins. Dent Mater. 2011;27:157-164.

28. Ogunyinka A, Palin WM, Shortall AC, et al. Photo initiation chemistry affects light transmission and degree of conversion of curing experimental dental resin composites. Dent Mater. 2007;23:807-813.

29. Decker C. Kinetic study and new applications of UV radiation curing. Macromol Rapid Commun. 2003;23:1067-1093.

30. Finan L, Palin WM, Moskwa N, et al. The influence of irradiation potential on the degree of conversion and mechanical properties of two bulk-fill flowable RBC base materials. Dent Mater. 2013;29:906-912.

31. Flury S, Peutzfeldt A, Lussi A. Influence of increment thickness on microhardness and dentin bond strength of bulk fill resin composites. Dent Mater. 2014;30:1104-1112.

32. Bhamra GS, Fleming GJP, Darvell BW. Influence of LED irradiance on flexural properties and Vickers hardness of resin-based composite materials. Dent Mater. 2010;26:148-155.

18

Antimicrobial Effect of Copper Oxide Nanoparticles on some Oral Bacteria and Candida Species

Amiri M[a], Etemadifar Z[b], Daneshkazemi A[a], Nateghi M[c*]

[a]Department of Operative Dentistry, Shahid Sadoughi University of Medical Sciences and Health Services, Yazd, Iran
[b]Department of Biology, University of Isfahan, Isfahan, Iran
[c]School of Dentistry, Shahid Sadoughi University of Medical Sciences and Health Services, Yazd, Iran

---

ARTICLE INFO

Key words:
Nanoparticle
Oral Streptococcus
Lactobacillus
Yeast
Dental Caries

Corresponding Author:
Mehrnoosh Nateghi
School of Dentistry, Shahid Sadoughi University of Medical Sciences and Health Services, Yazd, Iran.
Email: mehrnoosh.nateghi@yahoo.com

Abstract

Statement of Problem: Acid producing bacteria including Streptococcus mutans and lactobacilli cause tooth demineralization and lead to tooth decay. Also, oral colonization of the species of Candida has been reported in many studies that are resistant to antifungal agents.

Objectives: In this study, antibacterial and antifungal effects of nano-CuO were studied against some oral bacteria and yeast fungi.

Materials and Methods: The minimum inhibitory concentrations (MICs) of copper oxide nanoparticles (CuO NPs) for oral bacterial and fungal test strains were determined in 96-well microtiter plate technique. The agar diffusion test (ADT) was employed to assess the antifungal properties of nystatin.

Results: The MIC_{50} value of CuO NPs was determined at the range of 1–10 µg/ml for *S.* mutans, < 1 µg/ml for L. acidophilus, and 10 µg/ml for L. casei. Higher concentrations of CuO NPs (100-1000 µg/ml) were effective on the bacterial cell growth, resulting in 100% reduction in the optical density in TSB medium. The cells of Candida albicans, C. krusei and C. glabrata were treated with CuO NPs and the results showed a decrease in fungal growth at a concentration of 1-1000 µg/ml in TSB medium. The MIC_{50} value of CuO NPs was determined 1000 µg/ml for three species of Candida. The diameter of growth inhibition zones of 1100 µg/ml nystatin was obtained 15-21 mm for clinical isolates of three species of Candida.

Conclusions: With respect to the potential bactericidal activity of CuO NPs on various cariogenic bacteria examined in this study, these NPs could be introduce as a candidate control agent for preventing dental caries or dental infections. In our study, on the other hand, Nano copper oxide had a weak effect on the candida species.

Introduction

Antibiotic treatment of oral biofilms is inadequate, often leading to chronic oral infections and constrained tooth extraction or implant removal due to the development of antibiotic resistance [1,2]. Oral biofilms comprise a complex polymicrobial community in which oral streptococci are initial colonizers [3].

Tooth demineralization caused by acid producing bacteria including Streptococcus mutans, S. sobrinus, and Lactobacillus species, which can ferment dietary carbohydrates, leads to dental decay [4-6]. The bacterial gelatinous material adheres to tooth surfaces and becomes colonized by bacteria to form dental plaque. Several factors including dietary carbohydrates, cariogenic bacteria, and many host factors such as teeth and saliva result in tooth decay over time [4,5].

The most common etiological agent of candidiasis in compromised patients is known as Candida albicans. This organism can produce biofilm on the oral mucosa. The exopolymeric substance matrix surrounding the cells of Candida protects the yeast cells against harsh conditions and the antifungal antibiotics [7].

The use of nanoparticles, as new agents for inhibition of microbial growth, has developed due to the development of antibiotic resistance [8-10]. The particle with 1-100 nm size that behaves as a whole unit with respect to transport and properties is called nanoparticle [11-13]. These particles which have much higher surface area than conventional materials are currently considered as antimicrobial agents [8]. Among these nano-materials, nano-metals have been used more because of less toxicity [7,14].

The silver NPs were studied in most related research, exhibiting antibacterial effect at low concentrations [8,10,15].

Ionic nanopariculate metal oxides are among the potentially interesting antimicrobial agents, because of their extremely high surface areas and having unusual crystalline structures with high number of edges and corners and other reactive sites [16]. Copper oxide nanoparticle (CuO NP) is the simplest member of the Cu compounds that reveal a range of potential physical properties and is much cheaper than silver oxide. It can be mixed easily with polymers to provide the composites with unique physio-chemical properties. Also, these nanoparticles have high surface areas and unusual crystalline structures to give CuO NPs with antimicrobial activity that is dose dependent [17].

Metals NPs and other NPs are being combined with polymers (such as: dental composite) or coated onto surfaces which acquired the potential applications within the oral cavity [10,18].

In this study, the antimicrobial activity of CuO NPs against Streptococcus mutans, Lactobacillus acidophilus, L. casei and three species of oral Candida including C. albicans, C. krusei, and C. glabrata were investigated.

Materials and Methods

Preparation of microbial inoculums

Bacterial inoculums were prepared from cultured Streptococcus mutans (PTCC 1683), Lactobacillus casei (PTCC 1608), and L. acidophilus (PTCC 1643) on Tryptic Soy Agar (TSA) (236950 - BD Difco™) medium incubated at 37°C for 48 hours. The bacteria were transferred to Tryptic Soy Broth (TSB) (211825 - BD Difco™) media and incubated at 37 °C overnight. One ml from each overnight broth culture was inoculated to 10 ml broth medium and incubated at 37 °C on a rotary shaker with 180 rpm shaking until optical density adjusted to 0.5 McFarland standard.

Yeasts inoculums equivalent to 0.5 McFarland standard were prepared for antifungal assay of nystatin and CuO-NPs as explained for bacteria.

Preparation of nano-copper oxide solution

For preparation of stock nano-solution, 1 mg CuO NPs was dissolved in 1 ml sterilized double distilled water and kept in Ultrasonic Sonicator bath for 30 min.

MIC of nano-copper oxide

The minimum inhibitory concentrations (MICs) of CuO NPs for oral bacterial and fungal test strains were determined in 96-well microtiter plate technique as described by Padil and Cernik [19]. TSB medium was used for resistance experiments.

MIC values were detected by various concentrations of CuO NPs in the range of 1 µg/ml to 1000 µg/ml. As the first step, 50 µl aliquot of 0.5 McFarland microbial suspension was inoculated to the wells of microtiter plate; then, 50 µl of TSB supplemented with the considered concentrations of CuO NPs was added. The TSB medium without CuO NPs inoculated with the bacterium and TSB medium supplemented with CuO NPs without any bacterium were used as proper controls for these experiments. After incubation at 37

°C for 48 hours, the microtiter plates were scanned with an ELISA reader (Stat Fax -2100, Portland, ME, USA) at 600nm. All experiments were carried out in triplicates with proper blank.

Inhibition effect of nystatin
In this study, the inhibition effect of nystatin was experimented by agar diffusion test (ADT) method using the nystatin concentrations with a range of 0-1100 μg/ml dissolved in di-methyl sulfoxide (DMSO) as antifungal antibiotic for comparison by the CuO NPs. The inhibition zone diameter was measured after 48 hours of incubation at 37 °C.

CuO NPs with a size of 40 nm and purity of 98% were purchased from Nano Avijeh (Nanosav) Co.

Statistical Analysis
Data were analyzed by Excel 2013. All experiments were performed as triplicates. The means of data and standard deviations were analyzed by Excel.

Results

Growth inhibition of Bacteria by nano copper oxide in microtiter plate
Treatment of three oral bacteria including Streptococcus mutans, L. casei and L. acidophilus with CuO NPs resulted in a decrease in bacterial growth in the TSB medium (Figure 1). The MIC_{50} value of CuO NPs was determined at the range of 1–10 μg/ml for S. mutans, < 1 μg/ml for L. acidophilus, and 10μg/ml for L. casei (Figure 1). Higher concentrations of CuO

NPs (100-1000 μg/ml) were effective on the bacterial cell growth, resulting in 100% reduction of the optical density in TSB medium (Figure 1).

Inhibition of the growth of oral pathogen candida species by nano-copper oxide in microtiter plate
The cells of Candida albicans, C. krusei and C. glabrata were treated with CuO NPs, and the results showed a decrease in fungal growth at a concentration of 1-1000 μg/ml in TSB medium (Figure 2). The MIC_{50} value of CuO NPs was determined 1000 μg/ml for three species of Candida (Figure 2). In lower concentrations of CuO NPs (1-100 μg/ml), the yeast cells growth was slightly inhibited (almost 30-40% decrease) (Figure 2).

Diameter of growth inhibition zones of 1100 μg/ml nystatin was obtained from 15 mm till 21 mm for clinical isolates of the three species of Candida (Table 1). All the Candida species showed resistance to the concentrations of 0-55 μg/ml nystatin.

Discussion

The inhibition of oral bacteria, S. mutans and Actinomyces viscosus, with ZnO by concentrations of 78 - 312.5 μg/ml was reported by Hall-Stoodley et al. [20]. Also, EC50 value of CuO NPs was obtained as 78 μg/ml for Vibrio fischeri in their study. Khan et al. showed that CuO NPs in the concentration of 50 μg/ml had a higher biocide activity against growth and biofilm formation of oral microbiota than ZnO NPs [3]. Low concentrations (0.0001-1 μg/ml) of CuO

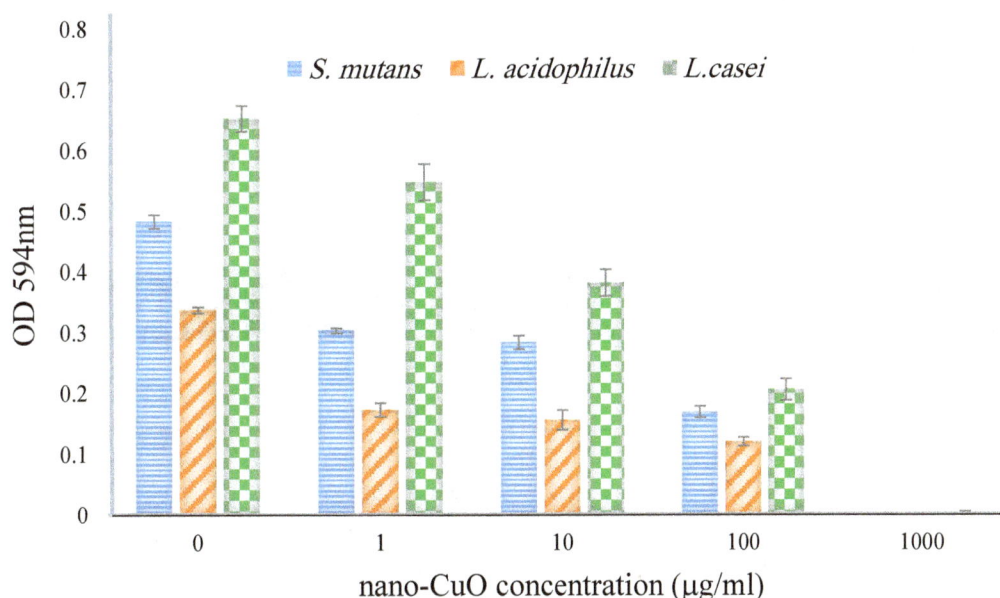

Figure 1: Effect of CuO NPs on the growth of oral bacteria: Streptococcus mutans, Lactobacillus casei, and L. acidophilus by microtiter plate technique in TSB medium incubated at 37 °C for 48 hours.

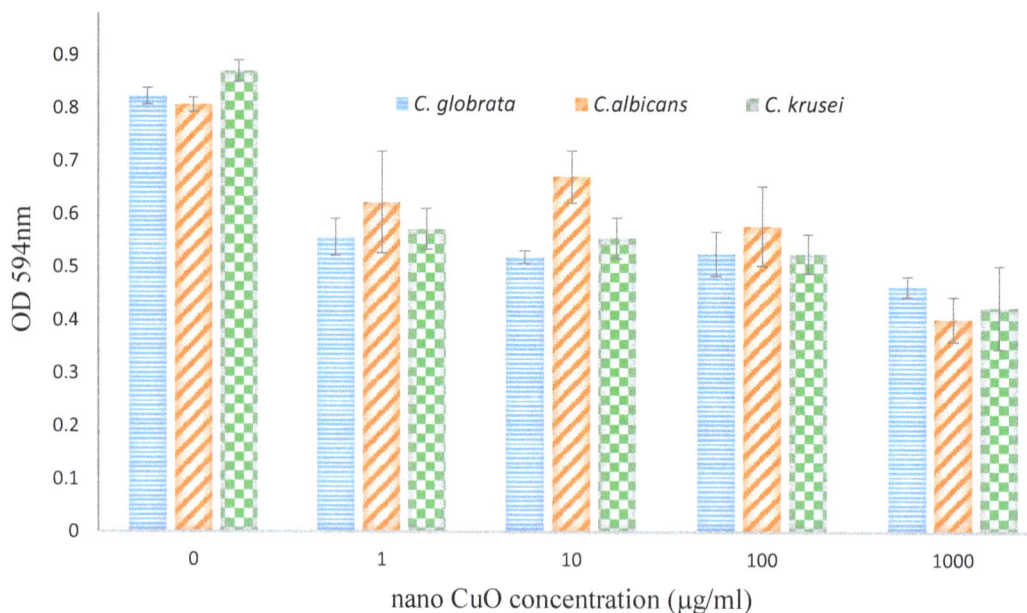

Figure 2: Antifungal activity of CuO NPs against Candida albicans, C. krusei, and C. glabrata by microtiter plate technique in TSB medium incubated at 37 °C for 48 hours.

NPs with 18-20 nm sizes were used by Eshed et al. for inhibition of Streptococcus mutans. The results showed that the growth was not inhibited, but biofilm formation was prevented in these low concentrations of CuO NPs [9].

The mechanism of antibacterial activity of nano-metal oxide is the production of different active oxygen species, like H_2O_2, which inhibit the growth of bacterial cells [21].

Alaker et al. showed that CuO NPs in a concentration of 100-5000 µg/ml had no toxic effect on human cells [8]. The micro- and nano-copper oxide up to 50 µg/ml showed no genotoxic and cytotoxic effects on Hella cells [22]. Thus, with respect to the potential bactericidal activity of CuO NPs on various oral bacteria examined in this study and also previous studies and no toxic effect on human cells, this NP could be introduce as a control agent for preventing dental caries or dental infections.

Most frequently isolated organisms from the oral cavity are from Candida species which are detected in 31-55% of healthy population [23]. The major yeast implicated in the esophagitis is C. albicans. C. glabrata or any other Candida species were rarely detected as infectious agents in these patients. Also, oral colonization of C. krusei and C. glabrata with antifungal resistance in vitro is described in compromised patients [23].

MIC_{50} value of Nano-CuO for Candida albicans was obtained 400 µg/ml by Karimiyan et al. [24]. The shape and size of nanoparticles can influence their antimicrobial activity [25], which led to different results in these experiments.

The antifungal activity of nystatin was studied on Candida albicans in previous studies. In one of them, the bioactivity of 30 µg/ml nystatin was obtained 18-24 mm in agar well diffusion test [26]. In another study, nystatin showed antifungal effectiveness against C. albicans, and MIC_{50} equal to 25 µg/ml was obtained. MIC50 standard of nystatin for sensitive Candida species is 4-7 µg/ml; thus, the experimented strains of candida in this study were resistant to

Table 1: Mean values and standard deviation (SD) of inhibition effect of nystatin on three species of *Candida* by well diffusion technique on Potato Dextrose Agar (PDA) medium after 48 hours of incubation at 37 °C.

Nystatin (µg/ml)	Inhibition zone (mm) ± SD		
	C. albicans	*C. glabrata*	*C. krusei*
0	0.0 ± 0.00	0.0 ± 0.00	0.0 ± 0.00
11	0.0 ± 0.00	0.0 ± 0.00	0.0 ± 0.00
55	10.5 ± 0.58	11.5 ± 0.58	0.0 ± 0.00
110	13 ± 1.15	14.5 ± 0.58	11 ± 1.15
550	18 ± 0.00	19 ± 1.15	13.5 ± 0.58
1100	21 ± 1.15	20.5 ± 0.58	15.5 ± 0.58

nystatin. In comparison with the inhibition effect of CuO NPs, the yeast strains showed resistance to nystatin.

The wide and indiscriminate use of antibiotics and different sensitivity of clinical strains of Candida toward the antifungal agents cause different values of drug inhibitory doses [27]. The results of this study showed that the examined yeast strains had considerable resistance to nystatin compared to those strains used by Khoshkholgh-Pahlaviani et al. [26]. Also, Amirrajab et al. showed high resistance of C. glabrata to some of antifungal antibiotics, such as amphotericin B (the MIC_{50} equal 1100 µg/ml) [28]. In our study, on the other hand, the growth of these strains decreased when treated by 1-1000 µg/ml of nano- copper oxide, and MIC_{50} was seen at a concentration of 1000 µg/ml of nanoparticles.

Compared to organic antibacterial agents such as antibiotics, inorganic substances with antimicrobial activity may have several advantages such as low possibility of resistance, and susceptibility of a broad range of microorganisms to these nano-materials.

Conclusions

Nano-copper oxide used in this study showed a high antimicrobial effect against the examined dental caries bacterial agents, and lower effect on three species of candida. Thus, this NP could be introduced as a candidate control agent for preventing dental caries or dental infections.

Conflict of Interest: None declared.

References

1. Martinez A, Guitián F, López-Píriz R, et al. Bone loss at implant with titanium abutments coated by soda lime glass containing silver nanoparticles: a histological study in the dog. PloS one. 2014;9: e86926.
2. Zitzmann NU, Berglundh T. Definition and prevalence of peri-implant diseases. J Clin Periodontol. 2008;35:286-291.
3. Khan ST, Ahamed M, Al-Khedhairy A, et al. Biocidal effect of copper and zinc oxide nanoparticles on human oral microbiome and biofilm formation. Mater Lett. 2013;97:67-70.
4. Agarwal R, Singh C, Yeluri R, et al. Prevention of Dental Caries-Measures beyond Fluoride. J Oral Hyg Health. 2014;2:1-6.
5. Selwitz RH, Ismail AI, Pitts NB. Dental caries. Lancet. 2007;369:51-59.
6. Hardie JM. Oral microbiology: current concepts in the microbiology of dental caries and periodontal disease. Br Dent J. 1992;172:271-278.
7. Lara HH, Romero-Urbina DG, Pierce C, et al. Effect of silver nanoparticles on Candida albicans biofilms: an ultrastructural study. J Nanobiotechnology. 2015;13:91.
8. Allaker RP. The use of nanoparticles to control oral biofilm formation. J Dent Res. 2010;89:1175-1186.
9. Eshed M, Lellouche J, Matalon S, et al. Sonochemical coatings of ZnO and CuO nanoparticlesinhibit Streptococcus mutans biofilm formation on teeth model. Langmuir. 2012;28:12288-12295.
10. Monteiro DR, Gorup LF, Takamiya AS, et al. The growing importance of materials that prevent microbial adhesion: antimicrobial effect of medical devices containing silver. Int J Antimicrob Agents. 2009;34:103-110.
11. Borzabadi-Farahani A, Borzabadi E, Lynch E. Nanoparticles in orthodontics, a review of antimicrobial and anti-caries applications. Acta Odontol Scand. 2014;72:413-417.
12. Weir E, Lawlor A, Whelan A, et al. The use of nanoparticles in anti-microbial materials and their characterization. Analyst. 2008;133:835-845.
13. Cushing BL, Kolesnichenko VL, O'Connor CJ. Recent advances in the liquid-phase syntheses of inorganic nanoparticles. Chem Rev. 2004;104:3893-3946.
14. Cioffi N, Rai M. Nano-antimicrobials: progress and prospects. 1st Edition. Springer Berlin Heidelberg: Berlin, Germany; 2012.
15. Cronholm P, Karlsson HL, Hedberg J, et al. Intracellular uptake and toxicity of Ag and CuO nanoparticles: a comparison between nanoparticles and their corresponding metal ions. Small. 2013;9:970-982.
16. Stoimenov PK, Klinger RL, Marchin GL, et al. Metal oxide nanoparticles as bactericidal agents. Langmuir. 2002;18:6679-6686.
17. Chang YN, Zhang M, Xia L, et al. The toxic effects and mechanisms of CuO and ZnO nanoparticles. Materials. 2012;5:2850-2871.
18. Hannig M, Kriener L, Hoth-Hannig W, et al. Influence of nanocomposite surface coating on biofilm formation in situ. J Nanosci Nanotech-

nol. 2007;7:4642-4648.

19. Padil VV, Černík M. Green synthesis of copper oxide nanoparticles using gum karaya as a biotemplate and their antibacterial application. Int J Nanomedicine. 2013;8:889-898.

20. Hall-Stoodley L, Costerton JW, Stoodley P. Bacterial biofilms: from the natural environment to infectious diseases. Nature Rev Microbiol. 2004;2:95-108.

21. Tavassoli Hojati S, Alaghemand H, Hamze F, et al. Antibacterial, physical and mechanical properties of flowable resin composites containing zinc oxide nanoparticles. Dent Mater. 2013;29:495-505.

22. Semisch A, Ohle J, Witt B, et al. Cytotoxicity and genotoxicity of nano-and microparticulate copper oxide: role of solubility and intracellular bioavailability. Part Fibre Toxicol. 2014;11:10.

23. Fidel PL Jr, Vazquez JA, Sobel JD. Candida glabrata: Review of epidemiology, pathogenesis, and clinical disease with comparison to C. albicans. Clin Microbiol Rev. 1999;12:80-96.

24. Karimiyan A, Najafzadeh H, Ghorbanpour M, et al. Antifungal effect of magnesium oxide, zinc oxide, silicon oxide and copper oxide nanoparticles against Candida albicans. Zahedan J Res Med Sci. 2015;17:29-31.

25. Khan MF, Hameedullah M, Ansari AH, et al. Flower-shaped ZnO nanoparticles synthesized by a novel approach at near-room temperatures with antibacterial and antifungal properties. Int J Nanomedicine. 2014;9:853-864.

26. Khoshkholgh-Pahlaviani MRM, Massiha AR, Issazadeh K, et al. Evaluation of antifungal activity of methanol extract of Acacia (Anagalisarvensis) leaves and nystatin against Candida albicans in vitro. Zahedan J Res Med Sci.2013;15:39-41.

27. AlSaidy HAM. Diagnosis of some types of yeasts associated with the human body and treated in the Garlic and Colocynthis extracts. Eur J Agric For Res. 2015;3:1-14.

28. Amirrajab N, Badali H, Didehdar M, et al. In vitro activities of six antifungal drugs against Candida glabrataisolates: An emerging pathogen. Jundishapur J Microbiol. 2016;9:e36638.

19

The Influence of Surface Polish and Beverages on the Roughness of Nanohybrid and Microhybrid Resin Composites

Sadeghi M[a], Deljoo Z[a], Bagheri R[b]

[a]Undergraduate Student, Shiraz Dental School, Shiraz University of Medical Sciences, Shiraz, Iran
[b]Dental Materials Department and Biomaterials Research Centre, Shiraz Dental School, Shiraz University of Medical Sciences, Shiraz, Iran

ARTICLE INFO

Key words:
Surface Roughness
Nanohybrid Composite
Microhtbrid Composite
Staining Solutions

Corresponding Author:
Rafat Bagheri,
Dental Materials Department
and Biomaterials Research
Centre, Shiraz Dental School,
Shiraz University of Medical
Sciences, Shiraz, Iran

Email: bagherir@yahoo.com

Abstract

Statement of the Problem: Surface roughness is a key factor in the aesthetics of restorative dentistry as it can determine the clinical quality and success of restorative materials. The chemical process of dissolution in the presence of mechanical forces can accelerate the surface roughness of tooth-coloured restorative materials.

Objectives: To determine the degree of surface roughness of a microhybrid and a nanohybrid resin composite after polishing and immersion in various solutions.

Materials and Methods: Two resin composites were used : a microhybrid (Gradia direct, GC), and a nanohybrid (Ice, SDI). A total of 54 disc-shaped specimens were prepared for each composite and immersed in distilled water incubated at 37 °C for 24 hours. After 24 h, the baseline measurement for surface roughness (Ra) was performed and the specimens were divided into 3 groups of 18 and tested with unpolished or after polishing with Sof-Lex disc and Enhance point systems. Specimens in each group were subdivided into 3 subgroups (n = 6) and immersed in 3 solutions (distilled water, coffee, and cola) for 7 days incubated at 37 °C. After 7 days, the specimens were rinsed with tap water for 10 seconds, dried with paper towel and Ra was measured again. Two randomly selected specimens of each group were sputter coated with gold and examined using a Field-Emission Scanning Electron Microscope (SEM).

Results: Gradia direct showed a greater R_a than ice in all solutions for all polishing systems ($p < 0.001$). Specimens polished with Enhance point revealed a significantly greater roughness than Sof-Lex discs and both showed greater R_a than unpolished specimens. Specimens immersed in coffee exhibited significantly greater surface roughness than that of distilled water ($p < 0.05$) and cola ($p < 0.001$).

Conclusions: Nano-hybrid composite showed a significantly smoother surface than microhybrid. Coffee exhibited the highest R_a compared to distilled water and cola. Enhance point revealed significantly greater R_a than Sof-Lex discs and unpolished group.

Introduction

One of the main advantages of resin composite is its gloss surface that is associated with its surface properties such as polishability. Due to its excellent aesthetic and surface characteristics, dental composite is frequently requested by patients even for restoration of the posterior teeth. Resin composites have grown fast since 50 years ago when the materials were first introduced to the market [1]. The most significant changes in the formulation of resin composites over the time are reduction of the filler particle sizes and increase in filler loading [2]. To achieve a better surface smoothness and optical properties nanofill and nanohybrid composites are introduced to the dental market [3,4].

Microfill resin composites with particles ranging from 0.02 to 0.04 μm represent excellent surface smoothness but they suffer functional durability due to having approximately 50 vol% resin matrix [5]. The combination of particles and nanoclusters reduces the interstitial spaces between the inorganic particles at the same time giving a possibility to have the maximum filler loading, thus providing better functional properties and polish maintenance [6].

On the other hand, discoloration of resin composite still remains a major disadvantage of the restorations. A survey of published studies showed that the highly polished and smooth surface restorations compared to rough surfaces have better aesthetics and less susceptibility to plaque accumulation and extrinsic discoloration [7].

The effect of polishing systems on the surface roughness of different types of resin composites has been reported. Some studies [8-10] that used polishing discs, wheels, and glaze materials indicated that the average roughness value of hybrid resin composites was the highest compared to microhybrid or nanohybrid resin composites [8-10]. It has been reported that after polishing procedures, nano-hybrids showed a similar or slightly lower roughness than micro-hybrids [11]. Although the smoothest surface is obtained when the resin composite polymerizes against a Mylar strip without further finishing or polishing [12,13], most restorations require finishing and polishing for final marginal adjustment. Moreover, the top surface polymerized against Mylar strip is a resin rich layer with low mechanical properties that require a proper polishing to not only increase the

wear resistance of the materials but also provide the smoothest possible surface [14,15].

It is reported that among different polishing systems, multi-step aluminum-oxide discs (Sof-Lex discs) exhibited the smoothest surface [9,16,17]. Antonson *et al.* [16] in their study evaluating the effect of polishing systems on different resin composites found that the baseline surface roughness (unpolished) of nanohybrid and hybrid differed significantly from each other whereas postoperatively there were no significance differences. The Sof-Lex discs provided the smoothest surface and microhybrid polished by Sof-Lex revealed lower gloss than the nanohybrid composite.

Although some studies have been conducted to assess the surface roughness of resin composites, the effect of different polishing systems exposed to common used beverages on the surface roughness of the microhybrid and nanohybrid resin composites are not widely studied. Therefore, this study aimed to assess the combined effect of mechanical and chemical factors on the surface property of resin composites. In this study, 3 polishing and finishing systems (Mylar strip, Sof-Lex disc and Enhance point systems) and 3 common drinks (distilled water, cola and coffee) were used to evaluate the effect of the combination of those on the surface roughness of nanohybrid and microhybrid resin composites. This study used profilometer to measure the surface roughness (R_a) and scanning electron microscope (SEM) to observe the surface roughness generated by all factors.

Materials and Methods

Specimen preparation

Two resin composites of shade A2 (Table 1), three polishing methods and three solutions were used in this study. A total of 108 disc-shaped specimens (54 for each composite) were prepared using a polyethylene mould of 10 mm diameter and 2 mm thickness. Resin composite was gently packed into the mould, and a clear Mylar strip was placed on the top and bottom surface to minimize oxygen inhibition layer. Then two glass slabs were placed over the strip and slight hand pressure was applied to extrude excess material. The top glass slide was removed and the specimen was cured for 20s each side using an LED curing unit with a wavelength range of 440-480 nm at an output

Table 1: Materials used in this study

Material	Manufacturer	Type	Composition	Lot number
Ice	SDI, Vic, Australia	Nanohybrid resin composite	(80 wt% / 61 vol%), SAS, AS (0.04 - 3 μm,) UDMA/ BisEMA/TEGDMA	2096SN
Gradia direct	GC Corporation, Tokyo, Japan	Microhybrid resin composite	(75 wt% / 59 vol%) FAS, Silica, prepolimerized filler Average 0.85μm UDMA dimethacrylate	1311063

UDMA = urethane dimethacrylate, TEGDMA=triethylene glycol dimethacrylate, SAS= Strontium alumino silicate, AS= amorphous , silica, BisEMA= bisphenol a Ethylmethacrylate

of 1500 mW/cm2 (Radii plus LED, SDI, Bays water, Vic, Australia). The specimen was removed from the mould and the edges were ground gently using 1000-grit silicon carbide paper. All the specimens were incubated in distilled water at 37ºC for 24 h.

After 24 h immersion, all the specimens of each material were divided into three groups of 18. One group was marked 'unpolished' and left undisturbed after removal of the matrix strip. Specimens in the second and third groups were polished using a low speed hand piece in a circular motion on just one side either with aluminum oxide-impregnated discs (Sof-Lex®, 3M/ESPE) or aluminum oxide-impregnated

silicon points (Enhance®, Dentsply). Details of the polishing procedures of both systems are explained in Table 2.

When all specimens were polished, each of the 3 groups was subdivided into 3 subgroups of 6 and immersed in distilled water, cola or coffee (Table 3) for 7 days incubated at 37ºC (n = 6). The staining solution was replaced with fresh solution every 48 h during the storage period.

Measurement of surface roughness

Surface roughness (R_a) of each specimen was measured after 24 h and before immersion into the

Table 2: Detail of polishing systems used in the study and instruction of use

Polishing systems	Manufacturer	Instruction of use	Lot number
Sof-Lex disc	3M /ESPE, USA	Applied coarse, medium, fine and superfine discs for 15, 30,45, and 70 circular motion respectively, finished with the same polishing paste mentioned below	N494170
Enhance polishing points(type:rubber points)	Dentsply,caulk, USA	Applied with 60 circular motion, finished with polishing paste (SDI) on rubber cap for 30 seconds at low speed and light pressure	1405271

Table 3: Solutions' information

Solutions	Manufacturer	pH	Concentration	Lot number
Cola	Canned underauthority of the Coca-cola company by khoshgovar mashad company,iran	2.47	10.6 gr carbohydrates, 10.6 gr total sugars, less than 10mgr sodium, per 100ml, 139 kcal per 330 ml	1A14W23
Coffee	Vittoriacoffee, Silverwater, NSW, Australia	5.41	(15 g/500 mL)	
Distilled water		6.8		

solutions for the unpolished group and after polishing for the 2 polished groups. After 7 days of immersion, the measurement procedures were performed again. A profilometer (Perthometer M2, Mahr, Germany) with a 0.25-mm cutoff value and 2-mm tracing length was used for the measurement. The roughness of three locations of each specimen was obtained and the average value was recorded. Before the measurement, each specimen was rinsed with tap water for 10 seconds and dried with paper towel. Two randomly selected specimens of each group were sputter coated with gold and examined using a Field-Emission Scanning Electron Microscope (SEM, CB1, Cambridge, England).

Statistical Analysis

SPSS version 18 (SPSS Inc., Chicago, IL., USA) was used for data analysis. Three-way ANOVA was used to assess the interaction between three factors: materials, polishing methods, and solutions. Due to significant interaction effects in the model, subgroup analysis using student's T-test and one-way ANOVA/ Tukey's HSD tests was applied. Paired T-test was used to compare the surface roughness between two time intervals (24 h and 7 days) in distilled water. A *p value of* < 0.05 was considered to be statistically significant.

Table 4: Analysis after 24 hours immersion in distilled water. A comparison between the surface roughness (Ra) of the composites with all polishing systems, and effect of time (24 versus 7 days) on the (Ra).

Solution	Composite	Unpolished	Sof-Lex	Enhance	Unpolished	Sof-Lex	Enhance
					Comparison of time (*P* value)		
Distilled Water	Gradia direct	.315 ± .005[Aa]	.620 ± .004[Ba]	.858 ± .004[Da]	7d > 24h (p = 0.001)	24h > 7d (p < 0.001)	24h > 7d (p < 0.001)
	Ice	.158 ± .003[Ab]	.320 ± .003[Bb]	.534 ± .005[Db]	7d > 24h (p < 0.001)	24h > 7d (p < 0.001)	24h > 7d (p < 0.001)

[A,B,D] letters show difference in the surface roughness between different polishing systems.

[a,b] letters show difference in the surface roughness between different types of resin composite.

Table 5: Analysis after 7 days immersion comparison of composites, 3 polishing systems and solutions

Solution	Composite	Unpolished	Sof-Lex	Enhance
Distilled water	Gradia direct	.320 ± .005^{Aa}	.610 ± .005^{Ba}	.842 ± .004^{Da}
	Ice	.162 ± .003^{Ab}	.310 ± .003^{Bb}	.522 ± .005^{Db}
Cola	Gradia direct	.310 ± .004^{Aa}	.600 ± .006^{Ba}	.892 ± .005^{Da}
	Ice	.152 ± .002^{Ab}	.340 ± .004^{Bb}	.540 ± .003^{Db}
Coffee	Gradia direct	.333 ± .006^{Aa}	.622 ± .004^{Ba}	.832 ± .005^{Da}
	Ice	.170 ± .004^{Ab}	.360 ± .003^{Bb}	.557 ± .004^{Db}

[A,B,D] letters show significant difference in the surface roughness between different polishing systems.
[a,b] letters show significant difference in the surface roughness between different types of resin composite.

Results

Three-way ANOVA revealed a significant interaction between all factors ($p < 0.001$). Table 4 shows that Gradia direct has a greater surface roughness (R_a) than Ice after 24 h immersion in distilled water and also after 7 days immersion in all solutions for all polishing systems ($p < 0.001$). Enhance point revealed significantly greater roughness than Sof-Lex discs and both showed greater R_a than Mylar strip (unpolished group).

Generally, the specimens of both resin composites of unpolished groups after 24 h of immersion in distilled water showed significantly lower Ra values than those of 7 days of immersion ($p < 0.001$), which is in contrast with the other 2 polishing groups in distilled water (Table 5). Table 5 compares the effect of staining solutions and distilled water on the surface roughness of resin composites based on different surface polishes which varies based on the material and polishing systems. Generally, for unpolished specimens, immersion in coffee after 7 days exhibited significantly greater surface roughness than in distilled water ($p < 0.05$) and cola ($p < 0.001$). Table 6 shows the significant pairwise result for solutions and compares the surface roughness cause by 3 solutions.

Discussion

A significant difference was found between the surface roughness of microhybrid and nanohybrid. Gradia direct showed a greater surface roughness

Table 6: Comparing the surface roughness between 3 solutions.

Resin composites	Polishing methods	Significant pairwise result for solutions
Gradia direct	Unpolished	coffee > distilled water > cola
	Sof-Lex	coffee > distilled water > cola
	Enhance	cola > distilled water > coffee
Ice	Unpolished	coffee > distilled water > cola
	Sof-Lex	coffee > cola > distilled water
	Enhance	coffee > cola > distilled water

than Ice. For both materials, using Mylar strip showed the smoothest surface; this is in agreement with many other previous studies [18-22]. However, resin rich layer in the restorations polymerized under Mylar strip is less resistant to abrasion and needs to be removed. Furthermore, all restorations need contouring adjustment, especially in the marginal area and occlusal surface, which needs to be polished that may end up with rough surfaces. Therefore, it is essential for a tooth-coloured restoration to be polished and finished with the best method to create the smoothest surface, hence prevents the plaque accumulation and staining.

The results of our study showed a significantly greater R_a when the Enhance point was used compared to Sof-Lex discs. This result is in agreement with those of other reported studies [23]. The authors speculated that the reason that Sof-Lex discs created smooth surfaces is related to their ability of removing the same amount of inorganic particles and organic matrix. The plane movement of the disc contributes to a smoother surface [23]. Despite the production of a rougher surface, Enhance polishing system is easier to form anatomic landmarks especially in the posterior teeth due to the rubber-like flexible material used in the system [24]. In contrast, the Soft-Lex disc has limitations for use in the proximal surfaces and posterior region of the mouth because of their rigidity; the discs are difficult to produce [25]. Therefore, the outcome of the polishing systems in the mouth may be different from the results obtained in the laboratory.

The results revealed that Ice (nanohybrid composite) performed significantly smoother than Gradia direct (microhybrid composite) in all solutions while using all polishing and finishing systems. This performance may be explained by the inorganic filler particles' hardness, volume percentage, shape, and size that are exposed after polishing [26]. It has been shown that solid filler particles in microhybrids are considerably larger than nanosized particles [27]. Moreover, Ice contains smaller filler particles and greater filler loading (61 vol %) in comparison to Gradia direct (59 vol %). This quantitative result was proven by qualitative examination (SEM images) shown in Figure 1. A few representative images of SEM in Figure 1 A-D present surface differences

of Ice and Gradia direct after immersion in coffee. The smoothest surface observed was for unpolished specimens of Ice immersed in coffee (Figure 1-A) and the roughest for Gradia polished with Enhance point immersed in coffee (Figure 1-D). After immersion in coffee, specimens polished by Sof-Lex discs, Ice (Figure 1-B) showed a smoother surface with less air bubbles than Gradia direct (Figure 1-C).

With regards to the effect of staining solutions on the surface roughness of resin composites, immersion in coffee (pH 5.41) resulted in a greater surface roughness than either cola (pH 2.47) or distilled water (pH 6.8) for both materials with almost all polishing systems. For unpolished specimens, immersion in coffee after 7 days exhibited significantly greater surface roughness than in distilled water ($p < 0.05$) and cola ($p < 0.001$). This is in agreement with the results of others [28,29] who found that coffee (pH 5.01) and tea (pH 5.38) stimulated the surface alteration of resin composites more significantly compared to red wine (pH 3.7). It is concluded that [30] increase in surface roughness in coffee may be associated with its acidic pH and a correlation between the type and quantity of load and the capacity of coffee to dissolve at a high temperature.

However, the other parts of the results of our study revealed that the surface roughness of both resin composites increased after 7 days of immersion in distilled water compared to 24 hours of immersion. It is speculated that the water uptake over the time could be a major reason for surface alteration of the materials rather than acidic pH or the temperature at which coffee is dissolved. Water softens the material [31] and, consequently, decreases the surface hardness [32]. Therefore, water sorption of these materials may have a significant outcome on the surface degradation of the materials.

Conclusions

Within the limitation of this study, the following conclusions were drawn: Gradia direct (microhybrid) showed significantly greater surface roughness than Ice (nanohybrid). Specimens immersed in coffee exhibited the highest R_a compared to distilled water and cola. Among the polishing systems, Enhance point revealed significantly greater surface roughness than Sof-Lex discs and both showed greater R_a than unpolished group.

Acknowledgments

The authors thank the Vice-Chancellor of Shiraz University of Medical Sciences for supporting this research (Grant# 9238) which is based on the thesis by Dr. Maryam Sadeghi. The authors also thank Dr. Mehrdad Vossoughi Statistician in Shiraz Dental School for his help with the statistical analysis, and SDI and GC for providing the materials used in this study.

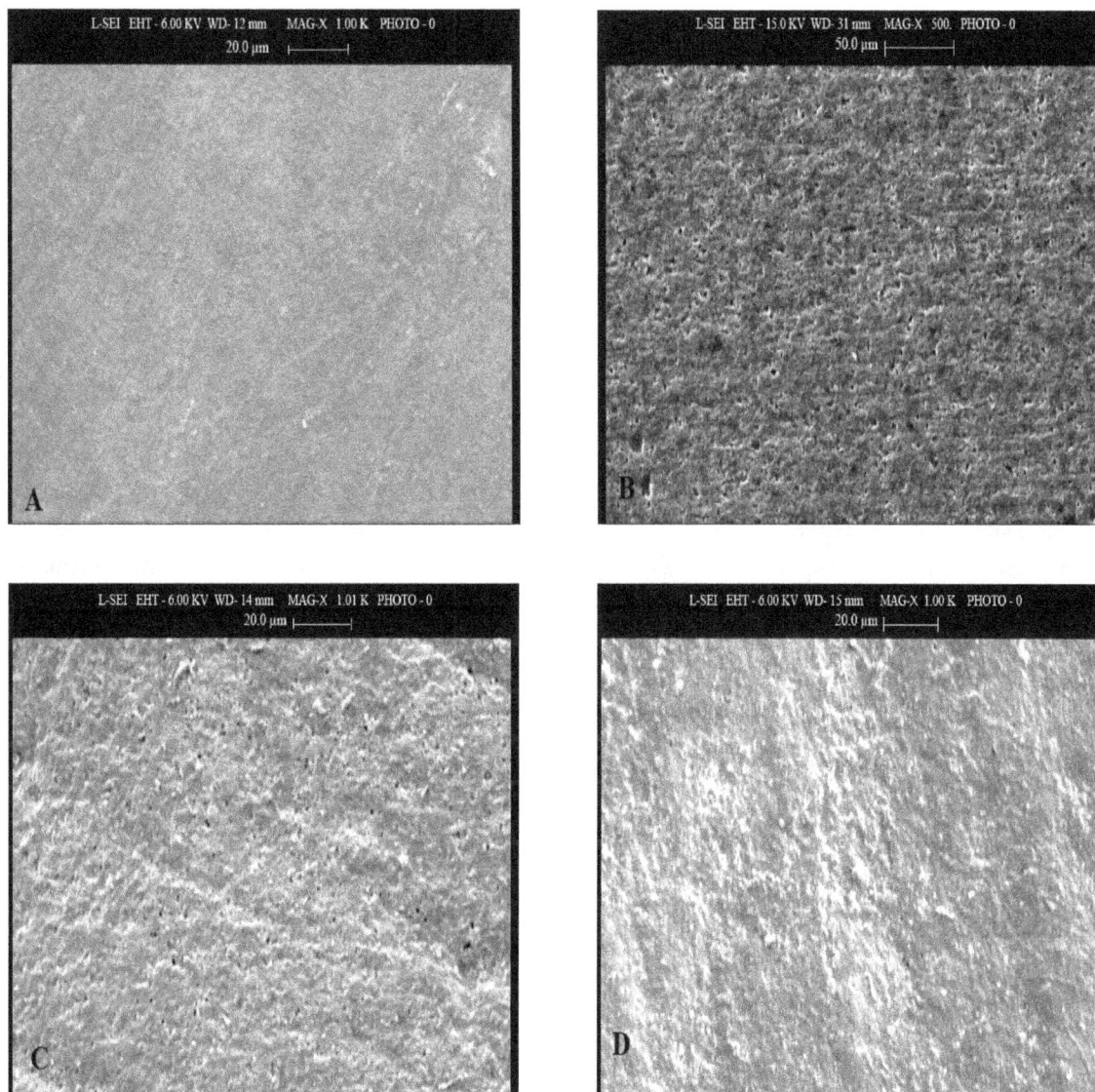

Figure 1: A- Ice unpolished after immersion in coffee, B- Ice polished with Sof-Lex after immersion in coffee, C- Gradia direct polished with Sof-Lex after immersion in coffee, D- Gradia direct polished with Enhance point after immersion in coffee

References

1. Ferracane JL. Resin compositestate of the art. Dent Mater. 2011;27:29-38.

2. Chen MH. Update on dental nanocomposites. J Dent Res. 2010;89:549-560.

3. Fortin D, Vargas MA. The spectrum of composites: new techniques and materials. J Am Dent Assoc. 2000;131:26S-30S.

4. St-Georges A, Bolla M, Fortin D, *et al*. Surface finish produced on three resin composites by new polishing systems. Oper Dent. 2005;30:593-597.

5. Da Costa J, Ferracane J, Paravina RD, *et al*. The effect of different polishing systems on surface

roughness and gloss of various resin composites. J Esthet Restor Dent. 2007;19:214-224.

6. Attar N. The effect of finishing and polishing procedures on the surface roughness of composite resin materials. J Contemp Dent Pract. 2007;8:27-35.

7. Endo T, Finger WJ, Kanehira M, et al. Surface texture and roughness of polished nanofill and nanohybrid resin composites. Dent Mater J. 2010;29:213-223.

8. Gulati G, Hegde R. Comparative Evaluation of two Polishing Systems on the Surface Texture of an aesthetic material (nano-composite): A Profilometric Study. People's Journal of Scientific Research. 2010;3:17-20.

9. Sarac D, Sarac YS, Kulunk S,et al. The effect of polishing techniques on the surface roughness and colour change of composite resins. J Prosthet Dent. 2006;96:33-40.

10. Schmitt VL, Puppin-Rontani RM, Naufel FS, et al. Effect of the polishing procedures on colour stability and surface roughness of composite resins. ISRN Dent. 2011;2011.

11. de Moraes R, Gonçalves Lde S, Lancellotti AC, et al. Nanohybrid resin composites: nanofiller loaded materials or traditional microhybrid resins? Oper Dent. 2009;34:551-557.

12. Ergücü Z, Türkün L. Surface roughness of novel resin composites polished with one-step systems. Oper Dent. 2007;32:185-192.

13. Janus J, Fauxpoint G, Arntz Y, et al. Surface roughness and morphology of three nanocomposites after two different polishing treatments by a multitechnique approach. Dent Mater. 2010;26:416-425.

14. Gordan V, Patel S, Barrett A, et al. Effect of surface finishing and storage media on bi-axial flexure strength and microhardness of resin-based composite. Oper Dent. 2003;28:560-567.

15. Ergücü Z, Türkün L, Aladag A. Colour stability of nanocomposites polished with one-step systems. Oper Dent. 2008;33:413-420.

16. Antonson SA, Yazici AR, Kilinc E, et al. Comparison of different finishing/polishing systems on surface roughness and gloss of resin composites. J Dent. 2011;39:9-17.

17. Lu H, Lee Y, Oguri M, et al. Properties of a dental resin composite with a spherical inorganic filler. Oper Dent. 2006;31:734-740.

18. Turkun L, Turkun M. The effect of one-step polishing system on the surface roughness of three esthetic resin composite materials. Oper Dent. 2004;29:203-211.

19. Barbosa SH, Zanata RL, Navarro MFdL, et al. Effect of different finishing and polishing techniques on the surface roughness of micro-filled, hybrid and packable composite resins. Braz Dent J. 2005;16:39-44.

20. Gedik R, Hürmüzlü F, Coskun A, et al. Surface roughness of new microhybrid resin-based composites. J Am Dent Assoc. 2005;136:1106-1112.

21. Çelik Ç, Özgünaltay G. Effect of finishing and polishing procedures on surface roughness of tooth-coloured materials. Quintessence Int. 2009;40:783-789.

22. Jefferies SR, Boston DW. Conventional polishing techniques versus a nanofilled surface sealer: preliminary findings regarding surface roughness changes and analysis. J Clin Dent. 2010;21:20-23.

23. Ritter AV. Posterior Resin-Based Composite Restorations: Clinical Recommendations for Optimal Success. J Esthet Restor Dent. 2001;13:88-99.

24. Yap A, Lye K, Sau C. Surface characteristics of tooth-coloured restoratives polished utilizing different polishing systems. Oper Dent. 1997;22:260-265.

25. Özgünaltay G, Yazici A, Görücü J. Effect of finishing and polishing procedures on the surface roughness of new tooth-coloured restoratives. J Oral Rehabil. 2003;30:218-224.

26. Taha NA, Ghanim A, Tavangar MS. A comparison evaluation of mechanical properties of resin modified glass ionomer with resin composite restoratives. J Dent Biomater. 2015;2:47-53.

27. Jung M, Sehr K, Klimek J. Surface texture of four nanofilled and one hybrid composite after finishing. Oper Dent. 2007;32:45-52.

28. Bagheri R, Burrow MF, Tyas M. Surface characteristics of aesthetic restorative materials–an SEM study. J Oral Rehabil. 2007;34:68-76.

29. Wongkhantee S, Patanapiradej V, Maneenut C, et al. Effect of acidic food and drinks on surface hardness of enamel, dentine, and tooth-coloured filling materials. J Dent. 2006;34:214-220.

30. de Gouvea C, Bedran LM, de Faria MA, et al. Surface roughness and translucency of resin

composites after immersion in coffee and soft drink. Acta Odontol Latinoam. 2011;24:3-7.

31. Bagheri R, Tyas MJ, Burrow MF. Comparison of the effect of storage media on hardness and shear punch strength of tooth-coloured restorative materials. Am J Dent. 2007; 20:329-334.

32. Bagheri R, Mese A, Burrow MF, *et al.* Comparison of the effect of storage media on shear punch strength of resin luting cements. J Dent. 2010;38:820-827.

20

Marginal Micro-leakage of Self-etch and All-in One Adhesives to Primary Teeth, with Mechanical or Chemo-Mechanical Caries Removal

Nouzari A[a], Zohrei A[a], Ferooz M[b], Mohammadi N[a]

[a]Department of Paediatrics, School of Dentistry, Shiraz University of Medical Sciences, Shiraz, Iran
[b]Melbourne Dental School, The University of Melbourne, Victoria, Australia

---

ARTICLE INFO	Abstract

Key words:
Marginal Micro-leakage
Primary Teeth
Carisolv
Conventional Method
Scotch Bond
Clearfil SE Bond

Corresponding Author:
Najmeh Mohammadi
Department of Paediatrics,
School of Dentistry,
Shiraz University of Medical
Sciences, Shiraz, Iran
Email:najmemohammadi64@
yahoo.com

Statement of Problem: Chemo-mechanical caries removal is an effective alternative to the traditional rotary drilling method. One of the factors that can influence micro-leakage is the method of caries removal.

Objectives: To compare the micro-leakage of resin composite in primary dentition using self-etch and all-in one adhesives following conventional and chemo-mechanical caries removal.

Materials and Methods: Sixty extracted human primary anterior teeth with class III carious lesions were collected. The selected teeth were divided randomly into two groups each consisting of 30 teeth. In group1 carious lesions were removed using Carisolv multi mix gel. In group 2, caries was removed using round steel burs in a slow–speed hand piece. Then, the specimens in each group were randomly divided into two subgroups (A and B) of 15 and treated by either Clearfil SE Bond (CSEB) or Scotch bond. All prepared cavities were filled with a resin composite (Estellite). All the specimens were stored in distilled water at 37°C for 24 hours and then thermocycled in 5°C and 55°C water with a dwell time of 20 seconds for 1500 cycles. The specimens were immersed in 1% methylene blue solution for 24 hours, removed, washed and sectioned mesiodistally. The sectioned splits were examined under a stereomicroscope to determine the micro-leakage scores. The data were analyzed using Kruskal-Wallis Test in SPSS version 21.

Results: There were no significant differences between micro-leakage scores among the four groups ($p = 0.127$). Score 0 of micro-leakage was detected for 60% of the specimens in group 1-A (Carisolv + CSEB), 73% of the group 2-A (hand piece + CSEB), 80% of the group 1-B (Carisolv + Scotch bond), and 93% of the group 2-B in which caries was removed using hand piece and bonded with Scotch bond.

Conclusions: Although caries removal using hand piece bur along with using Scotch bond adhesive performed less micro-leakage, it would seems that the use of Carisolv doesn't adversely affect the micro-leakage of composite restorations while using self-etch or all-in one adhesives.

Introduction

Dental caries which is one of the most prevalent chronic diseases causes localized dissolution and destruction of the calcified tooth tissue [1]. Traditionally, in most of the countries worldwide, rotary instrument has been used most commonly method to remove caries of children's teeth [2] Excessive loss of tooth structure occurs as the result of conventional caries removal with burs [3]. Moreover, restorative dental treatment in children, using conventional drill, is traumatic primarily mostly because of the children and their parents` fear and anxiety [4].

Other limitations of using rotary instruments include causing pain and need for anesthetics, which is unpleasant to many children [2]. Moreover, in some cases like allergy, anxiety or other diseases, the usage of anesthetics can be restricted [5]. The changing perception of cavity preparation and the introduction of variety of adhesive systems in the market, directed the clinician to the use another method of caries removal [2].

In chemo-mechanical caries removal (CMCR) method, carious lesions that have been solved by the solution is removed and followed by complete removal using gentle excavation. It has been proved that CMCR is a gentle method that removes only the infected tissues, thereby preserving the healthy dental structures, avoiding pulpal irritation and patient discomfort [2,5]. The latest CMCR system called Carisolv has been introduced to the European market (in 1980s) as a descendant to Caridex system. This method is suggested to be used for treatment of deciduous teeth, dental phobia and medically compromised patients [6].

Resin composite is increasingly the material of choice for the restoration of primary teeth and new materials with simplified procedures are being widely introduced to the market. Micro-leakage is one of the most common problems usually occurs at the gingival margin of the restorations which may causes postoperative sensitivity, recurrent caries, marginal deterioration, pulp injury, and enamel fracture [7].

One of the factors that can influence micro-leakage is the method of caries removal. Kubo et al. [8] in their study of comparing the nano-leakage of three dentin adhesive systems bonded to Carisolv treated dentin found that the use of chemo-mechanical caries removal does not adversely affect the bond to caries-affected dentin. The results of the study conducted by Coelho Okida and his colleagues [9] also reported that the method of caries removal did not influence the results of micro-leakage at any of the cavity margins. In the study by Ngujen et al. [10], the effect of Carisolv on the micro-leakage of composite restorations in the carious posterior human teeth was evaluated and no significant differences were observed between Carisolv and rotary instruments.

Dentin bonding agents also have an important role in reducing micro-leakage of the resin composite restorations. Self-etching adhesive has been a subject of interest especially with children due to simplifying the bonding procedure [11]. These bonding systems are being preferred over the traditional one since they eradicate the rinsing step, whereby the time of treatment and the need for patient compliance are reduced [12]. The new family of dental adhesives is also known as "universal" or "multi-mode" and represents the latest generation of adhesives on the market. They are designed under the "all-in one" concept [13].

The effect of Carisolv on the micro-leakage of composite restorations in primary dentition using all-in one adhesive has not been widely evaluated. The purpose of this study was to evaluate the effect of CMCR method on the micro-leakage of composite restorations in primary dentition using two recent popular self etch dentin bonding systems. The null hypothesis is that the method of caries removal and bonding system do not affect the micro-leakage of resin composites used in primary dentition.

Materials and Methods

To use the extracted teeth, we obtained the approval of ethics committee (Grant #5687) from Shiraz Dental School, Shiraz University of Medical Sciences. Sixty extracted human primary anterior teeth with class III carious lesions were collected, cleaned using scalpel and stored in 0.2% thymol solution. The selected teeth were divided randomly into two groups each consisting of 30 teeth. In group1, carious lesions were removed using Carisolv multi mix gel (Mediteam Dental AB, Savedalen, Sweden) according to the manufacturer's instruction. While applying pressure on the twin syringe mixing system, we mixed equal amounts of the two components. The mixed gel was applied to the carious dentin using special hand instrument and left for 30 seconds. The softened carious dentin was then removed by careful excavation with special non-cutting hand instrument. This procedure was repeated until the Carisolv gel

Table 1: Score criteria showing the amount of dye penetration; modified version of the method used by Di-wanji *et al.* [14].

0° = No leakage
1° = Less than or up to one-half of the depth of the cavity preparation
2° = More than one-half of the cavity preparation involved, but not up to the junction of the axial and occlusal or cervical wall
3° = Dye penetration up to the junction of the axial and occlusal or cervical wall, but not including the axial wall
4° = Dye penetration including the axial wall

was no longer cloudy and the dentin surface hardened when scraped with a blunt dental explorer.

In group 2, the caries was removed using round steel burs in a slow–speed hand piece. Specimens in each group were randomly divided into two subgroups of 15 and treated by either Clearfil SE Bond (CSEB) or Scotch bond according to the manufacturer's instruction. The subgroups were designated as A and B (n = 15). All prepared cavities were filled with a resin composite (Estellite, Tokuyama, Tokyo, Japan) and cured for 40 seconds using Coltolux 2.5 unit (Coltene, Germany) with 500mW/cm^2 output. The restorations were polished using sequences of Sof-lex discs (3M ESPE Co.; USA) from coarse to fine.

All the specimens were stored in distilled water at 37°C for 24 hours; the root apices were sealed using sticky wax named as model cement (Kem Dent, England). Then, they were thermocycled in 5 and 55 °C water with a dwell time of 20 seconds for 1500 cycles.

The tooth surfaces were covered using two coats of nail polish except for the surface of restorations and 1 mm around them. The specimens were immersed in 1% methylene blue solution for 24 hours and then removed from dye solution and washed under running water. The teeth were sectioned mesiodistally with a high-speed diamond saw (Isomet; buchler, USA).The corresponding sectioned splits were examined under a stereo-scope (wild M8, Wild Co. Model MMS 235, Swiss) at 40x magnification to determine the micro-leakage scores and penetrating micro-leakage. The score criteria used to show the amount of dye penetration was a modified version of the method

used by Diwanji *et al.* [14], as shown in Table 1. The data were analyzed using Kruskal-Wallis test in SPSS, version 21.

Results

The micro-leakage scores for all materials are shown in Table 2, and graphically in Figure 1. The lowest micro-leakage was obtained for group 2-B for the 93% scores 0, in which the caries was removed using round bur hand piece and resin composite bonded with Scotch bond (all-in one) system. The second lowest micro-leakage was of 80% score 0 that was found to be for the group 1-B (Carisolv + Scotch bond) followed by group 2-A and 1-A with 73% and 60% score 0 of micro-leakage respectively. The differences between micro-leakage scores among all four groups were not statistically significant (*p* = 0.127). The detailed result of Kruskal-Wallis Test is shown in Table 3.

Discussion

Marginal seal plays a major role in success of restorations. Marginal discoloration, recurrent caries, marginal deterioration and pulp damage can occur as a result of marginal leakage [15]. Method of caries removal may leave a particularly different amount of smear layer of the prepared dentin, which can affect the quality of bonding to the dentin and marginal seal [16].

Although there was no significant difference in the amount of micro-leakage between the four groups in the present study, the degree of micro-leakage in

Table 2: The frequency of micro-leakage scores in the tested groups

Groups		\multicolumn{5}{c}{Micro-leakage scores}				
		0	1	2	3	4
1-A	Carisolv + CSEB	9	2	2	2	0
1-B	Carisolv + Scotch bond	12	2	1	0	0
2-A	Hand piece Bur + CSEB	11	4	0	0	0
2-B	Hand piece Bur + Scotch bond	14	1	0	0	0

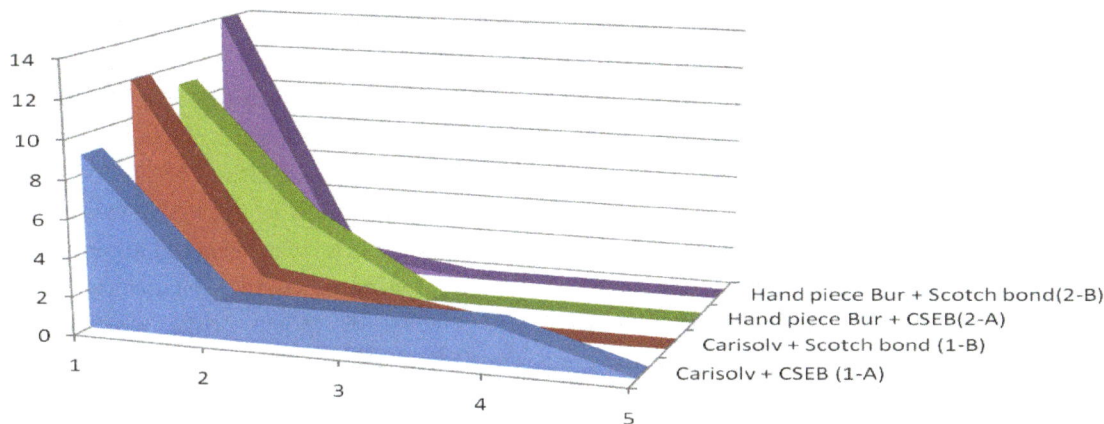

Figure 1: Micro-leakage scores in four groups of treatment

groups 1-A and 2-A seems to be more than that of groups 1-B and 2-B that may be due the remained Carisolv gel in the prepared cavity interloping with the adhesive systems. Other researches have shown the trace of Carisolv gel despite water irrigation [17,18]. In the study of Kubo *et al.* [8] the thickness of the hybrid layers was slightly greater in the rotary group than in the Carisolv group. Carisolv treatment probably allows for preservation of most of the caries-affected dentin. The composition and nature of the affected dentin is different form normal dentin. There are less mineral contents in the affected dentin compared to normal dentin causing demineralization due to caries process, also has less hardness than normal dentin. The dentinal tub tubules of the affected dentin have been filled with mineral crystals that are more resistant against etchant agents [19]. Another reason could be attributed to the remnants of the carious dentin, since Carisolv may not remove the carious dentin completely. However, this study demonstrated that the use of chemo-mechanical caries removal does not adversely affect the bond to the caries-affected dentin [8].

The results of our study also showed that there was no significant difference in the amount of leakage between the two methods of caries removal (CMCR and rotary instruments) this is in agreement with

the results reported by Ngujen *et al.* [10] and others [9,20]. The results of other studies also show that the bond strength of the resin composite to dentin surface created by chemo-mechanical and conventional methods is almost similar [21,22]. Mousavinenasab *et al.* [20] studied the micro-leakage of resin composite in the restorations of permanent posterior teeth following caries removal by Carisolv and rotary instruments. This study demonstrated that by applying etch and rinse adhesive system there was no significant difference in micro-leakage between conventional and chemo -mechanical caries removal methods.

In the present study, self-etch technique was used in primary teeth. The role of children`s compliance in success rate of bonded restorations that need proper isolation is definite. The self-etching adhesives eradicate the need of rinsing, therefore helps to reduce the time of treatment and the need for patient amenability especially in children [12]. Coelho Okida *et al.* [9] in a study compared the "etch and rinse" and "all-in one" adhesive systems after caries removal by CMCR and rotary instruments. They concluded that the adhesive system did not influence the rate of micro-leakage in the enamel margins and the techniques of caries removal did not affect the degree of marginal micro-leakage for enamel and dentin/cementum [9].

Results of our present study that is in agreement with those reported by Brandt *et al.* [23] revealed less micro-leakage in groups 2-B and 1-B than that of groups 1-A and 2-A (Table 2). A recent study indicated significantly higher bond strength for Carisolv than bur excavation using Clearfil SE bond on the primary caries affected dentin [24]. The better performance of scotch bond may be owing to its one step procedure decreasing the sensitivity of the usage

Group	Mean± SD	Median	Mean Ranks	p^* Value
1-A	0.80±1.1	.0000	36.40	
1-B	0.26±0.6	.0000	29.40	
2-A	0.26±0.4	.0000	30.83	0.127
2-B	0.06±0.2	.0000	25.33	

Table3: Description of micro-leakage score in the tested groups

*: Kruskal-Wallis H test

of Clearfil SE bond which has primer and bonding. In general, Carisolv® an effectively painless technique of caries removal performs to be of prospective complementary for use in clinical pediatric dentistry.

Conclusions

Based on the limitation of this study, the results showed that the use of Carisolv doesn't adversely affect the micro-leakage of composite restorations while using self-etch adhesives. The interactions between Carisolv treated dentin surface and different bonding systems, including self each adhesive should be evaluated in micro-tensile test. Further research is required to study the hybrid layer and characteristics of resin/dentin interface following chemo-mechanical caries removal method.

Acknowledgments

The authors thank the Vice-Chancellor of Shiraz University of Medical Sciences for supporting this research which is based on the thesis by Dr. Zohrei A (Grant#5687).

References

1. Lundeen TF, Roberson TM. In: Sturdevant's Art and science of operative dentistry. Roberson TM, Heymann HO, Swift EJ , editors. St Louis: Mosby Co; 2002. p. 60–128.

2. Pratap Kumar M, Nandakumar K, Sambashivarao P, *et al*. Chemo Mechanical Caries Removal - A New Horizon. Indian J Dent Adv. 2011;3:668-672.

3. Hannig M. Effect of Carisolv solution on sound, deminera-lized and denatured dentin–an ultrastructural investigation. Clin Oral Investig. 1999;3:155–159.

4. Scott DS, Hirschman R, Schroder K. Historical antecedents of dental anxiety. J Am Dent Assoc. 1984;108:42–45.

5. Balčiunienė I, Sabalaitė R, Juskiene I. Chemomechanical Caries Removal for Children. Stomatologija. 2005;7:40-44.

6. Beeley JA, Yip HK, Stevenson AG. Chemochemical caries removal: a review of the techniques and latest developments,conservative dentistry. Br Dent J. 2000;188:427-430.

7. Sharafeddin F, Yousefi H, Modiri SH, *et al*. Microleakage of Posterior Composite Restorations with Fiber Inserts Using two Adhesives after ging. J Dent (Shiraz). 2013;14:90–95.

8. Kubo S, Li H, Burrow MF, *et al*. Nanoleakage of dentin adhesive system bonded to Carisolv treated dentin. Oper Dent. 2002; 27:387-395.

9. Okida R, Martins T, Briso A. *In vitro* evaluation of marginal leakage in bonded restorations, with mechanical or chemical-mechanical (Carisolv) removal of carious tissue. Braz Oral Res. 2007;21:176-181.

10. Ngujen T, Doherty EH, Aboushala A, *et al*. Effect of chemomechanical caries removal system on microleakage available from:http// iadr.coonfex.iadr/2000/sundiego/techprogram/ index.html.

11. Perdigao J, Lopes, L, Lambrechts P, *et al*. Effects of self-etching primer on enamel shear bond strengths and SEM morphology. Am J Dent. 1997;10:141-146.

12. Peutzfeldt A, Nielsen LA. Bond Strength of a Sealant to Primary and Permanent Enamel: Phosphoric Acid Versus Self-etching Adhesive. Pediatr Dent. 2004;26:240-244.

13. Rosa WL, Piva E, Silva AF. Bond strength of universal adhesives: A systematic review and meta-analysis. J Dent. 2015;43:765-776.

14. Diwanji A, Dhar V, Arora R, *et al*. Comparative evaluation of microleakage of three restorative glass ionomer cements: An in vitro study. J Nat Sci Biol Med. 2014 ;5:373–377.

15. Summit JB, Robbins JW, Hilton TJ, *et al*. Fundamentals of Operative Dentistry. 2nd Edition. Chicago: Quintessence; 2001.

16. Yazici AR, Ozgunaltay G, Dayanagac B. A scanning electron microspic study of different caries removal techniques on human dentin. Oper Dent. 2002;27:360-366.

17. Arvidsson A, Liedberg B, Moller K, *et al*. Chemical and topographical analysis of dentin surface after Carisolv treatment. J Dent. 2002;30:67-75.

18. Kavaboura A, Elides G, Vougiouklakis G. Effect of Carisolv on the molecular composition of carious and sound dentin. JADAR and CED, Montpellier. 1999.

19. Ogawa K, Yamashita Y, Ichijo T, *et al*. The ultrastructure and hardness of the transparent layer of human carious dentin. J Dent Res. 1983;62:7-10.

20. Mousavinenasab SM. Microleakage of Composite

Restorations Following Chemo-mechanical and Conventional Caries Removal. J Tehran Univ Med Sci. 2004;1:12-17.

21. Frakenberger R, Oberschachtsiek H, Kramer N. Bond strength to dentin after mechanical and chemical removal of simulated caries. J Dent Res. 1999;78:322.

22. Haak R, Wicht MJ, Noack MJ. Does chemo-mechanical caries removal affect dentin adhesion:

Eur J Oral Sci. 2000;10:449-455.

23. Brandt PD, de Wet FA, du Preez IC. Self-etching bonding systems: in-vitro micro-leakage evaluation. SADJ. 2006;61:248,250-251.

24. Mohammadi N, Ferooz M, Eskandarian T, *et al.* Effect of Caries Removal Methods on the Shear Bond Strength of Resin and Glass IonomerAdhesives to Primary Dentin. J Dent Biomater, 2015;2:141-148.

21

Effect of Green Tea Extract as Antioxidant on Shear Bond Strength of Resin Composite to in-Office and Home-Bleached Enamel

Sharafeddin F[a], Farshad F[b], Azarian B[c], Afshari A[d]

[a]Department of Operative Dentistry and Biomaterial Research Center, School of Dentistry, Shiraz University of Medical Sciences, Shiraz, Iran
[b]Student Research Committee and Department of Operative Dentistry, School of Dentistry, Shiraz University of Medical Sciences, Shiraz, Iran
[c]Tohid high school, Shiraz , Iran
[d]Student Research Committee, School of Dentistry, Shiraz University of Medical Sciences, Shiraz, Iran

ARTICLE INFO

Key words:
Antioxidant
Green Tea
Shear Bond Strength
Tooth Bleaching
Composite Restoration

Corresponding Author:
Farnaz Farshad
Student Research
Committee and Department
of Operative Dentistry,
School of Dentistry, Shiraz
University of Medical
Sciences, Shiraz, Iran.
Email: farnazfarshad1@
yahoo.com

Abstract

Statement of Problem: Shear bond strength (SBS) of home and office bleached enamel will be compromised by immediate application of composite restoration. Antioxidant agent may overcome this problem.

Objectives: This in vitro study assessed the effect of green tea extract on shear bond strength of resin composite to in-office and home-bleached enamel.

Materials and Methods: In this experimental study, 40 extracted intact human incisors were embedded in cylindrical acrylic resin blocks (2.5 ×1.5 cm), with the coronal portion above the cemento enamel junction out of the block. Then, after bleaching labial enamel surfaces of 20 teeth with 15% carbamide peroxide 6 hours a day for 5 days, they were randomly divided into two groups: A1 and A2 (n = 10), depending upon whether or not they are treated with antioxidant. Labial enamel surfaces of the remaining 20 teeth were bleached with 38% hydrogen peroxide before being randomly divided into groups B1 and B2 (n = 10), again depending on whether or not the antioxidant was used in their treatment .

The experimental groups (A2,B2) were treated with 5% solution of green tea extract before resin composite restoration was done by a cylindrical Teflon mould (5×2 mm). Shear bond strength of the specimens was tested under a universal testing machine (Zwick/Roell Z020). The SBS data were analyzed by using One-way ANOVA and Tukey HSD tests ($p < 0.05$).

Results: There were no statistically significant differences between shear bond strength of the control group (A1) and treated group (A2) but there were statistically significant differences between the groups B1 and B2 ($p < 0.05$).

Conclusions: Application of antioxidant did not increase the shear bond strength of home-bleached enamel to resin composite but its application increased the shear bond strength of in-office bleached enamel to resin composite.

Introduction

Vital tooth bleaching generally involves the application of hydrogen peroxide on the tooth surface in an office technique or the application of carbamide peroxide in home technique [1,2].

Carbamide peroxide and hydrogen peroxide function as oxidative agents by forming free radicals, oxygen reactive molecules and hydrogen ions. These active molecules attack the pigments existing in the teeth and remove them; that is why, they are effective in whitening of the teeth [3-5]. In the home bleaching technique, carbamide peroxide is used based on its concentration 0.5-8 hours a day under a dentist's supervision [6]. Hydrogen peroxide or its derivatives are used in different concentrations in most in-office bleaching technique [7].

Bleaching treatment has some negative effects on the teeth which include decreasing the bonding ability, changing morphology of the enamel and dentin surface, decreasing the enamel wear resistance, causing surface roughness, increasing enamel porosity and changing the enamel and dentin mechanical features, such as fracture toughness which may reduce the tooth crack resistance and strength [8,9,10].

It has been shown that the shear bond strength (SBS) of resin composite to the tooth structure decreases immediately after using bleaching agent [7]. Residual peroxides which interfere with resin tag formation and the resin bond to the tooth is responsible for the reduction of shear bond strength. Oxygen is released after an appropriate time interval, i.e. from 24 hours to 2-4 weeks; the resin composite restores its shear bond strength again [7]. There are some techniques to improve the bond strength of resin composites after bleaching process, such as the removal of the superficial tooth surface and the application of adhesives containing organic solutions, alcohol or antioxidant agents on the bleached enamel surface [2,11-13].

It was reported that application of antioxidants had beneficial effects on SBS of resin composite restoration to the bleached enamel by its positive role against free radical reactions [14]. One type of antioxidant is green tea extract whose antioxidant activity is related to flanavols [15,16]. While it was reported that different concentration of green tea solution for especial time did not increase the SBS

of resin composite restoration to enamel bleached with 30% hydrogen peroxide [17], Sharafeddin et al. showed that the application of green tea solution on the bleached enamel by hydrogen peroxide increased the SBS of resin composite [18]. Sasaki et al. showed that 10% sodium ascorbate as an antioxidant neither reversed the oxidizing effect of 10% carbamide peroxide on enamel nor increased the SBS [14]. However, in one study, after the carbamide peroxide bleaching process, sodium ascorbate hydrogel application increased the SBS of bleached enamel surface. But this depended on the duration of the application of sodium ascorbate hydrogel [19].

To the best of our knowledge, there are few published studies comparing the effectiveness of green tea extract on SBS of in-office and home-bleached enamel. Hence, this in vitro study has been performed to evaluate the effects of green tea as an antioxidant on the SBS of in-office and home-bleached enamel.

Materials and Methods

In this experimental study, 40 recently extracted intact human maxillary incisors, without any defects, were collected and randomly divided into 4 groups (n = 10). The tooth roots were embedded in cylindrical shape of acrylic resin blocks (1.5 × 2.5 cm), the coronal part, above the cemento enamel junction, out of the block. The labial enamel surface of each tooth was polished (6 × 6 mm) with 600-grit silicon carbide paper (Moyco Precision Abrasives, Montgomeryville, PA, USA). The twenty sub- groups of prepared labial surfaces of the teeth surface were bleached with 15% carbamide peroxide gel (Opalescence, 15% PF, Ultradent Product Inc, South Jordan, UT, USA) 6 hours a day for 5 consecutive days. After completing the daily bleaching procedures, teeth were rinsed with water spray for 60 seconds and then kept them in distilled water at room temperature for one day. The remaining twenty prepared labial surfaces of the teeth were bleached with 38% hydrogen peroxide gel (Opalescence, Ultradent Product Inc., UT, USA) for 20 min according to the manufacturer instruction. The gel rinsed off thoroughly with water spray for 60 seconds and the process was repeated one more time.

The 5% green tea solution was prepared by dissolving a 5-mg green tea extract pill (Camgreen,

Giah Essence, Iran) into 100 mL of distilled water at room temperature [6]. The study groups were: A1, A2, B1, B2. In group A1 (control group), immediately after bleaching with 15% carbamide peroxide gel, composite restorative procedure was done after the application of adhesive. In group A2, immediately after bleaching, a 5% solution of green tea was applied on the carbamide peroxide bleached enamel surface for 10 minutes. Then, the samples were rinsed in water for 30 seconds and dried and resin composite buildup procedure was carried out.

In group B1 (control group), immediately after bleaching with 38% hydrogen peroxide gel, resin composite restorative procedure was carried out. In group B2, immediately after bleaching, a 5% solution of green tea was applied on the hydrogen peroxide bleached enamel for 10 minutes.

Then, the specimens were rinsed in water for 30 seconds and dried. Finally, resin composite restoration procedure was performed. Bleached enamel surfaces of specimens were etched by 37% phosphoric acid gel for 15 seconds (Total Etching Gel, IvoclarVivadent, Schaan, Liechtenstein). Then, they were rinsed with water spray for 15 seconds. Application of Adper Single Bond (3M ESPE, Dental Products, St Paul, MN, USA) was done and light-curing was performed by an LED unit (Demi Plus, Kerr, Switzerland) for 20 seconds at a light intensity of 1200 mW/cm². Finally, resin composite (Filtek Z350, 3M Dental Products) restoration procedure was carried out by using a Teflon mould measuring 5mm × 2mm in cured for 20 seconds.

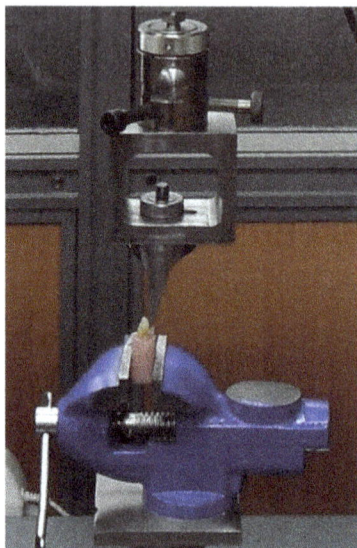

Figure 1: The specimen under the shear bond strength test using the Universal Testing Machine.

All the specimens were immersed in distilled water at room temperature for 24 hours. Then, the shear bond strength of the samples was measured by using a universal testing machine (Zwickroell Testing Mechine Z020, Germany) with a blade-shaped tip and the force was applied to the resin composite– enamel interface at a crosshead speed of 0.5 mm/min (Figure 1). Data was analyzed by SPSS version 18 (SPSS Inc, Chicago, IL., USA) using One-way ANOVA and *post-hoc* Tukey HSD tests ($p < 0.05$).

Results

The mean shear bond strength values and standard deviations in all of the 4 groups are presented in Table 1& Figure 2.

The results showed that there was no significant differences between the group A1 (carbamide peroxide)

Table 1: Descriptive Statistics of Shear Bond Strength (MPa) of the tested groups

Groups	Mean(±SD)
A1 (carbamide peroxide)	12.10 (2.30)[AB]
A2 (carbamideperoxide + green tea)	13.86(0.81)[A]
B1 (hydrogen peroxide)	10.52(1.23)[A]
B2 (hydrogen peroxide + green tea)	16.76(1.15)[B]

Mean values with at least a common letter in Superscript were not statistically different.

and group A2 (carbamide peroxide + green tea) treated with antioxidants, but there was a statistically significant difference between the group B1 (hydrogen peroxide) and B2 (hydrogen peroxide + green tea) ($p < 0.05$). Moreover, no statistical significant difference was found between groups A1 and B1 but reported significant differences between groups A2 and B2.

Discussion

The decrease in the shear bond strength of bleached tooth is related to residual peroxides which interfere with the process of resin tags formation and resin adhesion to the tooth structure, inhibiting the polymerization of resin monomers [5,20].

One study reported that the application of green tea solution for limited time did not increase the SBS of resin composite restoration to bleached enamel surface with 30% hydrogen peroxide [17]. In the

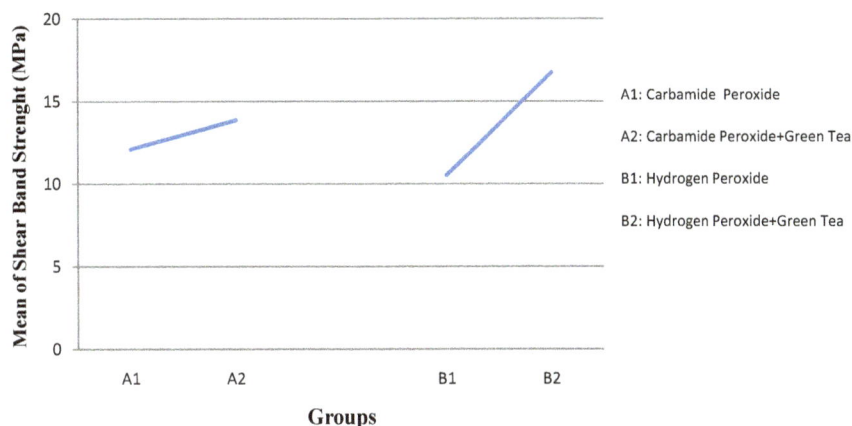

Figure 2: Comparison of shear bond strength (MPa) of all groups

present study, 15% carbamide peroxide bleaching gel was used in groups A1 (carbamide peroxide) and A2 (carbamide peroxide + green tea) and 38% hydrogen peroxide bleaching gel was used in groups B1(hydrogen peroxide) and B2 (hydrogen peroxide + green tea) and 5% green tea solution was applied for 10 minutes in groups A2 and B2. No significant increase in SBS of resin composite to home-bleached enamel was achieved in group A2 but significant increase in SBS was observed in group B2. This can be related to different concentration, composition and time of application of bleaching agents as well as different antioxidant and application time used.

Another study showed that the application of grape seed extract, pomegranate peel extract, sodium ascorbate, and green tea on enamel surface bleached with 38% hydrogen peroxide neutralized the effect of residual oxygen on the bleached enamel and increased the SBS of resin composite [18]. The concentration of green tea solution was the same as that used in this study but we used 15% carbamide peroxide for groups A1 and A2 as a bleaching agent that was weaker than (38% hydrogen peroxide) office bleaching agent, producing less residual oxygen molecules. We noticed that the effect of the antioxidant on SBS would decrease as the bleaching agent concentration decreased.

One study reported the effects of sodium ascorbate concentration as an antioxidant and the duration of application time on SBS of resin composite restoration to bleached enamel surface. The results revealed that the use of different concentration (10% and 20%) of sodium ascorbate hydrogel for 30, 60 and 120 minutes and bleaching with 17% carbamide peroxide gel increased the resin-enamel bond strength. The increased SBS of bleached enamel to resin composite

had a direct relation with the application time but there was no relation between these effects and different concentrations of sodium ascorbate [5].

In the present study, green tea solution was used as an antioxidant at 5% concentrations for 10 minutes. Significant increase was observed in SBS of resin composite to 38% hydrogen peroxide bleached enamel in group B2 (hydrogen peroxide + green tea), but there were no significant increase in SBS of resin composite to 15% carbamide peroxide bleached enamel in group A2 (carbamide peroxide + green tea). In the study mentioned above, the different types, concentrations and application times of antioxidant used might explain the differences noticed in the results. In the present study, 15% carbamide peroxide and 38% hydrogen peroxide were used as a bleaching agents but in the above mentioned study, 17% carbamide peroxide was used. This difference, i.e., 17% carbamide peroxide with 38% hydrogen peroxide, might be the underlying reason for producing more peroxide molecules and hence this could be the reason for greater effectiveness of antioxidants on the SBS of resin composite to the bleached enamel.

Another study investigated the effect of 10% sodium ascorbate and the effect of delaying the bonding procedure on the SBS of resin-modified glass-ionomer (RMGI) and SBS of resin composite. The enamel surface was bleached with 9.5% hydrogen peroxide for 6 hours a day for 7 days consecutively. They reported that the SBS decreased when the tested groups were restored with resin composite immediately after bleaching; also, RMGI did not bond to bleached enamel surface immediately after bleaching procedure. Therefore, application of 10% sodium ascorbate resulted in increasing the SBS of the restorations to enamel surface after bleaching with 9.5% hydrogen peroxide [20].

In the current study, in groups A1 and A2, carbamide peroxide 15% was used 6 hours a day for 5 consecutive days, and in groups B1 and B2, hydrogen peroxide 35% was used as a bleaching agent. In the study mentioned above and in our study, in groups B1 and B2, hydrogen peroxide was used as the bleaching agent which was stronger than carbamide peroxide in producing residual oxygen molecules and hence could significantly decrease SBS of resin composite. This was probably because of the significant effect of antioxidant material treatment in the groups that were bleached with hydrogen peroxide.

One study reported the positive effects of 10% sodium ascorbate gel as an antioxidant on the bonding capacity to enamel surface bleached with 10% carbamide peroxide;10% sodium ascorbate was applied for 10, 60, 120, 240, and 480 minutes on bleached enamel surface. This study reported that as the application time of the antioxidant increased, SBS of resin composite to enamel increased, too. For greater effectiveness, antioxidant gel should be applied to enamel surface for at least 60 minutes. Consistent with the results of the present study, no significant increase in shear bond strength was observed in the group that received the antioxidant for 10 minutes [12]. In the present study, in group A2, 15% carbamide peroxide was used, producing more oxygen reactive molecules than when 10% carbamide peroxide was used; the antioxidant was applied for 10 minutes. Therefore, based on the results of the current study, it seems that with increasing the concentration of bleaching agent, the application time of antioxidant should be increased.

Another study investigated the effects of 10% sodium ascorbate for 1 minute as an antioxidant on SBS of resin composite to enamel surface bleached with 35% hydrogen peroxide or with 16% carbamide peroxide gel and reported an increase of the SBS [21,22]. In the present study, 15% carbamide peroxide and 5% green tea were used for 10 minutes in group A2 but it did not show significant effects on SBS of resin composite to bleached enamel. Therefore, an increase of the concentration of antioxidant might be required.

It was reported that application of only 10% sodium ascorbate as an antioxidant resulted in an increase in shear bond strength of dual-cured resin cement to enamel surface bleached with carbamide peroxide gel but delaying the bonding procedure had no effects on increasing SBS of that of bleached enamel surface [23]. On the other hand, another study reported that application of 10% sodium ascorbate as an antioxidant and delaying the bonding process increased the bond strength [13,24].

One study assessed the neutralizing effect of 5% grape seed solution on the bond strength of enamel bleached with 38% hydrogen peroxide gel. They concluded that the use of 5% grape seed solution for 10 minutes completely neutralizes the effect of bleaching agents [8]. This study, in which 38% carbamide peroxide and 5% green tea solutions were used for 10 minutes, led to a similar result.

Another study showed that 6.5% grape seed solution as an antioxidant increased the shear bond strength of enamel bleached with 35% carbamide peroxide gel [25]. In the current study, using 15% carbamide peroxide and 5% green tea solution as an antioxidant; no significant increase was observed in SBS of resin composite to home-bleached enamel. But 35% carbamide peroxide gel produced more residual oxygen than 15% carbamid peroxide and this difference might be the underlying cause of the neutralizing effect of grape seed extract.

Further studies should be conducted to evaluate the effect of different application time, different concentrations and different types of antioxidants on shear bond strength of bleached enamel surface with different concentrations of bleaching agents.

Conclusions

Under the limitation of this in vitro study, it can be concluded that, surface treatment using green tea extract had no significant effects on the SBS of resin composite to enamel bleached with 15% carbamide peroxide gel but it had significant increasing effect on the shear bond strength of resin composite to enamel bleached with38% hydrogen peroxide gel.

Acknowledgements

The authors thank the Vice-Chancellory of Shiraz University of Medical Science and Biomaterial Research Center of Shiraz University of Medical Sciences for supporting this research (Grant# 7575). The authors also thank Dr. M. Vossoughi for the statistical analysis and Dr. Ehya Amalsaleh for improving the use of English in the manuscript.

Conflict of Interest: None declared.

References

1. Khoroushi M, Aghelinejad S. Effect of post-bleaching application of an antioxidant on enamel bond strength of three different adhesives. Med Oral Patol Oral Cir Bucal. 2011;16:990-996.

2. Tam LE, Abdool R, El-Badrawy W. Flexural strength and modulus properties of carbamide peroxide-treated bovine dentin. J Esthet Restor Dent. 2005;17:359-367.

3. Khoroushi M, Mazaheri H, Manoochehri A. Efeect of CPP-ACP application on fiexural strength of bleached enamel and dentin complex . Oper Dent. 2011:36:372-379.

4. Sharafeddin F, Varachehre M. Evaluation of microleakage in composite restoration by using self-etch and total etch adhesive after using 35% carbamide peroxide bleaching gel. J Isfahan Dent Sch. 2009;4:67-74.

5. Dabas D, Patil AC, Uppin VM. Evaluation of the Concentration and duration of application of sodium ascorbate hydrogel on the bond strength of composite resin to bleached enamel. J Conserv Dent. 2011;14:356-360

6. Sharafeddin F, Farshad F. The effect of aloe vera, pomegranate peel, grape seed extract, green tea, and sodium ascorbate as antioxidants on the shear bond strength of composite resin to home-bleached enamel. J Dent (Shiraz). 2015;16: 296-301.

7. Sharafeddin F, Zare S, Javanmardi Z. Effect of home bleaching on microleakage of fiber-reinforced and particle-filled composite resins. J Dent Res Dent Clin Dent Prospects. 2013;7:211-217.

8. Vidhya S , Srinivasulu S, Sujatha M, *et al* . Effect of grape seed extract on the bond strength of bleached enamel. Oper Dent. 2011;36:433-438.

9. Sharafeddin F, Koohpeima F, Palizian B. Evaluation of Microleakage in Class V Cavities Filled with Methacrylate-based versus Silorane-based Composites. J Dent Biomater. 2015;2:67-72.

10. Sharafeddin F, Darvishi F, Malekzadeh P. The

Effect of Incorporation of Polyethylene and Glass Fiber on the Microleakage of Silorane-based and Methacrylate-based Composites in Class II Restorations: An in Vitro Study. J Dent Biomater. 2015;2:39-46.

11. Ismail T, Sestili P, Akhtar S. Pomegranate peel and fruit extracts: a review of potential anti-inflammatory and anti-infective effects. J Ethnopharmacol. 2012 ;143:397-405.

12. Kaya AD ,Türkün M, Arici M. Reversal of compromised bonding in bleached enamel using antioxidant gel. Oper Dent. 2008; 33:441-447.

13. Bulut H, Kaya AD, Turkun M. Tensile bond strength of brackets after antioxidant treatment on bleached teeth. Eur J Orthod. 2005;27:466-471.

14. Sasaki RT, Flório FM, Basting RT. Effect of 10% sodium ascorbate and 10% alpha-tocopherol in different formulations on the shear bond strength of enamel and dentin submitted to a home-use bleaching treatment. Oper Dent. 2009;34:746-752.

15. Bornhoeft J, Castaneda D, Nemoseck T , *et al*. The protective effects of green tea polyphenols:lipid profile, inflammation, and antioxidant capacity in rats fed an atherogenic diet and dextran sodium sulfate. J Med Food. 2012 ;15:726-732.

16. Van Nederkassel AM, Daszykowski M, Massart DL, *et al*. Prediction of total green tea antioxidant capacity from chromatograms by multivariate modeling. J Chromatogr A. 2005;1096:177-186.

17. Arumugam MT, Nesamani R, Kittappa K, *et al*. Effect of various antioxidants on the shear bond strength of composite resin to bleached enamel: An in vito study. J Conserv Dent. 2014;17:22-26.

18. Sharafeddin F, Motamedi M, Modiri SH. Effect of Immediate Application of Pomegranate Peel, Grape Seed and Green Tea Extracts on Composite Shear Bond Strength of In-Office Bleached Enamel. Res J Biol Sci. 2013;8:83-87.

19. Muraguchi K, Shigenobu S, Suzuki S, *et al*. Improvement of bonding to bleached bovine tooth surfaces by ascorbic acid treatment. Dent Mater J. 2007; 26:875-881.

20. Danesh-Sani SA, Esmaili M. Effect of 10% sodium ascorbate hydrogel and delayed bonding on shear bond strength of composite resin and resin-modified glass ionomer to bleached

enamel. J Conserv Dent. 2011;14:241-246.

21. Kunt GE, Yılmaz N, Sen S, *et al*. Effect of antioxidant treatment on the shear bond strength of composite resin to bleached enamel. Acta Odontol Scand. 2011;69:287-291.

22. Lima AF, Fonseca FM, Freitas MS, *et al*. Effect of bleaching treatment and reduced application time of an antioxidant on bond strength to bleached enamel and subjacent dentine. J Adhes Dent. 2011;13:537-542.

23. Gökçe B, Cömlekoğlu ME, Ozpinar B, *et al*. Effect of antioxidant treatment on bond strength of a luting resin to bleached enamel. J Dent. 2008;36:780-785.

24. Bulut H, Turkun M, Kaya AD. Effect of an antioxidizing agent on the shear bond strength of brackets bonded to bleached human enamel. AM J Orthod Dentofacial Orthop. 2006;129:266-272.

25. Khamverdi Z, Rezaei-Soufi L, Kasraei S, *et al*. Effect of epigallocatechin gallate on shear bond strength of composite resin to bleached enamel: an in vitro study. Restor Dent Endod . 2013;38:241-247.

22

Shear Bond Strength of Porcelain to a Base-Metal Compared to Zirconia Core

Abrisham SM[a] MSD, DDS; Fallah Tafti A[a] MSD, DDS; Kheirkhah S[b] DDS; Tavakkoli MA[c*] DDS

[a]Department of Prosthodontics, Yazd University of Medical Sciences, Yazd, Iran
[b]School of Dentistry, Shahid Sadoughi University of Medical Sciences, Yazd, Iran.
[c]Department of Orthodontics, School of Dentistry, Shiraz University of Medical Sciences, Shiraz, Iran.

ARTICLE INFO

Key words:
Fixed Partial Denture
Dental Porcelain
Metal Ceramic Alloys
Zirconia
Computer-Aided Design
Shear Strength

Corresponding Author:
Mohammad Amin Tavakkoli
Department of Orthodontics,
School of Dentistry, Shiraz
University of Medical
Sciences, Shiraz, Iran.
Email: Tavakkolident@
gmail.com

Abstract

Statement of Problem: Recent clinical results for Zirconia all-ceramic restorations have revealed that the fracture rate 6-15% of the Zirconia framework is so low and the core of Zirconia has high stability. However, chipping-off fractures of porcelain are the most common reason for failures of Zirconia in the fixed partial dentures.

Objectives: The purpose of this study was to compare the shear bond strength (SBS) of porcelain in the porcelain fused to metal and all-ceramic crowns with Zirconia core.

Materials and Methods: Two groups were selected: porcelain fused to metal (PFM) and porcelain fused to Zirconia (PFZ) (n = 30).In the PFM group, a wax model (10 × 10 × 10mm)was used to cast metal base (Ni_Cr alloy). In the PFZ group, an acrylic cubic model (10 × 10 × 10mm) was made as Zirconia model for scanning.15 cubic Zirconia samples were milled by CAD-CAM. The procedure of porcelain veneering was conducted by the conventional layering technique up to 2 mm thickness (2.5 × 2.5 × 2 mm). All specimens were stored in water for 48 hrs. Thermal cycling was conducted for 20000 cycles between 55°C and 5°C alternatively for 30s.All samples were mounted in acrylic resin and the SBS test was performed, using a universal testing machine. The analysis of data was performed at a significance level of 0.05 using Kolmogorov-Smirnov and Mann-Whitney U-test.

Results: Mean of SBS in PFM and PFZ was 24.57 and 20.88, respectively. The results of Mann-Whitney test showed that there was no statistically significant difference between the two groups of porcelain fused to metal and Zirconia in item shear bond strength ($p = 0.455$).

Conclusions: There was no significant difference between the two groups of PFM and PFZ in the item SBS.

Introduction

In prosthodontics, the porcelain fused to metal (PFM) crowns has been considered a gold standard system in fixed partial dentures (FPDs) for 40 years [1]. This reliable choice can not only provide aesthetic characteristics similar to the natural teeth, but also enjoys mechanical features such as high flexural and shear bond strength (SBS). In recent years, the increasing requisition for aesthetic restorations as well as discussible toxic role of some dental alloys makes the development of another non-metal restoration justifiable [2].

Different studies revealed an excellent success rate for porcelain fused to zirconia (PFZ) crowns in comparison with PFM crowns [3,4].Yttria-stabilized Zirconia polycrystal (Y-TZP) has been used in recent years as a core material for all-ceramic restorations. It has high mechanical strength compared to other materials such as alumina and feldspathic porcelains (flexural strength of 900-1200 MPa, and fracture toughness of 9-10 MPa) [5]. Most of the mechanical strength is the result of transformation of monoclinic to a tetragonal structure due to its features of Y-TZP. It could tolerate occlusal loading. The conventional techniques (cupping) such as slip-casting and CAD-CAM ones are used for the frameworks of fixed-dental prostheses (FPDs) [6,7].

Recent clinical results for Zirconia all-ceramic restorations revealed that the fracture rate of the Zirconia framework is so low and Zirconia core has high stability [8,9]. However, chipping-off fractures of porcelain are the most common reason for failure of Zirconia in FPDs [8,9]. The rate of porcelain fracture in Zirconia in FPDs is extremely high in comparison with that in PFM [8]. It seems that the weakness in layered Zirconia-based porcelain is caused by the gap of bonding between the veneer material and the core of Zirconia. For longevity of restorations, this weakness has to be critically considered [9-10]. Long-term studies indicate that the fracture rates of porcelain in PFMs are 2.7-5.5% for a follow-up period of 10 to 15 years [11,12].

Clinical studies have revealed a high rate of fracture for porcelain-veneered zirconia-based restorations varying between 6% and 15% over a 3- to 5-year period. These are high values compared to the 4% fracture rate shown by conventional metal-ceramic restorations over 10 years [13].

The mechanism of adhesion between metal and porcelain is the micro-mechanical bond, van der Waals force, the coefficient of thermal expansion (CTE) match, and the interaction of ions between the metal and porcelain [14,15].Studies revealed that the bond strength of ceramic to metal layers was strong enough for functional load (54 - 71 MPa) [16-19].

Furthermore, the mechanism of bonding of zirconia to porcelain is still unknown, but based on few studies, the wettability of the ceramic and Zirconia surface, chemical bonding, and micromechanical interactions play a key role in this regard[17]. However, limited data exist on the bond strength of full ceramic crowns with Zirconia core [4,10].

The aim of this study was to compare the shear bond strength (SBS) of porcelain to a base metal compared to Zirconia.

Materials and Methods

Preparation of the Metal Core Specimens
At first, 15 wax cube-shaped specimens were prepared (10 × 10 × 10mm). Six layers of wax were superimposed to make a 10-mm thickness. Then, the cubes (10 × 10 × 10 mm) were casted in Nickel-chromium base metal alloy (4all,Ivoclar,Liechtenstein,Germany); they were sand-blasted and steam-cleaned(according to the standard ISO 6872). All specimens were fabricated by one dental technician.

Preparation of the Zirconia Core Specimens
A cubic shape silicone mould was filled with acrylic resin and then scanned. Fifteen cubic Zirconia samples (IPS e.max zirCAD) were milled by CAD-CAM (Amangirbach, Germany) with10 × 10 × 10 mm. They were sintered at 1,500 °C, dried, and sand-blasted with Al2O3 (120μ). The measurements were verified by the Digital Caliper Vernier. (Mitutoyo, Japan, 0.01mm). The cores were soaked in ultrasonic cleaner (Digital Ultrasonic Cleaner cd4820, Taiwan) for 10 minutes.

Porcelain Application for the Metal Group
At first, base metal copings were sand-blasted for each porcelain; then, degassing process was performed at 600 to 1000 °C for 18 min. (Auto therm 100, Koushafan Pars Co., Iran). They were sand-blasted by aluminum oxide (120 μ). The procedure of veneering was performed by the conventional layering technique according to manufacturers` instruction. First, two layers of opaque porcelain(E.Maxceram, Ivoclar, Liechtenstein) with 0.5 mm thickness were applied and fired; then, the dentin porcelain was compressed

Table 1: Descriptive results of comparison of shear bond strength of PFM & PFZ

Type\Item	Mean	95% CI		Median	IQR
		Lower	Upper		
PFM*	24.57	19.45	29.69	19.40	8.00
PFZ#	20.88	17.81	23.95	20.80	8.00

*Porcelain Fused to Metal
#Porcelain Fused to Zirconia

with 1.5 mm thickness by the vibration blotting technique and fired for glaze based on the manufacturer's instructions up to 2 mm thickness. Finally, the specimens were stored in water for 48 hrs.

Porcelain Preparation for the Zirconia Group
Zirconia core (e.maxceram, Ivoclar, Liechtenstein) was sintered at 1530°C for 12 hrs. (Programat, Ivoclar, Liechtenstein). Then, according to the manufacturer's instructions porcelain (E.Maxceram, Ivoclar, Liechtenstein) was applied up to 2 mm thickness and fired at 750°C for 19 min and glazed for 18 min.

All specimens were stored in water for 48 hrs. Thermal cycling (Thermocycler plus, Willytec, Grafelfing, Germany) was conducted for 20000 cycles between 55°C and 5°C alternatively for 30s to simulate the oral function for a two-year period for all samples of two groups.

Shear Bond Strength Test (SBS test)
All samples were mounted in acrylic resin. The SBS test was conducted using a piston in a universal testing machine (Zwick/Roll Z020; Zwick GmbH &Co, Germany) based on the ISO 6872 standards. The SBS test was conducted by placing the Zirconia/metal core at the side with a crosshead speed at 1 mm/min until failure. The maximum force at the time of

fracture was recorded; the SBS test was calculated using the formula below:

$$\text{Shear Stress (Mpa)} = \frac{\text{Load(N)}}{\text{Area(mm2)}}$$

Statistical Analysis
The analysis of data was performed at a significance level of 0.05 using the statistical software SPSS16.0 (SPSS, Inc., Chicago, IL). Kolmogorov-Smirnov test was used to assess the assumption of normality. Data were described using the median and interquartile range (IQR). Mann-Whitney U-test was used to compare the SBS between the two groups.

Results

Table 1 shows the descriptive statistics of the SBS measurements. The distribution of the SBS values in the groups was significantly deviated from normality ($p = 0.015$). Mann-Whitney U-test revealed that there were no significant differences between shear bond strength of porcelain to base metal alloy and Zirconia groups ($p = 0.455$)(Figure 1).

Discussion

The aim of this study was to compare the SBS to base

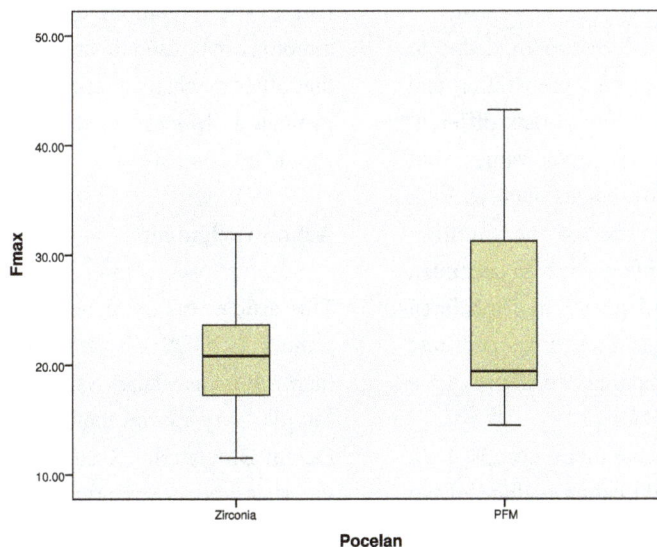

Figure 1: Results of the study in maximum force Shear Bond Strength for PFM & PFZ

metal (Nickel- chromium alloy) and Zirconia core. Nowadays, the usage of Zirconia core is controversial due to lack of evidence in comparison with gold standard choice (i.e. PFM) [20,21]. Many factors were discussed for the application of Zirconia core. One of the main factors to discuss is the SBS [20,22].

Based on the results, there were no significant differences between PFM and PFZ in the SBS. ($p = 0.455$).On the contrary, Turk *et al.* [23] stated that the SBS of the zirconia was significantly less than that of metal in pressing technique. However, the effect of different veneering techniques on the fracture strength of metal and zirconia frameworks was not significant.

In addition, the results of the studies by Aboushelib *et al.* [24] and Ansong *et al.* [25] were similar to those obtained by Subash *et al.* [26]. Nonetheless, Ishibe *et al.*[27] reported in their study that the mean shear bond strength for pressed Zirconia ceramic specimen ranged from 21.34 (24.30) MPa to 40.41 (10.28) MPa, ($p < 0.05$), while it ranged from 30.03 (9.49) MPa to 47.18 (12.99) MPa, ($p < 0.05$) for the layered Zirconia specimens, indicating the presence of higher bond strength value for layered samples than pressed specimens. Farzin said that conventional layering on base metal alloy had lower bond strength than heat press [28].

To meet ISO 9693 requirement, the mean debonding strength/crack initiation strength should be greater than 25 MPa. Owing to inherent brittleness of all-ceramic core materials, this test cannot be applied to the all-ceramic multi-layered system. There are still more choices among all bond strength test methods for these kinds of systems like three-four-point loading test, biaxial flexure test, and micro-tensile bond strength [19].

We decided to use the SBS test method due to its simplicity (the ease of specimen preparation and simple test protocol) and the ability to rank different products according to bond strength values, but the SBS test has some disadvantages such as high standard deviations, occurrence of non-uniform interfacial stresses, and the influence from specimen geometry. Therefore, the standardization of specimen preparation, cross-sectional surface area, and rate of loading application are important to improve the clinical usefulness of the SBS test.

Oh *et al.* showed that in the metal groups, both the core thickness and the fabrication method of the veneering porcelain significantly affected the fracture strength, while only the fabrication method affected the fracture strength in the zirconia groups [29].

Another factor influencing the bond strength is surface treatment. Different surface treatments of Zirconia, such as airborne-particle abrasion, application of a liner and creation of graded glass–Zirconia structures, sandblasting with Al2O3, grinding are proved to significantly improve the Zirconia–porcelain bond strength [21,22,30,31] But In our study no surface treatment was done.

On the other hand, Özkurt *et al.* revealed that the bond strength between Zirconia core and veneer was affected by the types of Zirconia and veneering materials used. Therefore, it is recommended that each type of Zirconia bonding should be used with manufacturer-recommended veneering ceramics [30].

All the five powders, Duceram Kiss, Vita VM13, Ceramco 3, Noritake EX-3, and Vintage, have bond strengths higher than the required 25 MPa minimum for Cr-Co alloy [28]. Moreover, due to its inherent properties such as high biocompatibility, chemical stability, aesthetics, and outstanding flexural strength, Zirconia may be the best substitute for PFM restorations. Nevertheless, Zirconia needs some improvements in these features to reach this goal [22,30].

Furthermore, as a limitation of our study, we suggest that further studies should be designed to evaluate and compare other comparable factors of each material such as color, and flexural strength. According to the available evidence, it is recommended that each material should be compared with different porcelain applying techniques.

Conclusions

Due to the limitations of our study, as to the SBS, zirconia can be used for crown core. It is recommended that other mechanical and aesthetic factors should be evaluated. Moreover, different porcelain powders should be compared.

Acknowledgments

This article was extracted from an original research project as DDS dissertation NO. (782). I should thank Sorayaneshaan Laboratory for fabricating the samples. My special thanks should also go to Shiraz Dental Biomaterial Research Center for performing the shear bond strength test. Finally, I appreciate Dr. M. Vossoughi's help in performing the required statistical analysis.

Conflict of Interest: None declared

References

1. Pjetursson BE, Tan K, Lang NP, *et al.* A systematic review of the survival and complication rates of fixed partial dentures (FPDs) after an observation period of at least 5 years. Clin Oral Implants Res. 2004;15:625-642.

2. Raigrodski AJ. Contemporary materials and technologies for all-ceramic fixed partial dentures: a review of the literature. J Prosthet Dent. 2004;92:557-562.

3. Ozer F, Mante FK, Chiche G, *et al.* A retrospective survey on long-term survival of posterior zirconia and porcelain-fused-to-metal crowns in private practice. Quintessence Int. 2014;45:31-38.

4. Diniz AC, Nascimento RM, Souza JC, *et al.* Fracture and shear bond strength analyses of different dental veneering ceramics to zirconia. Mater Sci Eng C Mater Biol Appl. 2014;38:79-84.

5. Guazzato M, Albakry M, Ringer SP, *et al.* Strength, fracture toughness and microstructure of a selection of all-ceramic materials. Part II. Zirconia-based dental ceramics. Dent Mater. 2004;20:449-456.

6. Tinschert J, Natt G, Mohrbotter N, *et al.* Lifetime of alumina-and zirconia ceramics used for crown and bridge restorations. J Biomedl Mater Res B Appl Biomater. 2007;80:317-321.

7. Sundh A, Sjögren G. A comparison of fracture strength of yttrium-oxide-partially-stabilized zirconia ceramic crowns with varying core thickness, shapes and veneer ceramics. J Oral Rehabil. 2004;31:682-688.

8. Sailer I, Pjetursson BE, Zwahlen M, *et al.* A systematic review of the survival and complication rates of all-ceramic and metal-ceramic reconstructions after an observation period of at least 3 years. Part II: fixed dental prostheses. Clin Oral Implants Res. 2007;18:86-96.

9. Sailer I, Feher A, Filser F, *et al.* Prospective clinical study of zirconia posterior fixed partial dentures: 3-year follow-up. Quintessence Int. 2006;37:685-693.

10. Raigrodski AJ, Chiche GJ, Potiket N, *et al.* The efficacy of posterior three-unit zirconium-oxide–based ceramic fixed partial dental prostheses: A prospective clinical pilot study. J Prosthet Dent. 2006;96:237-244.

11. Coornaert J, Adriaens P, De Boever J. Long-term clinical study of porcelain-fused-to-gold restorations. J Prosthet Dent. 1984;51:338-342.

12. Valderhaug J. A 15-year clinical evaluation of fixed prosthodontics. Acta Odontol Scand. 1991;49:35-40.

13. Augstin-Panadero R, Fons-Font A, Roman-Rodriguez JL, *et al.* Zirconia versus metal: a preliminary comparative analysis of ceramic veneer behavior. Int J Prosthodont. 2012;25:294-300.

14. Anusavice K. Phillips R. Phillips' science of dental materials. 11th Edition. St. Louis: Elsevier: 2003

15. Saito A, Komine F, Blatz MB, *et al.* A comparison of bond strength of layered veneering porcelains to zirconia and metal. J Prosthet Dent. 2010; 104:247-257.

16. Al-Shehri SA, Mohammed H, Wilson CA. Influence of lamination on the flexural strength of a dental castable glass ceramic. J Prosthet Dent. 1996;76:23-28.

17. Isgrò G, Pallav P, van der Zel JM, *et al.* The influence of the veneering porcelain and different surface treatments on the biaxial flexural strength of a heat-pressed ceramic. J Prosthet Dent. 2003;90:465-473.

18. De Jager N, Pallav P, Feilzer AJ. The influence of design parameters on the FEA-determined stress distribution in CAD–CAM produced all-ceramic dental crowns. Dent Mater. 2005;21:242-251.

19. ISO I. 9693: Metal-ceramic dental restorative systems. Switzerland: International Organization for Standardization. 1999.

20. Sevilla P, Sandino C, Arciniegas M, *et al.* Evaluating mechanical properties and degradation of YTZP dental implants. Mater Sci Eng C. 2010;30:14-19.

21. Chevalier J. What future for zirconia as a biomaterial? Biomaterials. 2006;27:535-543.

22. Denry I, Kelly JR. State of the art of zirconia for dental applications. Dent Mater. 2008;24:299-307.

23. Turk AG, Ulusoy M, Yuce M, *et al.* Effect of different veneeringtechniques on the fracture strength of metal and zirconia frameworks. J Adv Prosthodont. 2015;7:454-459.

24. Aboushelib MN, Kleverlaan CJ, Feilzer AJ. Microtensile bond strength of different components of core veneered all-ceramic restorations: Part II: Zirconia veneering ceramics. Dent Mater. 2006;22:857-863.

25. Ansong R, Flinn B, Chung K-H, *et al.* Fracture

toughness of heat-pressed and layered ceramics. J Prosthet Dent. 2013;109:234-240.

26. Subash M, Vijitha D, Deb S, *et al.* Evaluation of shear bond strength between zirconia core and ceramic veneers fabricated by pressing and layering techniques: In vitro study. J Pharm Bioallied Sci. 2015;7:612-615.

27. Ishibe M, Raigrodski AJ, Flinn BD, *et al.* Shear bond strengths of pressed and layered veneering ceramics to high-noble alloy and zirconia cores. J Prosthet Dent. 2011;106:29-37.

28. Farzin M, Khaledi AA, Malekpour B, *et al.* Evaluation of Bond Strength of Pressed and Layered Veneering Ceramics to Nickel-Chromi-um Alloy. J Dent. 2015;16:230-236.

29. Oh JW, Song KY, Ahn SG, *et al.* Effects of core characters and veneering technique on biaxial flexural strength in porcelain fused to metal and porcelain veneered zirconia. J Adv Prosthodont. 2015;7:349-357.

30. Özkurt Z, Iseri U, Kazazoglu E. Zirconia ceramic post systems: a literature review and a case report. Dent Mater J. 2010;29:233-245.

31. Mosharraf R, Rismanchian M, Savabi O, *et al.* Influence of surface modification techniques on shear bond strength between different zirconia cores and veneering ceramics. J Adv Prosthodont. 2011;3:221-228.

23

Comparative Study of Shear Bond Strength of Three Veneering Ceramics to a Zirconia Core

Aalaei Sh[a], Nematollahi F[b], Vartanian M[c], Beyabanaki E[d]

[a]Dental Caries Prevention Research Center, Qazvin University of Medical Sciences, Qazvin, Iran

[b]Department of Prosthodontics, Islamic Azad University, Dental Branch, Tehran, Iran

[c]General dentist, Qazvin, Iran

[d]Department of Prosthodontics, Faculty of Dentistry, Shahid Beheshti University of Medical Sciences, Tehran, Iran

ARTICLE INFO

Key words:
Ceramics
Dental Veneers
Shear Bond Strength
Zirconia

Corresponding Author:
Elaheh Beyabanaki,
Department of Prosthodontics,
Faculty of Dentistry, Shahid
Beheshti University of
Medical Sciences, Tehran, Iran

E-mail: e.beyabanaki@gmail.com

Abstract

Statement of Problem: Fracture of veneering porcelain has been described as the most frequent reason for the failure of zirconia-based fixed restorations.

Objectives: The purpose of this study was to evaluate and compare the shear bond strength of a zirconium oxide core material to three commercial veneering ceramics.

Materials and Methods: Three types of veneering ceramics were selected including IPS -emax Ceram, Vita VM9, and Cerabien. Thirty block specimens of zirconia core material were prepared in 4×4×9 mm dimensions. Three groups were created and the veneering ceramic was added to each of 10 blocks. Shear bond test was conducted with universal testing machine. Data were analyzed using one-way ANOVA ($p = 0.05$).

Results: Mean shear bond strength values and standard deviations were 26.03 MPa (6.32), 23.85 MPa (4.01), and 19.16 MPa (3.72) for Vita VM9, IPS emax Ceram, and Cerabien, respectively. Cerabien ceramic showed more failure as compared to the other ceramics. However, there was no significant difference among the three veneering groups.

Conclusions: Within the limitation of this study, it can be concluded that shear bond strength between zirconia core and three veneering ceramics was not significantly different.

Introduction

All-ceramic restorations have been dramatically improved during the recent decades. The reason for increasing the demand for such restorations is basically aesthetics and biological complications reported about traditional metal-ceramic restorations [1,2]. Among various all-ceramic materials introduced in the recent years, zirconium-oxide (zirconia; ZrO2) ceramic materials are one of the proper options for fixed restorations [3].

According to short and medium-term clinical studies, these materials are an appropriate option for frameworks in terms of stability and strength [4-7]. However, the main disadvantage of zirconia restorations is the chip off fracture of porcelain veneer which has been reported to be higher than that of metal-ceramic ones [8]. Therefore, bonding between veneer and core, and also the mechanical properties of the veneering ceramics play important roles in the success of these restorations [9].

Two types of fractures have been reported for zirconia restorations: cohesive and adhesive fractures. Cohesive failures indicate fractures within core or veneer, while adhesive failure refers to delamination of veneer off the core [10,11]. Factors affecting adhesion and cohesion mechanisms in zirconia restorations are coefficient of thermal expansion (CTE) compatibility between veneer and core, framework surface finish and pretreatments, wettability of veneer on the core, micromechanical retention, and firing process [10,12,13].

Different surface treatments have been suggested to improve veneer-core bonding in the zirconia restorations. Polishing, grinding, sandblasting, silica coating of zirconia surface and the use of laser are among the methods used to increase this bonding through chemical and/or mechanical retention [14-16]. Delamination of veneer off the core occurs as a result of residual stress developed during firing and cooling processes due to coefficient of thermal expansion (CTE) differences between veneer and core, and also incomplete heating of veneer on the core because of low thermal conductivity of zirconia [13,17-23].

The strength of the veneering ceramics, and also their bonding strength to the zirconia core are crucial factors for preventing the fracture of these restorations. There are different veneering ceramics in the market which are claimed they can safely be used with zirconia cores. However, there is not enough scientific data supporting their suitability for this purpose in terms of their bond strength to the zirconia cores. The aim of this study was to evaluate shear bond strength (SBS) of three brands of ceramics as veneering porcelains on zirconia cores. The null hypothesis was that there is no significant difference in the SBS of these veneering ceramics to the zirconia cores.

Materials and Methods

Thirty zirconia-based blocks (Zirkonzahn ,Steger, Ahrntal, Italy) with dimension of 4x4x12 mm were prepared using universal milling machine (Steger, Ahrntal, Italy) (Figure 1. A). The blocks were divided into three groups and placed in the sintering oven (Zirkonzahn, Italy) at room temperature which was raised to 1500 ℃ during 4 hours, and then remained in that temperature for 2 hours. Thereafter, the samples

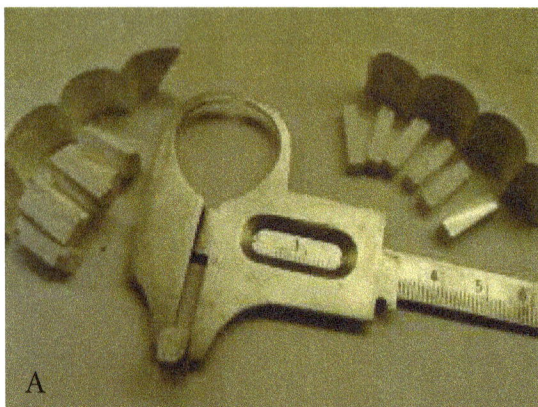

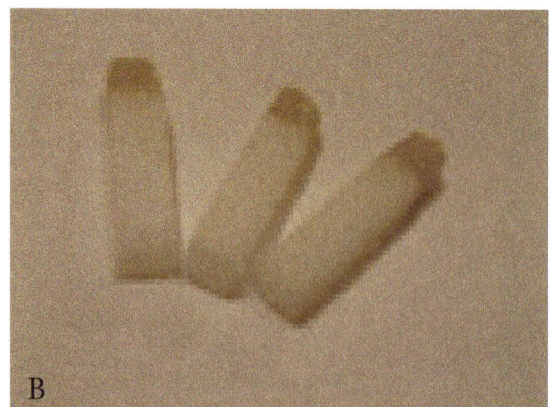

Figure 1: **A.** zirconia-based blocks (Zirkonzahn, Steger, Ahrntal, Italy) prepared at 4x4x12 mm dimensions. **B.** Three brands of veneering ceramics used for layering the zirconia cores.

were bench cooled to the room temperature during 10 hours. All the sintering procedure was followed according to the manufacturer's recommendation.

The bonding surface of the core blocks were finished using silicon carbide papers, grit 800 and then 1200 (Matador, Germany) in combination with water spray. Then, they were treated by 50 μm air-borne particles of aluminum oxide with 2 bar pressure, for 10 seconds with 10 mm distance to the blocks. Subsequently, the blocks were cleaned in the ultrasonic bath, with 10 ml of 70% methanol alcohol for 5 minutes, and then they were dried using an oil free air compressor (Nardi compressor model extreme; Italy) at the end [22].

One of three veneering ceramics was used in each group: IPS emax Ceram (Ivoclar-Vivadent, Schaan, Liehtenstien), Vita VM9 (Vita, Bad Sackingen, Germany), and Cerabien ZR (Noritake, Nagoya, Japan) (Table 1), (Figure 1.B). Each veneering ceramic was baked on ten zirconia cores (4x4x3 mm) at the manufacturer's recommended temperature. A thin layer of shade base (liner) was applied on the cores at first and preheated at 600 °C for 6 minutes

an appropriate amount of the respective liquid were mixed to form the sticky slurry, which was filled into the mould [22].

The same firing procedure was performed for firing the veneer ceramics according to the manufacturer's instruction, except for the firing temperature that was 930 °C. The samples were then mounted in the universal testing machine (Zwick Roell AG, Ulm, Germany) for measuring the shear bond strength between the veneers and the cores. The shear force at the crosshead speed of 1mm/min was applied vertically to the bonding interface until the fracture occurred. The resultant force (N) was divided by the bonding area (mm²) [Shear Stress (Mpa) = Load (N)/Area (mm²)]. One-way ANOVA was used to compare the mean shear bond strength between the groups. ZPV-test XPERT software V11.02 was used for statistical analysis. The level of significance was set to be 0.05.

Results

The mean and standard deviation (SD) of shear

Table 1: Presentation of the three veneering ceramics used in the study

Ceramics	Type	Liner lot No.	Liquid lot No.	Dentin lot No.	Manufacturer
Cerabien ZR	Feldespathic	OE720	OEY01	201611	Noritake, Nagoya, Japan
IPS e.max Ceram	Lithium disilicate	H30927	H33669	H24320	Ivoclar, Schaan
VM9	Feldsphatic	15420	7728	30580	Vita, BadSackingen, Germany

according to the manufacturer. Then, the oven temperature was raised to 950 °C for 4 minutes in the vacuum condition and maintained in this temperature for 1 minute with no vacuum. Thereafter, the oven door was opened when the temperature was decreased to 600 °C. The samples were bench cooled to the room temperature before applying the veneer ceramics. To standardize the porcelain veneer thickness, a plastic split mould cavity was used. Ceramic powder and

bond strength of each group is presented in Table 2. According to the results, Vita VM9 showed the highest bond strength to the zirconia cores (26.03 MPa). The lowest value of shear bond strength was observed in the group with Cerabien ceramic (19.16 MPa). The shear bond strength of IPS emax Ceram group was (23.85 MPa). However, there was no statistically significant difference between the three groups in terms of shear bond strength ($p > 0.188$).

Table 2: The mean values, standard deviation (SD), minimum and maximum of shear bond strength of the study groups

Core/Veneer	Mean SBS (MPa)	SD	Minimum (MPa)	Maximum (MPa)
Zirkonzah/Vita VM9	26.03	6.32	16.68	64.43
Zirkonzahn/IPS e.max Ivoclar	23.85	4.01	16.55	34.69
Zirkonzahn/Cerabien ZR Noritake	19.16	3.72	13.46	25.55

Discussion

The null hypothesis was supported since there was no statically significant difference between the shear bond strength of three tested veneering ceramics to the zirconia cores. The shear bond strength (SBS) test was used in the current study to measure the bond strength of three different veneering ceramics to the zirconia cores of one single brand (Zirkonzahn). Zirconium-based restorations are one of the popular aesthetic restorations that provide both esthetic and function as fixed restorations. However, one of the concerns about these restorations is the bond strength between the veneer and core which might result in debonding during function[13,17,18].

Despite the existence of a standard test of bond strength (three point bending test) and a minimum of 25 MPa bonding strength for veneering ceramic to the metal substructure in metal-ceramic restorations [24], there is no standardized test and a minimum vital bond strength for all-ceramic restorations yet [25]. There are different tests for evaluating the bond strength of veneer to the underlying ceramic core in all-ceramic restorations, including shear bond test [25], microtensile test [22], three and four point bending [26], and biaxial flexure strength tests [12]. The selected test in the current study was shear bond strength which is a simple and reliable test. However, this method may produce more non-uniform stresses at the interface in comparison to microtensile bond test [20]. Nevertheless, cracks at the adhesive zone may be induced during specimen preparation by the cutting and preparing the samples.

The reported core-veneer bond strength in all-ceramic samples reported by previous studies ranged from 9.4 MPa to 42 MPa. [10,17,22,25]. The mean SBS values in the present study (19.16, 23.85, 26.03) also comply with the range reported by other studies. However, none of the aforementioned studies have investigated the exact ceramic brands as veneering and core ceramics.

There are several factors that might have an effect on the bond strength of the veneer to the zirconia core, including cooling rate, polishing, sandblasting/silica coating of the zirconia surface, properties of veneer and core material, use of a liner material, use of colouring green stage zirconia, firing time duration, cooling rate, and thermo cycling, and thermal compatibility between core and veneer (CTE) [15-23]. Plastic and elastic deformations of the metallic frameworks could approximately compensate for the excessive stresses arising from coefficient of thermal expansion mismatch in metal-ceramic systems [27].

However, the zirconia framework has a higher rigidity and, therefore, can cause more destructive stresses in zirconia-based restorations [28]. Therefore, using veneering ceramics with the least coefficient of thermal expansion difference is crucial for success of all-ceramic restorations. In this study, we used veneering ceramics with acceptable thermal expansion coefficient ranges in relation to zirconia core ($9.1-10.2\times10^6$/K). According to Fischer et al. [19], the mean CTE of zirconia is 10.8/K, while the mean CTE of IPS emax Ceram, VM9, and Cerabien ZR are 10.4, 9.3, and 9.9/K, respectively.

The resultant mean SBS values of three different veneering ceramics to the zirconia cores were not significantly different which supported the null hypothesis. The small difference of CTE between the core and the veneering ceramics had minimal effect on the bond strength of the samples. This might explain the acceptable SBS of all the veneering ceramics to the zirconia core. Also, following manufacturer instruction in surface preparation and firing procedure ensures achieving the results claimed by the veneering ceramic manufacturer regarding the compatibility with a zirconia core. Furthermore, according to Aktas et al. [20], the veneering ceramic properties affected the results of shear bond strength to the zirconia core, although neither the zirconia core material nor colouring had significant effects on the results. However, they used different veneer and core materials in their study, except for IPS e.max Ceram as one of the veneering ceramics.

Also, Fazi et al. [21] showed that tensile strength of VitaVM9 veneer ceramic to the zirconia core was more than other veneering ceramics including Creation ZI and Lava ceram, although there was no significant difference between the three groups. This is in agreement with the findings of this study. However, Ozkurt et al. [17] observed that the SBS of VitaVM9 veneer ceramic to the Zirkonzahn cores was significantly greater than other groups in their study. However, Aboushelib et al. [22] revealed high SBS between a press-on ceramic and a Cercon zirconia core37.9) MPa). Although the veneering and core materials in their study was different, this finding might indicate that the press-on technique could result in a more strong bond between veneer and core ceramics as compared to the layering technique.

Nevertheless, the results of most of the studies that performed macro shear bond test showed that most fractures occurred in the veneering layer (cohesive failure) [25-28]. This finding implies that the feldspathic ceramics used with layering technique might not provide sufficient strength for veneering of zirconia cores in the final result. Therefore, comparing feldspathic and press-on ceramics in terms of their acceptability for usage with zirconia cores also need to be addressed in terms of the prevalence of cohesive and adhesive failures. It has also been shown that cyclic loading can be a cause of premature cracking and failure [15-23]. Feldspathic porcelain veneer is more sensitive to both static contacts and cyclic loading [29].

In order to perform a valid comparison between the studies, one should consider all the possible factors and conditions that might have an effect on the results. Some interfering factors such as storage conditions, type of specimen used, the preparation method, rate of load application, cross-sectional

surface area, and the operator experience are effective in the findings of the studies [17]. The limitations of the present study suggest that future studies should be performed under dynamic loadings, in a humid environment, simultaneous testing of the effect of modifying the core surface, and also considering the effect of core geometry on the final results. Also, other brands of zirconia cores and veneering ceramics need to be studied using other testing modalities before use in the clinical situations.

Conclusions

Within the limitation of the present study, there was no significant difference between three veneering ceramics (IPS emax Ceram, Vita VM9, and Cerabien ZR) to the zirconia cores (Zirkonzahn) in terms of shear bond strength.

Conflicts of interest: None declared.

References

1. Raigrodski AJ. Contemporary materials and technologies for all-ceramic fixed partial dentures: a review of the literature. J Prosthet Dent. 2004;92:557-562.
2. Blatz MB. Long-term clinical success of all-ceramic posterior restorations. Quintessence Int. 2002;33:415-426.
3. Denry I, Kelly JR. State of the art of zirconia for dental applications. Dent Mater. 2008;24:299-307.
4. Kim HJ, Lim HP, Park YJ, et al. Effect of zirconia surface treatments on the shear bond strength of veneering ceramic. J Prosthet Dent. 2011;105:315-322.
5. Raigrodski AJ, Chiche GJ, Potiket N, et al. The efficacy of posterior three-unit zirconium-oxide-based ceramic fixed partial dental prostheses: a prospective clinical pilot study. J Prosthet Dent. 2006;96:237-244.
6. Sailer I, Fehér A, Filser F, et al. Five-year clinical results of zirconia frameworks for posterior fixed partial dentures. Int J Prosthodont. 2007;20:383-388.
7. Roediger M, Gersdorff N, Huels A, et al. Prospective evaluation of zirconia posterior fixed partial dentures: four-year clinical results.

Int J Prosthodont. 2010;23:141-148.

8. Sailer I, Bjarni E, Pjetursson BE, *et al.* A Systematic review of the survival and complication rates of all-ceramic and metal-ceramic reconstructions after an observation period of at least 3 years. Part II: Fixed partial prostheses. Clin Oral Implants Res. 2007;18:86-96.

9. Guazzato M, Proos K, Sara G, *et al.* Strength, reliability, and mode of fracture of bilayered porcelain/core ceramics. Int J Prosthodont. 2004;17:142-149.

10. Choi BK, Han JS, Yang JH, *et al.* Shear bond strength of veneering porcelain to zirconia and metal cores. J Adv Prosthodont. 2009;1:129-135.

11. Anusavice KJ, Phillips RW. Phillips' science of dental materials. 11th Edition. St. Louis: W.B. Saunders: 2003.

12. Isgrò G, Pallav P, van der Zel JM, *et al.* The influence of the veneering porcelain and different surface treatments on the biaxial flexural strength of a heat-pressed ceramic. J Prosthet Dent. 2003;90:465-473.

13. Guazzato M, Walton TR, Franklin W, *et al.* Influence of thickness and cooling rate on development of spontaneous cracks in porcelain/zirconia structures. Aust Dent J. 2010;55:306-310.

14. Nishigori A, Yoshida T, Bottino MC, *et al.* Influence of zirconia surface treatment on veneering porcelain shear bond strength after cyclic loading. J Prosthet Dent. 2014;112:1392-1398.

15. Teng J, Wang H, Liao Y, *et al.* Evaluation of a conditioning method to improve core-veneer bond strength of zirconia restorations. J Prosthet Dent. 2012;107:380-387.

16. Liu D, Matinlinna JP, Tsoi JK, *et al.* A new modified laser pretreatment for porcelain zirconia bonding. Dent Mater. 2013;29:559-565.

17. Ozkurt Z, Kazazoglu E, Unal A. *In vitro* evaluation of shear bond strength of veneering ceramics to zirconia. Dent Mater J. 2010;29:138-146.

18. Swain MV. Unstable cracking (chipping) of veneering porcelain on all-ceramic dental crowns and fixed partial dentures. Acta Biomater. 2009;5:1668-1677.

19. Fischer J, Stawarzcyk B, Trottmann A, *et al.* Impact of thermal misfit on shear strength of veneering ceramic/zirconia composites. Dent Mater. 2009;25:419-423.

20. Aktas G, Sahin E, Vallittu P, *et al.* Effect of colouring green stage zirconia on the adhesion of veneering ceramics with different thermal expansion coefficients. Int J Oral Sci. 2013;5:236-241.

21. Fazi G, Vichi A, Ferrari M. Microtensile bond strength of three different veneering porcelain systems to a zirconia core for all ceramic restorations. Am J Dent. 2010;23:347-350.

22. Aboushelib MN, de Jager N, Kleverlaan CJ, *et al.* Microtensile bond strength of different components of core veneered all-ceramic restorations. Dent Mater. 2005;21:984-991.

23. Komine F, Saito A, Kobayashi K, *et al.* Effect of cooling rate on shear bond strength of veneering porcelain to a zirconia ceramic material. J Oral Sci. 2010;52:647-652.

24. International Organization for Standardization; ISO 9693 Metal-ceramic bond characterization (Schwickerath crack initiation test). Geneva, Switzerland.1999.

25. Al-Dohan HM, Yaman P, Dennison JB, *et al.* Shear strength of core-veneer interface in bi-layered ceramics. J Prosthet Dent. 2004;91:349–355.

26. White SN, Miklus VG, McLaren EA, *et al.* Flexural strength of a layered zirconia and porcelain dental all-ceramic system. J Prosthet Dent. 2005;94:125–131.

27. Anusavice KJ, Carroll JE. Effect of incompatibility stress on the fit of metal-ceramic crowns. J Dent Res. 1987;66:1341-1345.

28. Fischer J, Stawarczyk B, Hämmerle CH. Flexural strength of veneering ceramics for zirconia. J Dent. 2008;36:316-321.

29. Rueda AO, Anglada M, Jimenez-Pique E. Contact fatigue of veneer feldspathic porcelain on dental zirconia. Dent Mater. 2015;31:217-224.

Relevance of Micro-leakage to Orthodontic Bonding

Karandish M[a,b]

[a]Health Policy Research Center, Shiraz University of Medical Sciences, Shiraz, Iran
[b]Department of Orthodontics, Dental School, Shiraz University of Medical Sciences, Shiraz, Iran

ARTICLE INFO	Abstract

Key words:
Bonding
Orthodontic Brackets
Micro-leakage

Corresponding Author:
Maryam Karandish
Department of Orthodontics,
Dental School, Shiraz
University of Medical
Sciences, Shiraz, Iran.
Email: karandishm@sums.ac.ir

As it is seen, by passing the evolutionary process of banding of orthodontic attachments to the bonding ones, orthodontics have witnessed many developments, such as application of new adhesives, optimized base designs, new bracket materials, curing methods and more efficient primers. The studies often address the morphological, micro-leakage, and shear bond tests to evaluate bond efficacy. Among studies endeavored to develop the bond strength of brackets, some observed the reduction of micro-leakage of bracket-adhesive and enamel-adhesive interfaces. Owing to the importance of micro-leakage in orthodontics, this study aimed at reviewing the micro-leakage values directly relevant to the enamel decay and debonding of the brackets. To reach the best bond strength, the researchers tried to design different studies to evaluate the effect of variables and prevent any possible side effects in clinical situations. It is noticed that most studies have mainly focused on adhesives, enamel preparation and methods of curing which are discussed in this review. The literature was reviewed by searching databases, using micro-leakage and orthodontic bonding as the keywords. Having found the relevant studies, the researchers entered them into the database. After reviewing numerous studies conducted in this field, the type of adhesive or curing method was not found to have determinative role in the value of micro-leakage although more standardized studies are needed.

Introduction

One of the challenges in orthodontics is the bond strength between the bracket base and the enamel surface. In restorative dentistry discoloration of the restoration margins, caries, dental sensitivity and apparent failure of the restorations are mentioned as the results of micro-leakage [1]. The reduction in marginal integrity in this junction would causes debonding of brackets during orthodontic treatment [2-4]. Moreover, bacterial accumulation causes white spot lesions during the orthodontic treatment under the influence of unfavorable bond [1-4]. Polymerase shrinkage of bonding materials, in addition to intermittent thermal cycle of mouth [5] due to hot and cold meals and mechanical loads, reinforces the marginal gaps.

Different thermal expansion coefficients between Enamel ($\alpha = 12$ ppm/°C), adhesive ($\alpha = 20$–55 ppm/°C) and bracket base ($\alpha = 16$ ppm/°C) [6] will add a shear stress to the bond strength because of repeated expansion and contraction [7,8]. Fluid shift at the brackets-adhesive and enamel-adhesive interfaces and the lytic effect of water on the adhesive will form either large gaps or will cause debonding of brackets [5,7,9,10].

To reach the best bond strength, the researchers tried to design different studies to evaluate the effect of variables and prevent side effects in the clinical setting. Some of the studies focused on the effect of different adhesive materials, such as different self-etch primers [11-13], resin modified glass ionomers [14] and nanocomposites [15]. To reach the optimal bond , others applied different enamel preparations, such as application of brome-lain and papaein gel [16], calcium silicate-sodium phosphate salts or resin infiltration [17] laser beam [18-21], air and bur abrasion [22] and different curing methods [23,24]. Some other researchers emphasized using new bracket materials [25], coat-ing the bracket surface [26] and/or using optimized bracket base designs [27].

Having reviewed relevant studies performed, we noticed that after the banding of orthodontic attachments was replaced by the bonding ones, orthodontics underwent significant developments including the application of new adhesives, opti-mized base designs, new bracket materials, curing methods as well as more efficient primers. The studies often addressed the morphological, mi-cro-leakage, and shear bond tests to evaluate the efficacy of the bond [7,28].

Among studies conducted to develop bond strength of brackets, some observed the reduction of micro-leakage of bracket-adhesive and enamel-ad-hesive interfaces [29,30]. As numerous studies have been carried out to investigate the effect of micro-leakage in bracket debonding and white spot lesions during orthodontic treatment and as there, at times, has not been consensus among their find-ings, the current study has reviewed the parameters of micro-leakage value which are directly relevant to the enamel decay and debonding of the brackets.

Materials and Methods

Medline and EMBASE electronic database search-

es were undertaken. Search terms included ortho-dontic brackets and micro-leakage.

Results

With a simple search and after deleting the common papers, 35 papers were encountered. The papers with English full text were adopted. After a gross review on the title and abstracts, the more relevant studies comprising 32 articles were included. The papers discussing the micro-leakage of orthodontic bands were also excluded from the study

Discussion

Although there is some evidence showing no correlation between micro-leakage and clinical parameters in restorative dentistry [31], sever-al other studies insist on its adverse effects in orthodontics [5,7,9,10].

In order to investigate the micro-leakage accurately, the researchers have to use the related laboratory lab promptly. To accomplish this, each laboratory test in medical studies should fulfill some requirements- described for medical devices and compiled entitled "*Good Laboratory Practice*" by regulatory authorities such as the *Food & Drug Administration* (FDA) in Washington or the Eu-ropean authorities in Brussels in the 1970s and 1990s- respectively to be nominated internally valid [32]. The requirements are as follows: repro-ducible results, known parameters, acceptable and low variability of measured values and application of suitable devices for given purposes. On the other hand, the correlation of results with clinical find-ings addresses the external validity.

Considering this principle, we observed different methods used in evaluating micro-leakage beneath orthodontic brackets, as shown below.

The effect of adhesives on micro-leakage

The majority of studies conducted in this field were related to the application of different adhe-sives or modification of these materials. Although Buyuk *et al.* reported lower micro-leakage in low-shrinking composites, they found insufficient shear bond strength and adhesive remnant score [33] not clinically relevant. Kim *et al.* did not find significant differences between APC flash-free adhesive coated and PLUS adhesive coated system brackets [34]. Using a resin coat reduces the value of micro-leakage of orthodontic brackets [35].

Various studies were performed on the application of self-etch vs. acid-etch primers and its effect on the micro-leakage. Pakshir and Ajami, for example, did not find any statistically significant differences in micro-leakage using Transbond XT primer [36]. In a more comprehensive study [37] conducted on the effect of three self-adhesive resin cements, namely (Maxcem Elite, Relyx U 100 and Clearfil SA Cement), three two-step self-etch bonding system (Clearfil SE Bond, Clearfil Protecbond and Clearfil Liner Bond), three one-step self-etch bonding system (Transbond Plus SEP, Bond Force and Clearfil S3) and three total-etching bonding system (Transbond XT, GreenGlue and Kurasper F) on micro-leakage, it was not found to be directly related to the type of adhesive. To confirm the findings of these studies, Shahabi observed the same value for micro-leakage in spite of the lowest shear bond strength in self-etch primers (SEP) [38]. Uysal et al. adopted Transbond Plus Self-etching Primer vs Transbond XT. In contrast to previously addressed studies, they reported more micro-leakage in the application of self-etch primers [39].

Vicente et al. demonstrated that resin composites and flowable composites had poor performance after thermocycling [40]. Resin modified glass ionomers (RMGI) resulted in more micro-leakage especially at the enamel-adhesive interface [41]. The study performed on rebonding brackets found no differences in micro-leakage using various adhesive removal methods [42].

In comparison with direct and indirect bonding techniques, it was observed that applying different adhesives had no effects on micro-leakage [43]. This finding was verified by Ozturk et al. [44]. Canbek et al. compared human and bovine teeth for the evaluation of micro-leakage beneath the brackets. They reached the conclusion that unlike the thermocycled specimens, the value of micro-leakage in human teeth was less in the absence of thermocycling [7].

The effect of enamel preparation on micro-leakage
Some other studies applied different enamel preparations to investigate the differences in

micro-leakage. Toodehzaeim et al., for instance, found no differences between 1.5 and 2.5 watt Er:YAG laser and acid-etch preparation [19] although in a previous study, acid-etching appeared to have superior properties than laser preparation [45]. Furthermore, application of NaF 2% was reported to decrease micro-leakage on hypomineralised enamel [46].

The effect of contamination on micro-leakage
In a number of studies, the effect of contamination was addressed. Kustarci et al. found no differences in micro-leakage value between chlorhexidine gluconate, Clearfil Protect Bond and KTP laser [47]. Micro-leakage caused by enamel erosion increased in the presence of drinks. This might imply that these drinks could cause loss of adhesive materials [48]. Effect of saliva contamination in deteriorating the micro-leakage value was reported to be more evident in enamel adhesive interface [49]. Thus, debonding of brackets was more likely than decay on enamel surface.

The effect of light curing on micro-leakage
Having compared LED with Plasma arc units, Davari et al. observed that LED led to more micro-leakage value [23]. Ulker, however, found no differences in micro-leakage value of high and low- intensity curing units [50]. Micro-leakage beneath ceramic brackets was less with the protocol of curing with LEDs than with conventional curing unit [51].

Modules for evaluation of micro-leakage
Sample preparation
Almost all studies share a common method in preparation of samples for micro-leakage studies. After preparation of tooth surfaces and immersing them in a dye solution, the researcher began testing them. However, because of the ability of fluorescent dye to penetrate into the tubules, distorting results are inevitable [52,53]. In most studies conducted in this field, methylene blue is the optional choice [49,54]. The organic base of this molecule is combined with acid and its size is somehow smaller than the size of bacteria, helping the methylene blue to penetrate the tubules [6,54,55]. Unlike some other researchers, Ozturk et al. applied silver nitrate solution [44]. They could not detect

penetration of dye because the particle could not penetrate into mini gaps.

Microscopic evaluation methods

The efficiency of microscopic evaluations can be determined through assessing the penetration depth, the quality and thickness of the hybrid layer [31]. After adhesive marked with a fluorescent dye, the researchers evaluated the specimen microscopically with a scanning electron microscope (SEM), a fluorescence microscope, the light microscope [34] or a confocal laser scanning microscope (CLSM).

On the other hand, most researchers [49-51,56,57] adopted stereomicroscope as an aid to evaluate the micro-leakage beneath orthodontic brackets. Arhun *et al.* reported more leakage at adhesive-bracket interface of metal brackets [56]. In addition, most researchers evaluated both the gingival and incisal margins [51]. Generally speaking, the stereomicroscope has the advantage of greater depth perception and allowing viewers to see objects in three dimensions but with low magnification.

The light microscope and SEM can qualitatively measure micro-leakage but they are dependent on a software program [58]. Some researchers adopted dye penetration light microscope evaluation. Kim *et al*, for instance, evaluated micro-leakage beneath ceramic brackets [34]. Although not statistically significant, they found higher median micro-leakage in the Flash-Free group. In addition, Canbek *et al.* evaluated the cervical and incisal bracket surfaces for excess bonding material using this technique [7]. They also analyzed dye penetration and adhesive-bracket and adhesive-enamel micro-leakage. However, Chapra *et al*, by adding surface-penetrating sealants, reached different results [29]. They found better marginal integrity both in unsealed and sealed groups. Buyuk [33] and Vicente [40] also applied this method. Vicente evaluated micro-leakage with the image analysis equipment to interpret the data. Navarro used SEM to evaluate the micro-leakage value [48] but Ozturk adopted micro CT [44]. To reduce the variability in the subjective evaluation of micro-leakage value, it is strictly recommended to increase the reproducibility of the results with the help of one examiner. The intra-operator variability (2-8%) is significant-

ly less than inter-operative one (10-20%) [31].

Conclusions

Micro-leakage is one of the challenging topics in orthodontics. Scientific evidence has focused on the indispensable role of micro-leakage in bracket debonding and white spot lesions during orthodontic treatment. Generally, it seems that the type of adhesive or curing method does not have determinative role in the value of micro-leakage. Less micro-leakage is seen at the bracket-adhesive interface of the ceramic brackets. The most popular method to evaluate the micro-leakage is the analysis under a stereomicroscope.

Conflict of Interest: None declared.

References

1. Youssef MN, Youssef FA, Souza-Zaroni WC, *et al*. Effect of enamel preparation method on in vitro marginal microleakage of a flowable composite used as pit and fissure sealant. Int J Paediatr Dent. 2006;16:342-347.
2. Oesterle LJ, Newman SM, Shellhart WC. Comparative bond strength of brackets cured using a pulsed xenon curing light with 2 different light-guide sizes. Am J Orthod Dentofacial Orthop. 2002;122:242-250.
3. James JW, Miller BH, English JD, *et al*. Effects of high-speed curing devices on shear bond strength and microleakage of orthodontic brackets. Am J Orthod Dentofacial Orthop. 2003;123:555-561.
4. Sabzevari B, Ramazanzadeh BA, Moazzami SM, *et al*. Microleakage under Orthodontic Metal Brackets Bonded with Three Different Bonding Techniques with/without Thermocycling. J Dent Mater Tech. 2013;2:21-28.
5. Bishara SE, Ajlouni R, Laffoon JF. Effect of thermocycling on the shear bond strength of a cyanoacrylate orthodontic adhesive. Am J Orthod Dentofacial Orthop. 2003;123:21-24.
6. Mahal RS. A Standardized Approach to Determine the Effect of Thermocycling and Long Term Storage on the Shear Bond Strength of Orthodontic Brackets Cemented to Bovine Enamel. National Library of Canada: Univer-

sity of Toronto; 2000.

7. Canbek K, Karbach M, Gottschalk F, *et al*. Evaluation of bovine and human teeth exposed to thermocycling for microleakage under bonded metal brackets. J Orofac Orthop. 2013;74:102-112.

8. Bishara SE, Ostby AW, Laffoon JF, *et al*. Shear bond strength comparison of two adhesive systems following thermocycling. A new self-etch primer and a resin-modified glass ionomer. Angle Orthod. 2007;77:337-341.

9. Arnold RW, Combe EC, Warford JH Jr. Bonding of stainless steel brackets to enamel with a new self-etching primer. Am J Orthod Dentofacial Orthop. 2002;122:274-276.

10. Causton BE, Johnson NW. Changes in the dentine of human teeth following extraction and their implication for in-vitro studies of adhesion to tooth substance. Arch Oral Biol. 1979;24:229-232.

11. Schauseil M, Blocher S, Hellak A, *et al*. Shear bond strength and debonding characteristics of a new premixed self-etching with a reference total-etch adhesive. Head Face Med. 2016;12:19.

12. Ousehal L, El Aouame A, Rachdy Z, *et al*. Comparison of the efficacy of a conventional primer and a self-etching primer. Int Orthod. 2016;14:195-205.

13. Atram H, Jakati SV, Aley M, *et al*. Clearfil Protect Bond(™) versus Uni-Etch(™) antibacterial self-etchant: A war of giants against shear bond strength. Indian J Dent Res. 2016;27:54-60.

14. Elnafar AA, Alam MK, Hasan R. The impact of surface preparation on shear bond strength of metallic orthodontic brackets bonded with a resin-modified glass ionomer cement. J Orthod. 2014;41:201-207.

15. Uysal T, Yagci A, Uysal B, *et al*. Are nano-composites and nano-ionomers suitable for orthodontic bracket bonding? Eur J Orthod. 2010;32:78-82.

16. Pithon MM, Campos MS, Coqueiro Rda S. Effect of bromelain and papain gel on enamel deproteinisation before orthodontic bracket bonding. Aust Orthod J. 2016;32:23-30.

17. Costenoble A, Vennat E, Attal JP, *et al*. Bond strength and interfacial morphology of orthodontic brackets bonded to eroded enamel treated with calcium silicate-sodium phosphate salts or resin infiltration. Angle Orthod. 2016.

18. Zhang ZC, Qian YF, Yang YM, *et al*. Bond strength of metal brackets bonded to a silica-based ceramic with light-cured adhesive : Influence of various surface treatment methods. J Orofac Orthop. 2016.

19. Toodehzaeim MH, Yassaei S, Karandish M, *et al*. In vitro evaluation of microleakage around orthodontic brackets using laser etching and Acid etching methods. J Dent (Tehran). 2014;11:263-269.

20. Aglarci C, Demir N, Aksakalli S, *et al*. Bond strengths of brackets bonded to enamel surfaces conditioned with femtosecond and Er:YAG laser systems. Lasers Med Sci. 2016;31:1177-1183.

21. Karandish M. The efficiency of laser application on the enamel surface: a systematic review. J Lasers Med Sci. 2014;5:108-114.

22. Charles A, Senkutvan R, Ramya RS, *et al*. Evaluation of shear bond strength with different enamel pretreatments: an in vitro study. Indian J Dent Res. 2014;25:470-474.

23. Davari A, Yassaei S, Karandish M, *et al*. In vitro evaluation of microleakage under ceramic and metal brackets bonded with LED and plasma arc curing. J Contemp Dent Pract. 2012;13:644-649.

24. Heravi F, Moazzami SM, Ghaffari N, *et al*. Evaluation of shear bond strength of orthodontic brackets using trans-illumination technique with different curing profiles of LED light-curing unit in posterior teeth. Prog Orthod. 2013;14:49.

25. Foersch M, Schuster C, Rahimi RK, *et al*. A new flash-free orthodontic adhesive system: A first clinical and stereomicroscopic study. Angle Orthod. 2016;86:260-264.

26. Cao B, Wang Y, Li N, *et al*. Preparation of an orthodontic bracket coated with an nitrogen-doped TiO(2-x)N(y) thin film and examination of its antimicrobial performance. Dent Mater J. 2013;32:311-316.

27. Shyagali TR, Bhayya DP, Urs CB, *et al*. Finite element study on modification of bracket base and its effects on bond strength. Dental Press J Orthod. 2015;20:76-82.

28. Lopes MB, Consani S, Gonini-Junior A, et al. Comparison of microleakage in human and bovine substrates using confocal microscopy. Bull Tokyo Dent Coll. 2009;50:111-116.

29. Chapra A, White GE. Leakage reduction with a surface-penetrating sealant around stainless-steel orthodontic brackets bonded with a light cured composite resin. J Clin Pediatr Dent. 2003;27:271-276.

30. Wilson RM, Donly KJ. Demineralization around orthodontic brackets bonded with resin-modified glass ionomer cement and fluoride-releasing resin composite. Pediatr Dent. 2001;23:255-259.

31. Heintze SD. Clinical relevance of tests on bond strength, microleakage and marginal adaptation. Dent Mater. 2013;29:59-84.

32. FDA. Good laboratory practice (GLP); 1978 [PART 58 52 FR 33780, 1978, last revision 2004].

33. Buyuk SK, Cantekin K, Demirbuga S, et al. Are the low-shrinking composites suitable for orthodontic bracket bonding? Eur J Dent. 2013;7:284-288.

34. Kim J, Kanavakis G, Finkelman MD, et al. Microleakage under ceramic flash-free orthodontic brackets after thermal cycling. Angle Orthod. 2016.

35. Abdelnaby YL, Al-Wakeel EE. Influence of modifying the resin coat application protocol on bond strength and microleakage of metal orthodontic brackets. Angle Orthod. 2010;80:378-384.

36. Pakshir H, Ajami S. Effect of Enamel Preparation and Light Curing Methods on Microleakage under Orthodontic Brackets. J Dent (Tehran). 2015;12:436-446.

37. Alkis H, Turkkahraman H, Adanir N. Microleakage under orthodontic brackets bonded with different adhesive systems. Eur J Dent. 2015;9:117-121.

38. Shahabi M, Ahrari F, Mohamadipour H, et al. Microleakage and shear bond strength of orthodontc brackets bonded to hypomineralized enamel following different surface preparations. J Clin Exp Dent. 2014;6:110-115.

39. Uysal T, Ulker M, Ramoglu SI, et al. Microleakage under metallic and ceramic brackets bonded with orthodontic self-etching primer systems. Angle Orthod. 2008;78:1089-1094.

40. Vicente A, Ortiz AJ, Bravo LA. Microleakage beneath brackets bonded with flowable materials: effect of thermocycling. Eur J Orthod. 2009;31:390-396.

41. Ramoglu SI, Uysal T, Ulker M, et al. Microleakage under ceramic and metallic brackets bonded with resin-modified glass ionomer. Angle Orthod. 2009;79:183-143.

42. Tudehzaeim MH, Yassaei S, Taherimoghadam S. Comparison of Microleakage under Rebonded Stainless Steel Orthodontic Brackets Using Two Methods of Adhesive Removal: Sandblast and Laser. J Dent (Tehran). 2015;12:118-124.

43. Yagci A, Uysal T, Ulker M, et al. Microleakage under orthodontic brackets bonded with the custom base indirect bonding technique. Eur J Orthod. 2010;32:259-263.

44. Ozturk F, Ersoz M, Ozturk SA, et al. Micro-CT evaluation of microleakage under orthodontic ceramic brackets bonded with different bonding techniques and adhesives. Eur J Orthod. 2016;38:163-169.

45. Hamamci N, Akkurt A, Basaran G. In vitro evaluation of microleakage under orthodontic brackets using two different laser etching, self etching and acid etching methods. Lasers Med Sci. 2010;25:811-816.

46. Moosavi H, Ahrari F, Mohamadipour H. The effect of different surface treatments of demineralised enamel on microleakage under metal orthodontic brackets. Prog Orthod. 2013;14:2.

47. Kustarci A, Sokucu O. Effect of chlorhexidine gluconate, Clearfil Protect Bond, and KTP laser on microleakage under metal orthodontic brackets with thermocycling. Photomed Laser Surg. 2010;28:57-62.

48. Navarro R, Vicente A, Ortiz AJ, et al. The effects of two soft drinks on bond strength, bracket microleakage, and adhesive remnant on intact and sealed enamel. Eur J Orthod. 2011;33:60-65.

49. Toodehzaeim MH, Rezaie N. Effect of Saliva Contamination on Microleakage Beneath Bonded Brackets: A Comparison Between Two Moisture-Tolerant Bonding Systems. J Dent (Tehran). 2015;12:747-755.

50. Ulker M, Uysal T, Ramoglu SI , et al. Microleakage under orthodontic brackets using

high-intensity curing lights. Angle Orthod. 2009;79:144-149.

51. Arikan S, Arhun N, Arman A, *et al*. Microleakage beneath ceramic and metal brackets photopolymerized with LED or conventional light curing units. Angle Orthod. 2006;76:1035-1040.

52. Watson TF. Fact and artefact in confocal microscopy. Adv Dent Res. 1997;11:433-441.

53. Van Meerbeek B, Vargas M, Inoue S, *et al*. Microscopy investigations. Techniques, results, limitations. Am J Dent. 2000;13:3-18.

54. Yavuz I, Aydin H, Ulku R, *et al*. A new method: measurement of microleakage volume using human, dog and bovine permanent teeth. Elec J Biotech. 2006;9:8-17.

55. Lopes MB, Sinhoreti MA, Gonini Junior A,*et al*. Comparative study of tubular diameter and quantity for human and bovine dentin at different depths. Braz Dental J. 2009;20:279-283.

56. Arhun N, Arman A, Cehreli SB, *et al*. Microleakage beneath ceramic and metal brackets bonded with a conventional and an antibacterial adhesive system. Angle Orthod. 2006;76:1028-1034.

57. Uysal T, Ramoglu SI, Ulker M, *et al*. Effects of high-intensity curing lights on microleakage under orthodontic bands. Am J Orthod Dentofacial Orthop. 2010;138:201-207

58. Heintze SD, Ruffieux C, Rousson V. Clinical performance of cervical restorations--a meta-analysis. Dent Mater. 2010;26:993-1000.

Concentration of Calcium, Phosphate and Fluoride Ions in Microbial Plaque and Saliva after Using CPP-ACP Paste in 6-9 Year-old Children

Poureslami HR[a], Hoseinifar Ra[b], Hoseinifar Re[c], Sharifi H[d], Poureslami P[e]

[a]Oral and Dental Diseases Research Center AND Kerman Social Determinants on Oral Health Research Center AND Department of Pediatric Dentistry, School of Dentistry, Kerman University of Medical Sciences, Kerman, Iran
[b]Department of Operative Dentistry, School of Dentistry, Kerman University of Medical Science. Kerman, Iran
[c]Department of Pediatric Dentistry, School of Dentistry, Kerman University of Medical Sciences, Kerman, Iran
[d]Regional Knowledge Hub, and WHO Collaborating Centre for HIV Surveillance, Kerman University of Medical Sciences, Kerman, Iran
[e]School of Dentistry, Mashhad University of Medical Sciences, Mashhad, Iran

ARTICLE INFO	Abstract
Key words: Dental Plaque Fluoride Calcium *Corresponding Author:* Reihaneh Hoseinifar Department of Pediatric Dentistry, School of Dentistry, Kerman University of Medical Sciences, Kerman, Iran Email: reihanehosseinifar@ gmail.com	***Statement of Problem:*** Dental caries is one of the most common chronic diseases in children. The balance between demineralization and remineralization of the decayed teeth depends on the calcium and phosphate content of the tooth surface. Therefore, if a product such as casein phospho peptides - amorphous calcium phosphate (CPP-ACP) which can significantly increase the availability of calcium and phosphate in the plaque and saliva should have an anti-caries protective effect. ***Objectives:*** The purpose of this study was to evaluate the concentration of calcium, phosphate and fluoride in the plaque and saliva of children before and after applying the CPP-ACP paste. ***Materials and Methods:*** A total of 25 children aged between 6-9 years were selected for this clinical trial study. At first, 1 ml of unstimulated saliva was collected and then 1 mg of the plaque sample was collected from the buccal surfaces of the two first primary molars on the upper jaw. In the next step, CPP-ACP paste (GC Corp, Japan) was applied on the tooth surfaces and then the plaque and saliva sampling was performed after 60 minutes. The amount of calcium ions was measured by Ion meter instrument (Metrohm Co, Swiss) and the amounts of phosphate and fluoride ions were measured by Ion Chromatography instrument (Metrohm Co, Swiss). Data were analyzed using paired *t*-test at a $p < 0.05$ level of significance. ***Results:*** There were statistically significant differences in the calcium and phosphate concentration of the saliva and plaque before and after applying the CPP-ACP paste. There were also statistically significant differences in the fluoride levels of the plaque before and after applying the CPP-ACP paste. However, there were no statistically significant differences in the fluoride levels of the saliva before and after applying the CPP-ACP paste. ***Conclusions:*** In this study, the use of the CPP-ACP paste significantly increased the fluoride levels of the plaque and the calcium and phosphate levels of both saliva and plaque. Hence, CPP-ACP paste can facilitate the remineralization of tooth surfaces and is useful for protecting the primary teeth.

Introduction

Dental caries is the most common chronic infectious disease in children [1]. A recent study [2] reported that the prevalence of caries in 6-9 year old Iranian children was 89-90%, with a mean dmft score ranging about 3.3-4.8. While the mean dmft scores among children in Saudi Arabia (2010), Brazil (1996), China (2002), Palestine (2007) and Philippines (1998) were 5,3.9,4.5,6.5 and 4.6 respectively [3-6].

Dental caries can affect the children's quality of life. In most small children (less than 2 years old), dental decay lead to reduced weight gain and reduced growth [7]. Impaired speech development and reduced self-esteem have been reported to be associated with early tooth loss caused by dental caries [8].

The current focus of researches conducted in this field is the development of non-invasive treatment approaches [9], and casein phospho peptides-amorphous calcium phosphate(CPP-ACP) has been introduced by Eric Reynold and coworkers as a therapeutic approach to enhance the remineralization [10]. CPP-ACP is a bioactive substance basically made from milk products and is composed of two parts: casein phospho peptides (CPP) and amorphous calcium phosphate (ACP) [11].

CPP has a great potential to stabilize calcium and phosphate in "nanocluster" forms of ions in solution and to remarkably enhance the level of calcium and phosphate in dental plaque [11]. CPP can bind to the biofilm, enamel and soft tissues, thereby delivering the calcium and phosphate ions exactly to the sites where they are needed. The free calcium and phosphate ions move out of the CPP, enter the enamel prisms, and restore the apatite crystals [12].

CPP-ACP has been shown to have anticariogenic properties in laboratory, and also in animal and human in situ experiments. The anticariogenic mechanism of CPP-ACP is incorporating ACP in dental plaque, which buffers the free calcium and phosphate ions and creates a state of supersaturated level of calcium and phosphate regarding the tooth enamel; this reduces the enamel demineralization and promotes remineralization [11].

CPP-ACP is useful in the treatment of dental caries, white spot lesions, hypocalcified enamel, dentin hypersensitivity, mild fluorosis, and erosion. CPP-ACP can also prevent demineralization around the brackets and other orthodontic appliances and facilitate a normal post-eruptive maturation process [11].

CPP-ACP properties such as inhibition of demineralization, enhanced remineralization and its bacteriostatic/bactericidal effect are similar to the single most useful anticaries agent, fluoride, while CPP-ACP demonstrates none of the adverse effects of fluoride such as fluorosis at moderate doses and toxicity at higher doses [13,14].

Sufficient amounts of calcium and phosphate ions must be available for net remineralization to occur, but this process is normally restricted by the amount of available calcium and phosphate [15]. Therefore, if a product such as CPP-ACP can significantly increase the availability of calcium and phosphate in plaque, it should have an anti-caries protective effect by decreasing demineralization, enhancing remineralization, or probably a combination of both [13].

In the previous studies, only the calcium and phosphate concentrations of the saliva after chewing the CPP-ACP containing gum were evaluated, and there is no report about the fluoride concentrations of the saliva and plaque and also calcium and phosphate concentrations of the plaque after applying the CPP-ACP paste. Therefore, the aim of this study was to evaluate the concentration of calcium, phosphate and fluoride in the plaque and saliva of children aged between 6-9 years before and after applying the CPP-ACP paste.

Materials and Methods

A total of 25 students aged between 6-9 years, with good oral hygiene, no active caries and no systemic disease, and resident in a charity educational center in Kerman/Iran, was selected to take part in this clinical trial study.

Ethical approval for this study was obtained from the Ethics Committee of Kerman University of Medical Sciences (IR.Kmu.REC.1394.594). After taking the informed consent, the bacterial plaque was removed using a slow-speed hand piece and a soft rubber cup without using any other substances. The subjects were asked to avoid brushing teeth, using dental floss or fluoride and other medical substances for 48 hours, and then sampling of the plaque and saliva was performed as follows:

Collecting and preparing saliva samples

Saliva sampling was done prior to dental plaque sampling. The subjects were instructed to expectorate a minimum of 1 ml of unstimulated saliva over 5 minutes into a sterile plastic container and then the samples were immediately transferred to the laboratory. Then, 1 ml of salivary samples was transferred to the coded micro-tubes using a sampler. For the preparation of the samples, 900 µl of the saliva sample was mixed with 100 µl of 1 M HClO$_4$ solution and after 2 hours, 100 µl of 90% TISAB III solution (JENWAY, England) was added to the mixture; then, the samples were centrifuged at 12000 rpm for three minutes.

Collecting and preparing plaque samples

Before plaque sampling, the subjects were asked to swallow to remove any pooled saliva. Using sterile applicators (Kerr, USA), we collected the plaque samples from the buccal surfaces of the two first primary molars on the upper jaw and then 1 mg of the sample was transferred into a coded microtube containing 1.5 ml of mineral oil. In order to increase the sensitivity of the measurements, plaque samples were weighted with a digital scale with the sensitivity of 10^{-4} g. All micro-tubes were centrifuged at 12000 rpm for 5 minutes. Subsequently, the collected samples were mixed with 200 µl of 1 M HClO$_{4\ solution}$ and diluted with 1800 µl of TISAB III solution for stability and recording ionic power. All plaque and saliva samples were filtered by a 0.2µ filter. The preparation of the plaque and saliva samples was performed according to the previously described technique by Vogel *et al.* [16].

The amount of calcium ions of the plaque and saliva samples was measured by Ion meter instrument (Metrohm Co, Swiss) and a calcium specific electrode, and the amount of phosphate and fluoride ions was measured by Ion Chromatography instrument (Metrohm Co. Swiss) using their specific columns.

After the first stage of the research, the children followed their usual oral health habits and diet for 14 days. Subsequently, bacterial plaque from the surfaces of the teeth was removed and they were asked to avoid brushing the teeth, using dental floss, fluoride and other medical substances for 48 h. Subsequently, the CPP-ACP paste (GC Corp, Japan) was applied by a sterile swap on the buccal surfaces of the two first primary molars of the upper jaw and then plaque and saliva sampling was performed after 60 minutes. The subjects were asked to avoid eating, drinking and rinsing of the mouth in the period between the application of CPP-ACP paste and collection of the samples. The procedures were repeated similar to the first stage. Data were analyzed by SPSS (v.13.5) software package using paired *t*-test at a $p < 0.05$ level of significance.

Results

The mean calcium, phosphate and fluoride concentrations of the plaque and saliva before and after applying CPP-ACP paste are shown in Table 1. The results showed that the use of CPP-ACP paste significantly increased the calcium, phosphate and fluoride concentrations of the plaque. ($p < 0.001$,

Table 1: The mean calcium, phosphate and fluoride concentrations of the plaque and saliva before and after application of the CPP-ACP paste

Group			Mean	Std.Deviation	*p* value
Saliva	Calcium(µg/ml)	Control	19.04	10.1	< 0.001
		CPP-ACP	43.87	24.7	
	Fluoride(ppm)	Control	0.65	0.15	0.512
		CPP-ACP	0.68	0.15	
	phosphate(µg/ml)	Control	0.33	0.06	< 0.001
		CPP-ACP	0.92	0.26	
plaque	calcium(µg/ml)	Control	22.17	9.1	< 0.001
		CPP-ACP	48.8	23.2	
	Fluoride(ppm)	Control	0.79	0.15	0.029
		CPP-ACP	0.98	0.3	
	phosphate(µg/ml)	Control	0.65	0.26	< 0.001
		CPP-ACP	1.88	0.56	

SD: Standard deviation

$p < 0.001$, $p = 0.029$, respectively).

The results also showed that the use of the CPP-ACP paste significantly increased the calcium and phosphate concentrations of the saliva. ($p < 0.001$, $p < 0.001$, respectively). However, the use of the CPP-ACP paste did not significantly increase the saliva fluoride levels ($p = 0.512$).

Discussion

Several studies have reported an inverse association of plaque Calcium, Phosphate levels and caries experience [17,18].

The results of this study showed that the use of CPP-ACP paste significantly increased the saliva and plaque calcium and phosphate levels. This is consistent with the results of the previous studies.

For example, Kakatkar *et al.* [19] evaluated the impact of CPP–ACP containing gum on the salivary concentration of calcium and phosphate and indicated that CPP-ACP containing chewing gum increased the calcium concentration of the saliva significantly; however, a significant decrease was observed in the phosphate concentration of the saliva for up to 1 hour after chewing the gum, as compared to the baseline. They concluded that this pseudo decrease in the salivary concentration of phosphate could be attributed to the increase in the salivary flow rate after chewing the CPP–ACP containing gum [19].

Reynolds *et al.* [20] evaluated the retention ability of CPP-ACP in supragingival plaque when delivered in a chewing gum or mouth rinse and reported that CPP-ACP-containing mouth rinse significantly increased the level of calcium and inorganic phosphate in supragingival plaque and demonstrated that CPP-ACP could still be detected on the plaque 3 hours after chewing the gum. Moreover, electron microscopic analysis of the supragingival plaque samples indicated that the CPP-ACP was bound to the intercellular matrix of the plaque and on the surface of the bacterial cells [20], confirming the work of Rose who demonstrated that CPP-ACP binds tightly to Streptococcus mutans and model plaque[13,14]. In the mentioned studies, only the calcium and phosphate concentrations of the plaque and saliva after chewing the CPP-ACP containing gum were evaluated, while in the current study the fluoride concentrations of the saliva and plaque were also examined. Moreover, in the current study the studied subjects were children.

In the present study, the mean concentrations of calcium and phosphate (in both the plaque and saliva)

after applying CPP-ACP paste were more than two times and three times (respectively) as much as that in the baseline. Fluoride ions can promote the remineralization of previously demineralized enamel if adequate amounts of plaque or salivary calcium and phosphate ions are available when the fluoride is applied (For every two fluoride ions, six phosphate ions and ten calcium ions are needed to form one unit cell of fluorapatite ($Ca10(PO4)6F2$)) [21]. Additionally, it is reported that high extracellular free calcium concentrations may have bacteriostatic or even bactericidal effects. Hence, it is possible that due to the maintenance of high free calcium, CPP-ACP may have an additional anti-plaque effect [13,22]. These results highlight the importance of the availability of plaque or salivary calcium and phosphate ions.

In a physiologic condition, the buffering potential of the saliva and its content of ions retains the PH of the oral cavity close to the saturation state [23]. However, due to various reasons, this balance may move towards demineralization of tooth structure. Srinivasan *et al.* [24] observed that no remineralization occurred in the eroded enamel which was immersed in the saliva compared to groups treated with CPP-ACP and CPP-ACPF. In many cases, saliva cannot shift towards remineralization by itself because of the presence of mature bacterial plaques or active caries; therefore, remineralizing agents are necessary for shifting towards remineralization [24].

Morgan *et al.* [25] evaluated the effect of CPP-ACP containing gum on the approximal caries. In this two year study, the children were assigned to either a test (CPP–ACP containing gum) or control (sugar-free gum without CPP-ACP) groups. All subjects received accepted preventive procedures, including fluoridated dentifrice, fluoridated water and access to professional care. But the CPP-ACP gum (the tested group) significantly slowed progression and enhanced remineralization of approximal caries relative to the control gum after 24-months. Moreover, the analyses of the sections of remineralized enamel by the CPP-ACP demonstrated that the deposited mineral was hydroxyapatite with higher Calcium: Phosphate ratio than normal hydroxyapatite; therefore, the remineralized enamel was more resistant to acid challenge [25].

In the current study, the use of the CPP-ACP paste significantly increased the fluoride concentrations of the plaque. Some researchers believe that the accumulation of fluoride on the plaque depends on the presence of calcium ions. They attributed this fact to the role of salivary calcium in the bacterial cell wall bonding of fluoride[26,27]. Therefore in the current study, the significant increase in the fluoride concentration of the plaque is related to the availability of high amounts of calcium ions. Reynolds *et al.* [21] also evaluated the ability of CPP-ACP to enhance the incorporation of fluoride into the plaque, indicating that the addition of 2% CPP-ACP to the 450-ppm-fluoride rinse increased the fluoride incorporation into supragingival plaque significantly, where the fluoride concentration of the plaque was over double that obtained with the fluoride rinse alone. CPP-ACP also increased the fluoride incorporation into subsurface enamel and substantially increased the enamel subsurface remineralization compared with fluoride alone. Moreover, the dentifrice containing 2% CPP-ACP plus 1100-ppm-F' produced a more homogenous remineralization throughout the body of the lesion [28].

Fluoride was introduced into dentistry over 70 years ago [29]. Fluoride ions play several significant roles in caries-prevention; these include the formation of fluorapatite crystals, which are more acid resistant than hydroxyapatite, interference with ionic bonding during plaque and pellicle formation, the enhancement of remineralization and the inhibition of the microbial growth and metabolism [30].

Conclusions

In this study, the use of the CPP-ACP paste significantly increased the fluoride levels of the plaque and calcium and phosphate levels of both saliva and plaque. Hence, CPP-ACP paste can facilitate the remineralization of tooth surfaces and is useful for protecting the primary teeth, especially when oral hygiene is not desirable.

Conflict of Interest: None declared.

Refrences

1. Shammukha G, Jethmalani SB, Basavaraj N, *et al.* Evaluation of changes in salivary concentration calcium by CPP-ACP containing chewing gum–A clinical trial. Int J Adv Res Oral Sci. 2012;1:1-7.

2. Pakshir HR. Oral health in Iran. Int Dent J. 2004;54:367-372.

3. Al Agili DE. A systematic review of population-based dental caries studies among children in Saudi Arabia. Saudi Dent J. 2013;25:3-11.

4. Bagramian RA, Garcia-Godoy F, Volpe AR. The global increase in dental caries. A pending public health crisis. Am J Dent. 2009;22:3-8.

5. Wang HY, Petersen PE, Bian JY, *et al.* The second national survey of oral health status of children and adults in China. Int Dent J .2002;4:283-290.

6. Bajali M, Sgan-Cohen HD, Abdulgani E, *et al.* Oral health status of Palestinian children in the West Bank-Preliminary Data. Middle East J Oral Health. 2007;1:10-12.

7. Petersen PE, Estupinan-Day S, Ndiaye C. WHO's action for continuous improvement in oral health. Bull World Health Organ. 2005;83:642.

8. Çolak H, Dülgergil ÇT, Dalli M, *et al.* Early childhood caries update: A review of causes, diagnoses, and treatments. J Nat Sci Biol Med. 2013;4:29-38.

9. Rezvani MB, Karimi M, Rasoolzade RA, *et al.* Comparing the Effects of Whey Extract and Casein Phosphopeptide-Amorphous Calcium Phosphate (CPP-ACP) on Enamel Microhardness. J Dent. 2015;16:49-53.

10. Walsh LJ. Contemporary technologies for remineralization therapies: A review. Int Dent SA. 2009;11:6-16.

11. Reema SD, Lahiri PK, Roy SS. Review of casein phosphopeptides-amorphous calcium phosphate. Chin J Dent Res. 2014;17:7-14.

12. Jayarajan J, Janardhanam P, Jayakumar P, *et al.* Efficacy of CPP-ACP and CPP-ACPF on enamel remineralization-An in vitro study using scanning electron microscope and DIAGNOdent®. Indian J Dent Res. 2011;22:77-82.

13. Rose RK. Binding characteristics of Streptococcus mutans for calcium and casein phosphopeptide. Caries Res. 2000;34:427-431.

14. Rose RK. Effects of an anticariogenic casein phosphopeptide on calcium diffusion in streptococcal model dental plaques. Arch Oral Biol. 2000;45:569-575.

15. Hegde MN, Devadiga D, Jemsily PA. Comparative evaluation of effect of acidic beverage on enamel surface pre-treated with various remineralizing agents: An In vitro study. J Conserv Dent. 2012;15:351-356.

16. Vogel G, Zhang Z, Chow L, *et al.* Changes in lactate and other ions in plaque and saliva after a fluoride rinse and subsequent sucrose

administration. Caries Res. 2002;36:44-52.

17. Moreno E, Margolis H. Composition of human plaque fluid. J Dent Res. 1988;67:1181-1189.

18. Shaw L, Murray J, Burchell C, *et al.* Calcium and phosphorus content of plaque and saliva in relation to dental caries. Caries Res. 1983;17:543-548.

19. Kakatkar G, Nagarajappa R, Bhat N, *et al.* Evaluation of Salivary Calcium and Phosphorous Concentration Before and After Chewing CPP-ACP Containing Chewing Gum. Acta stomatologica Croatica. 2012;46:117-125.

20. Reynolds E, Cai F, Shen P, *et al.* Retention in plaque and remineralization of enamel lesions by various forms of calcium in a mouthrinse or sugar-free chewing gum. J Dent Res. 2003;82:206-211.

21. Reynolds E. Calcium phosphate-based remineralization systems: scientific evidence? Aust Dent J. 2008;53:268-273.

22. Kobayashi H, Van Brunt J, Harold FM. ATP-linked calcium transport in cells and membrane vesicles of Streptococcus faecalis. J Biol Chem. 1978;253:2085-2092.

23. Heshmat H, Banava S, Abdian H, *et al.* Effects of Casein Phosphopeptide amorphous Calcium Phosphate and casein phosphopeptide amorphous Calcium Phosphate Fluoride on alterations of

dental plaque pH following sucrose consumption. J Islamic Dent Assoc IRAN. 2014;26:274-279.

24. Srinivasan N, Kavitha M, Loganathan S. Comparison of the remineralization potential of CPP–ACP and CPP–ACP with 900ppm fluoride on eroded human enamel: An in situ study. Arch Oral Biol. 2010;55:541-544.

25. Morgan M, Adams G, Bailey D, *et al.* The anticariogenic effect of sugar-free gum containing CPP-ACP nanocomplexes on approximal caries determined using digital bitewing radiography. Caries Res. 2008;42:171-184.

26. Cochrane N, Cai F, Huq N, *et al.* New approaches to enhanced remineralization of tooth enamel. J Dent Res. 2010;89:1187-1197.

27. Kato K, Nakagaki H, Arai K, *et al.* The influence of salivary variables on fluoride retention in dental plaque exposed to a mineral-enriching solution. Caries Res. 2002;36:58-63.

28. Reynolds E, Cai F, Cochrane N, *et al.* Fluoride and casein phosphopeptide-amorphous calcium phosphate. J Dent Res. 2008;87:344-348.

29. Buzalaf MA, Pessan JP, Honório HM, *et al.* Mechanisms of action of fluoride for caries control. Mongor Oral Sci. 2011;22:97-114.

30. Niessen L, Gibson G. Oral health for a lifetime: Preventive strategies for the older adult. Quintessence Int. 1997;28:626-630.

26

Vickers Hardness of Composite Resins Cured with LED and QTH Units

Alaghemand H[a], Ramezani M[b], Abedi H[c], Gholamrezaee Saravi M[c], Zarenejad N[c]

[a]Department of Restorative Dentistry, Head of the Dental Materials Research Center, Faculty of Dentistry, Babol University of Medical Sciences, Babol, Iran
[b]Department of Endodontics, Faculty of Dentistry, Mazandaran University of Medical Sciences, Sari, Iran
[c]Department of Restorative Dentistry, Faculty of Dentistry, Mazandaran University of Medical Sciences, Sari, Iran

ARTICLE INFO

Key words:
Resin Composite
Hardness
Light-curing
LED
QTH

Corresponding Author:
Nafiseh Zarenejad,
Department of Restorative
Dentistry, Faculty of Dentistry,
Mazandaran University of
Medical Sciences, Sari, Iran

Email: zarenejadn@yahoo.com

Abstract

Statement of Problem: One of the factors affecting the degree of polymerization of light-cured composites is the type of light-curing unit used. In addition, physicomechanical properties of the composite resins depend on the degree of conversion and polymerization.

Objectives: Since the type of initiator in new composite resins is not explained by manufacturers, this study is an attempt to compare the depth of hardening, with two LED and QTH light-curing units.

Materials and Methods: Fifteen samples prepared from Gradia Direct and Filtek Z250, both of which being universal, were cured with QTH (Astralis 7) and LED (Bluephase C8) light-curing units. All the samples were molded in polyester resin and cut from the middle by a disk. The hardness of the cut area was evaluated at 0, 0.5, 1, 1.5, 2, 2.5, 3, 3.5 and 4-mm depth intervals and also at the same interval as the width of the sample, with Vickers hardness machine, while the samples were placed in a darkroom. Data were statistically analyzed using one-way ANOVA, two-way ANOVA, t-test and post Hoc Tukey's tests in SPSS, version 16.

Results: Filtek Z250 was harder than Gradia Direct at all the depth with both light-curing units. The hardness of Filtek Z250 sample cured with Astralis 7 was higher than that cured with LED, but with Gradia Direct the LED unit resulted in higher hardness. Curing depth was not significantly different between the groups ($p = 0.109$).

Conclusions: Vickers hardness number for both composites used in this study is in an acceptable range for clinical implications. The composites' composition is important to be considered for selection of light unit. Based on the findings of the present study, LED did not present more curing depth compared with QTH.

Introduction

Light-cured composite resins are widely used [1-5] and have advantages over self-cured composite resins [2,3]. Today, there are basically four main sources for polymerization of light-cured composite resins [2,6,7]: Quartz-tungsten-halogen (QTH), Plasma Arc (PAC), Light-emitting diode (LED), and Laser.

For years, QTH unit, the output light intensity of which is 400–800 mW/cm^2, was the gold standard for composite resin polymerization [2,4,6,8-11]. The majority of QTH units used in dental offices have output light intensities lower than the least recommended values. Furthermore, slow curing and limited depth of curing are some other disadvantages [2,4,8-13].

The technique used to produce light in LED units is different from that in QTH units. Hot filaments are used for heat production in halogen lamps, but in gallium nitride LEDs, electron moving in a direction between positive and negative areas under an adequate voltage leads to the production of blue light. Hence the emitting spectrum of LED covers the absorbed spectrum by camphorquinone without filtering. The latest documents released indicate that LED lamps result in the highest polymerization and have lower energy consumption in comparison to QTH units. Previous LED units had output light intensities around 300 mW/cm^2, but the new models of LED units with high light intensity are claimed to have shorter exposure time and deeper curing. Based on the advantages mentioned, today LED units are widely accepted [1,2, 14,15].

The following are some of the important factors affecting the adequate polymerization of a composite resin and consequently favorable depth of curing:

a. The specification of light source, including wavelength of the output light and its intensity, the duration of light exposure and distance from the light source. b. Composition of composite resin and type of the initiator. c. The volume of the cured composite resin.

The depth of cure is the depth at which composite resin preserves 80% of its surface hardness and after that the composite resin has no sufficient polymerization [11].

The most common light initiator used in the composite resin materials is camphorquinone, the absorption spectrum of which is around 468 nm [1,2,15,16]. However, it is possible to use the other light initiators such as phenyl propanedione (PPD) with an absorption spectrum of 410 nm or bisacyl phosphine oxide and triacil phosphine oxide with an absorption spectrum of 320–390 nm [1,8,10,15].

Because the output spectrum of LED units is limited and it is closer to the absorption spectrum of camphorquinone, it is unlikely to have a sufficient depth of cure when other initiators are used. Manufacturers claim that the acceptable curing depth in dark-shade composite resins is achieved in shorter times with LED than QTH. There are still some questions about the depth of cure regarding the LED [16,17,18-22]. Evaluation of curing depth and also the degree of monomer conversion and composite resin polymerization is carried out using two direct methods with Fourier Transform Infrared Spectroscopy (FTIR) or Raman Spectroscopy, assessing the carbonic double bonds and an indirect method assessing composite resin hardness in different depths with Vickers device [2,7,17].

As the physical and mechanical properties of the composite resins are directly related to the degree of monomer conversion and the extent of polymerization, and that ever-increasing numbers of new composite resins are marketed with different light initiators, this study was designed to identify and compare the depth hardness of two composite resins cured with LED and QTH units. The null hypothesis stated that there would be no difference in curing depth and hardness between the two composite resins cured with two different units.

Materials and Methods

Two types of composite resin (Table 1), Filtek Z250 and Gradia Direct, both in A2 shade and universal, were light-cured with two different light-curing units, i.e. Bluphase C8 Light-emitting diode-LED (Ivoclar Vivadent, Austria) and Astralis 7 Quartz-tungsten-halogen-QTH (Ivoclar Vivadent, Austria) (Table 2).

Filtek Z250 has been used in most of previous researches as an acceptable composite in case hardness assessment of newly-introduced composites with. On the other hand, Gradia Direct as a microfil composite is now widely used in esthetic restoration, either anterior or posterior zone.

A total of 60 samples were prepared for four 15-sample groups. Composite resin samples were

Table 1: Specifications of composite resins used

Resin Composite	Manufacturer	Organic ingredient	Filler	Particle size
Filtek Z250	3M ESPE, USA	BisGMA, UDMA, BisEMA	68 vol%: Zr/Si	0.01-3.5
Gradia	GC dental Corp. Japan	UDMA	Trimodal filler system (60 vol %): PPF-Pre polymerized filler FP-Aluminoborosillicate glass NP- Sillica	0.005-0.01

prepared in rubber moulds, measuring 6 mm in internal diameter and 5 mm in depth; then two groups were cured with LED Bluphase C8 and two others with QTH Astralis 7. To avoid sample porosity and air bubble entrapment, on 2.5 mm sample were put in the mould. The samples were protected from the preventing effect of the air at both sides of the mould with a thin glass and then they were stored for 24 hours in darkness, water and room temperature for completion of polymerization. All the samples were wrapped in an epoxy resin and cut in the middle and polished using 400-, 800-, 1000-, 1500-, 2000- and 2500-grit abrasive paper. The hardness of the sectioned areas was assessed at 0, 0.5, 1, 1.5, 2, 2.5,

Table 2 : Specifications of light curing units used in the study

Light Unit	Intensity (cm/mw^2)	Radiation Time	Wavelength (nm)
LED Bluphase C8	800	20 s	360-540
QTH Astralis 7	400	40 s	400-500

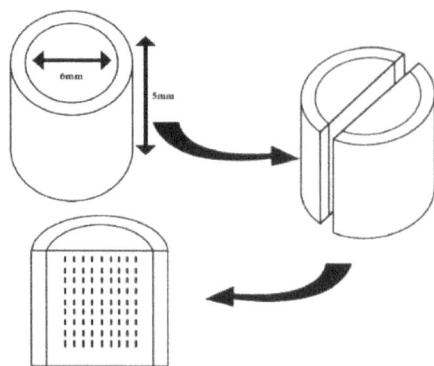

Figure 1: Schematic representation of sample fabricated (81 VHNs obtained by multiplying) points in horizon (each 0/5 mm away from the next one) into 9 points in depth (each 0/5 mm away from the next one)

3, 3.5, and 4-mm distances from the surface using Vickers device (MH2 Model, Coopa Corp., Iran) while the samples had been kept in darkness (Figure 1). The load used with the device was 500 gr for 10 seconds. Data were analyzed statistically using one-way ANOVA, two-way ANOVA and Tukey HSD tests (Table 3).

Results

Filtek Z250 was harder than Gradia Direct in all the depths with both light-curing units. The hardness of Filtek Z250 cured with Astralis 7 QTH unit was higher than that cured with Bluephase C8 LED, but

Table 3: Statistical difference of VHNs Hardness between the two composites (according to the distance from the surface)

Distance from the surface (mm)	0	0.5	1	1.5	2	2.5	3	3.5	4
Sig.		0.000	0.000	0.000	0.000	0.000	552.	0.418	0.043	0.021

for Gradia Direct the Bluephase C8 LED unit resulted in higher hardness than Astralis 7 QTH. In all the groups, 80% of the surface hardness was obtained at 2-mm depth. Curing depth was not significantly different between all the groups ($p = 0.109$). Filtek Z250 cured with each unit preserved its hardness at 3-mm depth to a level which could be identified with Vickers microhardness Device. After 3 mm, the composite could be easily removed with a scalpel blade. Gradia Direct with Bluephase C8 up to 3.5 mm and with Astralis 7 QTH had measurable hardness up to 2.5 mm, beyond which it could easily be removed with a scalpel blade. To compare the hardness of all the samples cured with the two units in all the groups, from the surface up to 2-mm depth, the hardness of the four groups was significantly different but from 2-mm up to 4-mm depth , there was no significant different as shown in Table 3.

Figure 2 shows that surface hardness of the two composites is significantly different. Surface hardness

of Filtek Z250 is two times more than that of Gradia direct, whereas at 2.5 mm depth hardness drop of Filtek Z 250 is more obvious than that of Gradia direct.

Discussion

The null hypothesis was rejected. The light-curing units are of paramount importance since sufficient polymerization is necessary to achieve acceptable physical properties. There is controversy over defining the depth of cure for QTH units in comparison to LED units. Based on previous studies, the LED is superior to QTH due to its higher curing depth; hence more polymerization occurs on the composite resin. A possible explanation for this quality might be the proximity of emitted wave spectrum of LED to the absorption spectrum of camphorquinone.

Clinically speaking, the composite is added incrementally, because the maximum depth of cure is 2

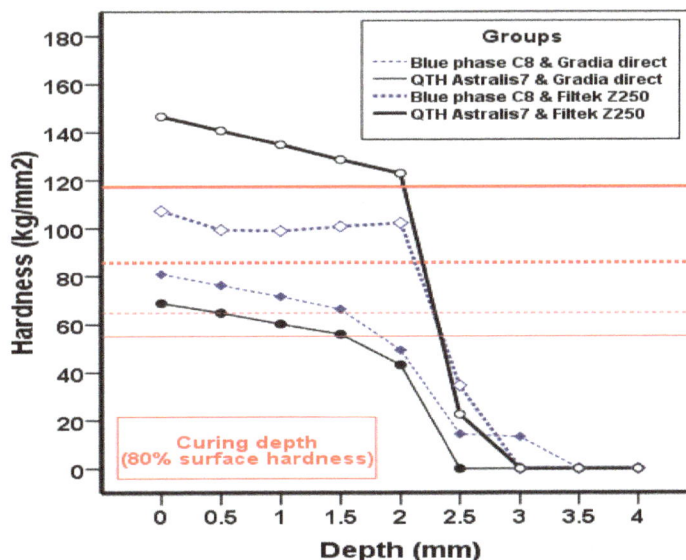

Figure 2: Comparison of four groups based on 80% of surface VHNs hardness

millimeter, but in this experimental study the samples were used in one 5-mm diameter, since it was to check the ability of LED units to provide curing depth more than 2 mm and in clinic the distance from light cure tip is more than 2mm (5mm or more). Previous studies implemented the proportion of superficial hardness to underlying hardness and accepted that the polymerization is good if the mentioned proportion is at least 80%. According to 80% limit of hardness, two QTH Astralis 7 and LED Bluephase C8 light-curing units were used to cure two composite resin types; Filtek Z250 and Gradia Direct had almost similar curing depths. The superficial hardness of Filtek Z250 was higher than that of Gradia Direct, which is not in line with the results of Torno et al. because they concluded that the composite resins which were closer to the surface were cured more efficiently with all the light sources used [17].

Differences between light-curing units and exposure times can be considered as reasons for such discrepancy. In the present study, the hardness of Filtek Z250 was higher when it was cured with QTH unit compared to when it was cured with LED unit; this is consistent with the results of Sadeghiyani et al. and Polydorou et al., who used two translucent composite resins exposed to QTH and LED units [1,18]. Sadeghiyani used Astralis 7 as QTH. In both studies, the results mentioned for better results of QTH was noticeable heat produced with light unit. Composite resin hardness after polymerization is affected by some factors, including composition of composite resin, type of light initiator, light unit, and the amount of light energy with a suitable wavelength [3].

Energy density of QTH is higher than that of LED because power density of QTH, as one factor affecting the energy density is higher than that of LED. Moreover, Filtek Z250 has a higher percentage of filler than Gradia Direct, which itself is effective in higher hardness. Based on the results reported by Price et al., hardness obtained with Ultralum 2 LED was higher in all the sections compared to QTH, which is different from the results of the present study [20]. They attributed their findings to the LED light source, as QTH delivers a wide spectrum whereas the Ultralum 2 with 440-480 nm wavelength focuses on the most appropriate spectrum for polymerization that is 440-490 nm [23-26]. The reasons which can be mentioned for low hardness of Gradia Direct

are the composition of composite resin itself which is microhybrid and the lower content of fillers compared to Filtek Z250; that is why it needs longer exposure time which has been recommended by the manufacture as well, although both composite resins were A2 shade. Interestingly, although the exposure time was longer for Gradia Direct, its hardness was much lower than that of Filtek Z250.

On the other hand, Gradia Direct composite resin is a microhybrid with higher percentage of microfil fillers. Phenyl propane accompanying dimetacrylate in the composition of Gradia Direct can be considered for its different behavior from Filtek Z250. Some manufacturers use lower amounts of camphorquinone in combination with other initiators like phenyl propanedione (PPD) with an absorption spectrum of 410 nm. Gomes et al. reported in 2006 that these two initiators have synergistic interactions [19]. Probably absorption wavelength of PPD is closer to the output light of LED Bluephase C8, resulting in higher curing depth of Gradia Direct with this light-curing unit.

Light intensity decreases while passing through the composite resin, especially with microfil composite resins like Gradia Direct. Totally, light intensity decreases when it passes through composite resins due to absorption, refraction and reflection. That is why composite hardness decreases from surface to deep layers, and that according to manufacturers the majority of composite resins have curing depths of 2 mm. This claim was verified in this study as well. According to Figure 2, the lower hardness of Gradia direct rather than Filtek Z 250 at the surface can be the result of having microfil texture.

As shown in Figure 2, the Gradia Direct has more VHNs with Bluphase C8 LED rather than Astralis 7 QTH. It might be due to consistency of light emitted from Bluphase C8 LED with the composition of Gradia Direct, a fact that must be considered clinically.

On the contrary, Filtek Z 250 is more consistent with Astralis 7 QTH. In fact with increasing depth, both light-curing units exhibited rather similar functions, which might be attributed to a decrease in light intensity due to refraction and absorption. Another explanation for this phenomenon is the fact that a high percentage of short waves is absorbed close to the composite resin surface, so they cannot activate the co-initiator [4]. Refraction of these wavelengths occurs more than the longer wavelengths. Therefore, when facing the new brands of composite resins on the market, their different properties must be addressed carefully.

Suggestion

It is suggested that the mentioned composite should be cured with the other kinds of LED units to see if there are findings different from those obtained from the present study.

Limitation

It was difficult and time consuming to evaluate such high number of points. .

Conclusions

VHNs hardness for both composites used in this study is in an acceptable range for clinical implications. The composite composition is important to be considered for selection of light unit. Based on the findings of the present study, LED did not present more curing depth compared with QTH.

References

1. Polydorou O, Manolakis A, Hellwig E, *et al*. Evaluation of the curing depth of two translucent composite materials using a halogen and two LED curing units. Clin Oral Investig. 2008;12:45-51.

2. Manojlovic D, Dramicanin MD, Lezaja M, *et al*. Effect of resin and photoinitiator on colour, translucency and colour stability of conventional and low-shrinkage model composites. Dent Mater. 2016;32:183-191.

3. Aravamudhan K, Floyd CJ, Rakowski D, *et al*. Light-emitting diode curing light irradiance and polymerization of resin-based composite. J Am Dent Assoc. 2006;137:213-223.

4. Rode KM, de Freitas PM, and Lloret PR, *et al*. Micro-hardness evaluation of a microhybrid composite resin light-cured with halogen light, light - emitting diode and argon ion laser. Lasers Med Sci. 2009;24:87-92.

5. Rahiotis C, kakaboura A, Loukidis M, *et al*. Curing efficiency of various types of light curing units. Eur J Oral Sci. 2004;112:89-94.

6. Strydom C. Prerequisites for proper curing. J Dent Assoc S Afr. 2005;60:254-255.

7. Ceballos, L, Fuentes MV, Tafalla H, *et al*. Curing effectiveness of resin composites at different exposure times using LED and halogen units. Med Oral Patol Oral Cir Bucal. 2009; 14:51-56.

8. Yazici AR, Kugel G, Gul G. The knoop hardness of a composite resin polymerized with different curing lights and different modes. J Contemp Dent Pract. 2007;8:52-59.

9. Tak O, Altintas SH, Ozturk N, *et al*. Effect of three types of light-curing units on 5-year colour changes of light-cured composite. Clin Oral Investig. 2009;13:29-35.

10. Dunn WJ, Bush AC. A Comparison of polymerization by light-emitting diode and halogen-based light-curing units. J Am Dent Assoc. 2002;133:335-341.

11. Komori PC, de Paula AB, Martin AA, *et al*. Effect of light Energy Density on conversion Degree and hardness of dual-cured Resin cement. Oper Dent. 2010;35:120-124.

12. Mills RW, Uhl A, Jandt KD. Optical power outputs, spectra and dental composite depths of cure, obtained with blue light emitting diode (LED) and halogen light curing units (LCUS). Br Dent J. 2002;193:459-463.

13. Burgess JO, Walker RS, Rorche CJ, *et al*. light curing: An update. Compend Contin Educ Dent. 2002;23:889-892,894-896.

14. Leonard DL, Charlton DG, Roberts HW, *et al*. Polymerization efficiency of LED curing lights. J Esthet Restor Dent. 2002;14:286-295.

15. Correr AB, Sinhoreti MA, Sobrinho LC, *et al*. Effect of the increase of Energy Density on knoop hardness of Dental composites light-cured by conventional QTH, LED and xenon plasma Arc. Braz Dent J. 2005;16:218-224.

16. Yazici AR, Celik C, Dayangac B, *et al*. Effects of different light-curing units/modes on the microleakage of flowable composite resin. Eur J Dent. 2008;2:240-246.

17. Torno V, Soares P, Martin JM, *et al*. Effects of irradiance, wavelength and thermal emission of different light-curing units on the Knoop and Vickers Hardness of a composite resin. J Biomed Mater Res B Appl Biomater. 2008;85:166-171.

18. Hubbezoglu I, Bolayir G, Dogan OM, *et al*. Microhardness evaluation of resin composite polymerized by three different light sources. Dent Mater J. 2007;26:845-853.

19. Gomes GM, Calixto AL, Santos FA, *et al*.

Hardness of a bleaching shade resin composite polymerized with different light-curing sources. Braz Oral Res. 2006;20:337-341.

20. Price RB, Felix CA. Effect of delivering light in specific narrow bandwidths from 394 to 515 nm on the microhardness of resin composites. Dent Mater. 2009;25:899-908.

21. Dsouza R, Subhash H, Neuhaus K, *et al*. Assessment of curing behavior of light-activated dental composites using intensity correlation based multiple reference optical coherence tomography. Lasers Surg Med. 2016;48:77-82.

22. Khan AA, Siddiqui AZ, Mohsin SF, *et al*. Influence of mouth rinses on the surface hardness of dental resin nano-composite. Pak J Med Sci. 2015;31:1485-1489.

23. EL-Mowfy O, EL-Badrawy W, Wasef M, *et al*. Efficacy of new LED light-curing units in hardening of Class II composite restorations. J Can Dent Assoc. 2007;73:253-253e.

24. Guilardo RD, Consani S, Xediek Consani RL, *et al*. Effect of different light curing units on Knoop hardness and temprature of resin composite. Indian J Dent Res. 2009;20:308-312.

25. Price RB, Fahey J, Felix CM. Knoop microhardness mapping used to compare the Efficacy of LED, QTH and PAC curing lights. Oper Dent. 2010;35:58-68.

26. Cerveira GP, Berthold TB, Souto AA, *et al*. Degree of conversion and hardness of an orthodontic resin cured with a light-emitting diode and a quartz-tungsten-halogen light. Eur J Orthod. 2010;32:83-86.

27

Comparison of Microtensile Bond Strength of Silorane-Based Composite with the Conventional Methacrylate Composite to the Dentin of Primary Teeth

Sharifi Mª, Khoramian Tusi Sᵇ*

ªDepartment of Paediatric Dentistry, School of Dentistry, Rafsanjan University of Medical Sciences, Rafsanjan, Iran

ᵇDepartment of Paediatric Dentistry, School of Dentistry, Alborz University of Medical Sciences, Karaj, Iran

---

ARTICLE INFO

Key words:
Microtensile Bond Strength
Silorane Adhesive System
Methacrylate Composite
Self-etch Primer

Corresponding Author:
Somayeh Khoramian Tusi
Department of Paediatric
Dentistry, School of
Dentistry, Alborz University
of Medical Sciences, Karaj,
Iran
Email:So_khoramian@
yahoo.com

Abstract

Statement of Problem: The bond strength between restorative material and tooth structure is so important for conduction of durable restoration. Considering the recent attention to low shrinkage composite resins, evaluation of micro tensile bond strength of these materials would be valuable.

Objectives: To compare the microtensile bond strength of silorane composite resin (Filtek P90) with the conventional methacrylate composite (Filtek Z250) with and without applying acid etch before application of bonding system.

Materials and Methods: In this experimental study, 24 intact primary canines were used. After the dentin was exposed, the teeth were randomly divided into four groups as follows: the first group (silorane bond system + composite Filtek P90); the second group (etch + silorane bond system + composite Filtek P90); the third group (Single bond + composite Filtek Z250); and the fourth group (etch + Single bond + composite Filtek Z250). The teeth were cut on the longitudinal axis and the interface between the composite and dentin were grinded buccolingually and mesiodistally. The samples were subjected to a microtensile force until breakage. The obtained values were recorded in MPa; data were analyzed using One-way ANOVA and Tamhane's T2 statistical tests.

Results: The average microtensile bond strength in all groups had a statistically significant difference with each other (all $p < 0.05$). The highest bond strength belonged to the second group (etch + silorane bond system + composite Filtek P90) and the lowest value was related to the third group (Single bond + composite Filtek Z250).

Conclusions: As the second group (etch + silorane bond system + composite Filtek P90) exhibited higher microtensile bond strength, it may prove that using composite Filtek P90 is preferable to be used in primary dentin in comparison with composite Filtek Z250, and using etch + silorane bond system is more advantageous than single bond system.

Introduction

Extensive research continues to create a better restorative material and the more advanced and applicable techniques in the restorative dentistry. The highest recent efforts in response to the growing needs and expectations are the usage of composite resin. The resin composite restorations have been accepted due to their great beauty and having other benefits such as low heat transfer ability, and tooth structure protection during cavity preparation [1,2]. Physical properties of composite dental material have been improved during decades, but bond strength, specially to the dentin, has still remained a challenge [3,4].

If the bond between the restoration and tooth fails, recurrence caries occurs and higher destruction of dental tissue is seen [5]. Micro-leakage poses a particular problem for the teeth in the paediatric patient because the floor of the cavity preparation may be close to the pulp. Added insult to the pulp is caused by the seepage of the irritants that penetrate around the restoration and through the thin layer of dentin, or a microscopic pulpal exposure may produce irreversible pulp damage [2].

The volumetric shrinkage for traditional methacrylate-based composites ranges from 2% to 6%. Similarly, the marginal gap rate in the clinical assessment of the resin composite restorations based on the material type and clinical application method has a range of 14% to 54% [5]. The volumetric shrinkage of the composite resins is mainly dependent on the chemical composition of the resin matrix. Therefore, the efforts have been made to reduce the polymerization shrinkage with the change in the resin composition, including strengthening of the conventional composite resins Bis-GMA *via* the addition of the new monomers such as the UEDMA and Bis-EMA and or utilization of the longer resin molecules such as EMA6 in Filtek Z250 [6]. The other facts of these efforts are to change the monomeric phase matrix structure with the use of the ring-opening monomers [7].

The conducted researches [8,9] have shown that the reinforced formula with Oxirane/Polyol had a determined reduction in the polymerization shrinkage and cusp deflection in relation to the conventional methacrylate composite resins. The polymerization contraction reduction was in association with the cationic-ring-opening monomers. Concerns about cytotoxicity and mutagenicity of the resins with the

Oxirane/Polyol base existed in the clinical application. In order to solve the raised problems, a new resin formula was obtained from the Oxirane and Silorane molecule reaction that was entitled 'Silorane' [8].

The silorane had very good tissue compatibility and its cytotoxicity is equivalent or less than the conventional methacrylate monomers. Silorane is insoluble and stable in the biological solutions. Even in comparison to the composite resins with methacrylate base, it causes less cusp deflection. In the conducted studies, it has been shown that silorane possesses optimal mechanical characteristics as a restorative material. The ring-opening reaction present in the silorane has reduced the polymerization shrinkage volumetric rate to less than 1% [8-10].

In the recent years, numerous researches have studied the characteristics of this new resin composite and its clinical application; many of these researches have focused on the application of this kind of resin composite on the permanent teeth [10-12]. Yet, sufficient laboratory or clinical studies showing usefulness of this new resin composite in the primary teeth have not been conducted. In the primary teeth, in contrast to the permanent teeth, the thickness of the dental material is less and that of the prismless enamel is high; therefore, the results of the resin composite application and the bond system in the permanent teeth cannot be generalized to the primary teeth [11].

Contemporary dental adhesive systems can be classified according to application techniques as etch and rinse or self-etching adhesive systems. Manufacturers combine together either primer and bonding resin or etchant and primer agent to reduce the number of bottles and clinical steps. Also they simplify the bonding protocol by producing all-in-one systems. An important indicator of an adhesive systems' effectiveness is bond strength; Because the bonding layer must support composite shrinkage stress and occlusal forces to avoid gap formation which leads to micro-leakage, secondary caries, and postoperative sensitivity [9,13].

Therefore, there is a need to conduct a study assessing the silorane application to the primary teeth dentin is felt. Numerous methods are used for evaluating the bond strength rate of the restorative materials and bonding system, among which the shear and tensile bond test can be addressed [14].

For the measurement of the tensile bond strength, recently the Micro Tensile Bond Strength (µTBS) technique has been introduced *via* Sano [15]. This new method has many advantages over standard methods for measuring the bond strength; they include:

1-It provides the possibility to prepare several resin cylinders joint to the dentin in a dental sample. 2-It provides the possibility to test the dental levels with different clinical characteristics such as decayed dentin, dentinal tubule sclerosis and enamel surfaces. 3-With the reduction of experiment surface, the superficial defects and distinctiveness reduces and causes prevention of inappropriate distribution of force and premature bond collapse. 4- It provides the possibility for testing the localized differences in the bond strength in the tooth [7,8].

The present study was conducted aiming at comparing micro- tensile bond strength of the silorane composite Filtek P90 with the conventional methacrylate composite Filtek Z250 to the primary teeth dentin.

Material and Methods

In this experimental study, 24 primary canines without decay, fracture, and cracks which were extracted due to orthodontics treatment were used. For teeth disinfection, after cleaning of the tissue wastes with scaler, they were placed in 10% formaldehyde solution (Dr. Mojalali, Tehran, Iran) for a period of 24 hours. Using diamond grinding fissure bur number 012 (Tizkavan, Tehran, Iran) we removed the coronal part of the canine teeth and exposed the dentin surface. Then, the surfaces were investigated under steriomicroscop for pulp horns or microscopic pulp exposure. If there was no microscopic pulp exposure, the teeth were randomly divided into the four groups (n = 6). The prepared teeth surface was washed with water and air aspirator for a period of 15 seconds and dried and after that in each group the dentin surface was covered with the following composite, respectively. The composite with an incremental technique was placed in the two layers of two millimetres [16,17].

Group A: Composite Filtek P90 with an individual self etch bond system

In this group, according to the manufacture's instructions the primer existing in the special composite kit; Silorane Filtek P90 (3M ESPE, MI, USA) was `brushed' on the sample surface for a period of 15 seconds and diffused for five seconds with a gentle air aspiration; then, it was cured for a period of 10 seconds *via* light curing machine QTH

(Coltolux 75, OH, USA) with 1000mw/cm^2 light intensity. Later the special composite bonding Filtek P90 was applied to the samples' surface and after the diffusion with the gentle air aspiration was cured for a period of 10 seconds. Eventually, the composite Filtek P90 was conformed in two layers of two millimeters on the dentin surface and each layer was cured for a period of 40 seconds.

Group B: Composite Filtek P90 with the use of acid etching and an individual bond

In this group, the work stages were similar to Group A with a difference that before the primer use, the dentin surface was etched with the use of 37% phosphoric acid (3M ESPE, MI, USA) for 15 seconds, washed for a period of 10 seconds and dried.

Group C: Composite Filtek Z250 with the self etch bond system:

In this group, the self etch bonding system, Single bond, as per the manufacturing company's instruction was used for bonding. Then, the composite Filtek Z250 similar to the earlier groups was conformed to the dentin surface and cured for a period of 40 seconds.

Group D: Composite Filtek Z250 with the use of acid etching and self-etch bond system:

In this group, the dentin surface was etched for 15 seconds with the use of 37% phosphoric acid and then washed for a period of 10 seconds and dried. Then, the self etch bonding system, Single bond, (3M ESPE, MI, USA) was used for bonding based on the manufacturer's instruction. Then, the composite Filtek Z250 similar to the earlier groups was conformed to the dentin surface and cured for a period of 40 seconds.

All samples were maintained for a week at room temperature in the physiologic serum and then cut buccolingually parallel to the longitudinal axis of the tooth *via* Universal Cutting Machine (Zwick, Ulam, Germany) sothat at least two samples were obtained from each tooth (12 samples in each group).

Then, the interface between the dentin and restoration was grinded buccolingually and mesiodistally with the diamond grinding fissure bur number 012 (Tizkavan, Tehran, Iran) till the hourglass shape was created with 9μm dimentions in the buccolingual and mesiodistal sides to create a surface segment at the micron level in the area of tensile force implementation. Then, the samples were adhered with cyanoacrylate adhesive (Zapit, Dental, USA) to the arms of Universal Testing Machine (model Π60185, BISCO, Schaumburg, USA). The samples were subjected to 0.55 mm in a minute tensile force until they broke.

The microtensile strength was calculated using the following formula: With the calculation of force value (according to Newton's law) and its division of the segment surface (based on the mm^2), the results were reported in MPa. If the prepared samples were broken before the test conduction, number zero was recorded in the flowchart.

For a blind study, the person who conducted the tensile bond test only recorded the considered group number and was unaware of the types of application material in different groups. The assumption of normality was approved with the use of the Kolmogorov-Semirnov test (all $p > 0.05$) while the homogeneity of variance was not approved via Levene's test ($p < 0.01$), so One-way ANOVA and Tamhane's T2 tests were used for comparison of the groups; A $p < 0.05$ was considered as statistically significant.

Results

The One-way ANOVA test showed that there was a significant difference between the composite resin microtensile bond strength to the dentin among the groups ($p < 0.001$). The average composite resin microtensile bond strength to the dentin is presented in Table 1.

As shown in Table 1, the highest micro-tensile bond strength (31.86 ± 6.25 MPa) pertaining to group 2 where composite Filtek P90 was used with etch and bond on the dentin surface and the lowest was related to group 3 in which the composite Filtek Z250 was used with only bond and without etch on the dentin surface (11.95 ± 2.08). Tamhane's T2 test showed

that there was a significant difference between the micro-tensile bond strength of all other groups ($p < 0.05$), except for between the first and fourth groups ($p = 0.994$) (Table 1).

Discussion

For the microtensile bond strength conduction, the two methods of the sample construction beam and hourglass are used [18]. In the present study, the samples were prepared in the form of an hourglass and the reason for selection of this form was that beam preparation with accessible equipment and tools was not possible. Besides, in the case of the existence of the required equipment, also it seemed that beam preparation with a sufficient length in the primary teeth despite the pulp extent was difficult since in most of the samples the distance of the pulp to interphase was 3mm or less. On the other hand, hourglass form provides more attachment surface in the upper and lower areas of the designed arms of the test machine which reduces premature debond of the samples from the test machine arms [19-22].

In the present study, the microtensile bond strength test was used to assess the bond strength of the composites Filtek P90 and Filtek Z250 to the dentin of the primary teeth. For the comparison of the silorane composite, Filtek P90, with the methacrylate composites, Filtek Z250 had been used in a usual manner, which possesses a long record in relation to the newer methacrylate composites. Filtek Z250 is a micro-hybrid composite resin with 60% filler volume that has a polymerization contraction equivalent to 2.7 [23].

In order to investigate the surface etch effect on the micro tensile bond strength in one of the investigated groups, the dentin surface was etched with 37% acid phosphoric before applying silorane bonding system. For equivalence of the bonding factors, two kinds of

Table 1: Mean value, standard deviation and *p*-Value of micro-tensile bond strength (MPa) of resin composite to dentin in different groups

Groups	Mean ± SD	*p*-value[*]		
		1	2	3
1=(Siloran bond + composite Filtek P90)	17.23 ± 3.47	-	-	-
2=(Etch + siloran bond + Composite Filtek P90)	31.86 ± 6.25	0.001	-	-
3=(single bond + Composite Filtek Z250)	11.95 ± 2.08	0.001	0.001	-
4=(Etch + single bond + Composite Filtek Z250)	16.65 ± 2.50	0.994	0.001	0.002

*: Pairwise comparisons using Tamhane's T2 post-hoc test

composites, for the Filtek Z250 composite the Single Bond, self etch bonding was used and in one of the investigated groups also the same bonding with the use of acid etch was adopted [22].

The present study results also showed that there was a significant statistical difference between the first and second groups in a manner that in the G_2 in which acid etch was used before silorane bonding system, the microtensile bond strength was higher in comparison to the G_1 in which only the silorane bonding system was used [23].

This fact can be explained in regard to the silorane bonding system to the teeth which has a two-bottle self-etch. The first stage was the use of a hydrophilic primer. Contrary to the primer systems of the two-step self-etch which are polymerized after bonding enforcement, in this primer the polymerization occurs in the first stage itself and prior to the bonding application; therefore, the bonding to enamel and dentin and formation of the hybrid layer take place in the first stage of the primer application similar to the one-step self etch systems [24-27].

pH of the silorane primer is 2.7 till stability of the existing monomers in the primers and their half-life increases. This high pH of the primer classified silorane primer in the very weak (ultra-mild) group and silorane bonding contain two polar molecules attach from its hydrophilic front with hydrophilic primer and from its hydrophobia front to the silorane hydrophobia composite [28].

In the studies conducted by Mine et al. [29] on silorane bonding system, it was shown that the hybrid layer had a maximum of few hundred nanometers' thickness that could be due to the high pH of the primer. In the grinded dentin with a very low agile, the hybrid layer thickness is in the extent of a few hundred nanometers.

Similarly, the resin tags are not seen due to the high pH of the primer; the smear plug is not removed from the inside of the dentin tubules. Therefore, in case the primer is implemented on a thicker layer from the smear layer which is produced via a quick diamond abrasive, the bond is created only in the superficial layer. So, the efficiency of the silorane bond is essentially in the first stage of the implementation of the primer and depends on the characteristics of the left smear layer.

Similarly, the composite Filtek Z250 with etch usage prior to the self etch bonding system showed better results because in the self etch systems with the use of the calcium and phosphoric ions primer that are

separated from the apatite, the hydroxyl crystals will remain suspended in the alcohol and or the water that exists as a solvent in the primer. When this solution is evaporated with the use of the air aspiration, this calcium and phosphate content could reduce the execution solvency of the primer and lead to their sedimentation in the primer. This causes a decrease in the permeation ability of the bonding material to the surface prepared with a primer and eventually the bonding strength decreases [28].

The use of 'acid etch' prior to the primer implementation with elimination of a part of the calcium and phosphate ions prevents this from happening. Even though it is mentioned in some studies, that the strength of the bond systems, self etch and total etch does not have a statistically significant difference with each other, but the present study findings are not in the same line with this point [29].

Even the significant difference for the second and third groups can be related to the difference of the bond characteristics and the weaker bond of the self etch composite Filtek Z250 bond system in comparison to the silorane bond system after the acid etch usage. This can also be used to justify the structural difference of the two composites and a lower polymerization contraction of the silorane composite Filtek P90 in comparison to the methacrylate composite Filtek Z250 [30-31].

The recorded silorane polymerization shrinkage rate in the experimental studies [32-34] is lower than the entire methacrylate composites. Therefore, a lower force is imposed due to the contraction of the material during the strengthening on the interface of the material and dentin and this can be the reason for a closer contact of silorane with the surface and a better bond establishment [32-34].

Moreover, the other case that can have an effect on the bond strength to a dentin is the characteristics of dentin itself that is influenced by the age, tooth kind, decay rate, restorative or reaction dentin production and intermediate environment. For elimination of these variables in this study, the intact primary canines lacking decay in which less than 1/3 of their root length was eroded and had an equal intermediate level (serum) in the environment were used [35].

Conclusions

Considering the conducted study, the silorane resin composite (Filtek P90) had a higher micro-tensile bond strength to the primary dentin compared with the methacrylate composite Filtek Z250, and etching the dentin surface prior to applying the primer and silorane bonding system leads to a better outcome.

Acknowledgements

The authors thank the Vice-Chancellory of Rafsanjan University of Medical Sciences for supporting this research.

Conflict of Interest: None declared.

References

1. Mcdonald R, Avery D, Stookey G, *et al*. Dental caries in the child and adolescent. In: Mcdonald R, Avery D, Dean J. Dentistry for child and adolescent. 9th Edition. ST.Louis: Mosby M: 2011;177-204.

2. Moore K. Dental materials. In: Mcdonald R, Avery D, Dean J. Dentistry for child and adolescent. 9th Edition. ST. Louis: Mosby M: 2011;296-312.

3. Donly K, Segura A. Dental materials. In: Pinkham J, Casamassimo P, McTigue D, Fields H, Nowak A. Pediatric dentistry infancy through adolescence. 5th Edition. St. Louis: Elsevier Saunders WB: 2013;325-340.

4. Dewaele M, Truffier-Boutry D, Devaux J, *et al*. Volume contraction in photocured dental resins: the shrinkage-conversion relationship revisited. Dent Mater. 2006;22: 359-365.

5. Charton C, Colon P, Pla F. Shrinkage stress in light-cured composite resins: influence of material and photo-activation mode. Dent Mater. 2007;23:911-920.

6. Cadenaro M, Biasotto M, Scuor N, *et al*. Assessment of polymerization contraction stress of three composite resins. Dent Mater. 2008;24:681-685.

7. Ilie N, Kunzelmann KH, Hickel R. Evaluation of micro-tensile bond strengths of composite materials in comparison to their polymerization shrinkage. Dent Mater. 2006;22:593-601.

8. Palin W, Fleming G, Burke F, *et al*. The influence of short and medium-term water immersion on the hydrolytic stability of novel low-shrink dental composites. Dent Mater. 2005;21:852-863.

9. Ilie N, Hickel R. Macro-, micro- and nanomechanical investigations on silorane and methacrylate-based composites. Dent Mater.

2009;25:810-819.

10. Van Ende A, Munck J, Mine A, *et al*. Does a low-shrinkage composite induce less stress at the adhesive interface? Dent Mater. 2009;25:825-833.

11. Nozaka K, Suruga Y, Amari E. Micro-leakage of composite resins in cavities upper primary molars. Int J Paediatr Dent. 1999;9:185-194.

12. Al-Boni R, Raja OM. Microleakage evaluation of silorane based composite versus methacrylate based composite. J Conserv Dent. 2010;13:152-155.

13. John R, Christense W, Henry W, *et al*. Space maintenance in the primary dentition. In: Pinkham J, Casamassimo P, Mctigue D, Fields H, Nowak A. Pediatric Dentistry Infancy Through Adolescence. 5th Edition. St. Louis: Elsevier Saunders: 2013. p. 379-384.

14. Stangel I, Nathanson D, Hsu CS. Shear strength of the composite bond to the etched porcelain. J Dent Res. 1987;66:1460-1465.

15. Sano H, Shono T, Sonoda H, *et al*. Relationship between surface area for adhesion and tensile bond strength evalution of micro tensile bond strength of micro tensile bond test. Dent Mater. 1994;10:236-240.

16. Santos M, Podorieszach A, Rizkalla AS, *et al*. Microleakage and microtensile bond strength of silorane-based and dimethacrylate-based restorative systems. Compend Contin Educ Dent. 2013;34:19-24.

17. Kranjangta N, Sirsawasdi S. Micro tensile bond strength of silorane-based resin composite and corresponding adhesive in class I occlusal restoration. Am J Dent. 2011;24:346-353.

18. Cabrera E, Macorra JC. Micro tensile bond strenght distributions of three composite material with different polymerization shirinkages to dentin. Adhes Dent. 2010;13:39-48.

19. Giacobbi MF, Vandewalle KS. Microtensile bond strength of a new silorane-based composite resin adhesive. Gen Dent. 2012;60:148-152.

20. 20. Poureslami HR, Sajadi F, Sharifi M, *et al*. Marginal micro leakage of low shirinkage composite silorane in primary teeth. J Dent Res Dent Clin Dent Prospect. 2012;6:94-97.

21. Soldo M, Simeon M, Matijevic J, *et al*. Marginal leakage of class V cavities restored with silorane-based and methacrylate-based resin systems. Den Mater. 2013;32:853–885.

22. Snomez SI, Akbay oba A, Almzm M. Micro

tensile bond strength of different adhesive system to dent. KutipFak Derg. 2012;14:191-199.

23. Badr S, Atef-Ibrahim M, El-Seoud H. Silorane-based composite bond to primary and permanent teeth. Dent Mater. 2007;23:911-920.

24. Almeida e Silva JS, Rolla JN, Baratieri LN, *et al*. The influence of different placement techniques on the microtensile bond strength of low-shrink silorane composite bonded to Class I cavities. Gen Dent. 2011;59:233-237.

25. Pereira JDS, Dias CTS. Bond strength between silorane-based composite resin and dentin substrate. Am J Dent. 2013;4:90-94.

26. Fruits TJ, Duncanson MG Jr, Miller RC. Bond strength of fluride releasing restorative materials. Am J Dent. 1996;9:219-222.

27. Daneshkazemi AR, Davari AR, Ataei E, *et al*. Effect of mechanical and thermal load cycling on micro tensile bond strength of clearfil SE bond to superficial dentin. Dent Res J. 2013;10;202-209.

28. Lien W, Vandewalle KS. Physical properties of a new silorane-based restorative system. Dent Mater. 2009;10:18-20.

29. Mine A, De Munck J, Van Ende A, *et al*. TEM characterization of a silorane composite bonded to enamel/dentin. Dent Mater. 2010;26:524-532.

30. Neelima L, Sathish ES, Kandaswamy D, *et al*. Evaluation of microtensile bond strength of total-etch, self-etch and glass ionomer adhesive to human dentin: An *invitro* study. Indian J Dent Res. 2008;19:129-133.

31. Koliniotou-Koumpia E, Kouros P, Dionysopoulos D, *et al*. Bonding strength of silorane based composite to Er-YAG laser prepared dentin. Lasers Med sci. 2013; 13:240-252.

32. Lowe RA. The search for a low-shrinkage direct composite. Inside Dent. 2010;1: 78-84.

33. Thalacker C, Heumann A, Weinmann W, *et al*. Marginal integrity of class V silorane and methacrylate composite restorations. J Dent Res. 2004;83:A1364.

34. Bagis YH, Baltacioglu IH, Kahyaogullari S. Comparing microleakage and the layering methods of silorane-based resin composite in wide Class II MOD cavities. Oper Dent. 2009;34:578-585.

35. Ramos JC, Perdigao J. Bond strength and SEM morphology of dentin amalgam adhesives. Am J Dent. 1997;10:152-158.

Permissions

All chapters in this book were first published in JDB, by Shiraz University of Medical Sciences; hereby published with permission under the Creative Commons Attribution License or equivalent. Every chapter published in this book has been scrutinized by our experts. Their significance has been extensively debated. The topics covered herein carry significant findings which will fuel the growth of the discipline. They may even be implemented as practical applications or may be referred to as a beginning point for another development.

The contributors of this book come from diverse backgrounds, making this book a truly international effort. This book will bring forth new frontiers with its revolutionizing research information and detailed analysis of the nascent developments around the world.

We would like to thank all the contributing authors for lending their expertise to make the book truly unique. They have played a crucial role in the development of this book. Without their invaluable contributions this book wouldn't have been possible. They have made vital efforts to compile up to date information on the varied aspects of this subject to make this book a valuable addition to the collection of many professionals and students.

This book was conceptualized with the vision of imparting up-to-date information and advanced data in this field. To ensure the same, a matchless editorial board was set up. Every individual on the board went through rigorous rounds of assessment to prove their worth. After which they invested a large part of their time researching and compiling the most relevant data for our readers.

The editorial board has been involved in producing this book since its inception. They have spent rigorous hours researching and exploring the diverse topics which have resulted in the successful publishing of this book. They have passed on their knowledge of decades through this book. To expedite this challenging task, the publisher supported the team at every step. A small team of assistant editors was also appointed to further simplify the editing procedure and attain best results for the readers.

Apart from the editorial board, the designing team has also invested a significant amount of their time in understanding the subject and creating the most relevant covers. They scrutinized every image to scout for the most suitable representation of the subject and create an appropriate cover for the book.

The publishing team has been an ardent support to the editorial, designing and production team. Their endless efforts to recruit the best for this project, has resulted in the accomplishment of this book. They are a veteran in the field of academics and their pool of knowledge is as vast as their experience in printing. Their expertise and guidance has proved useful at every step. Their uncompromising quality standards have made this book an exceptional effort. Their encouragement from time to time has been an inspiration for everyone.

The publisher and the editorial board hope that this book will prove to be a valuable piece of knowledge for researchers, students, practitioners and scholars across the globe.

List of Contributors

Movahhedian N
Assistant Professor, Department of Oral and Maxillofacial Radiology, Faculty of Dentistry, Shiraz University of Medial Science, Shiraz, Iran

Shahidi Sh
Professor, Department of Oral and Maxillofacial Radiology, Biomaterials Research Center, School of Dentistry, Shiraz University of Medical Sciences, Shiraz, Iran

Jozari S
Student Research Committee, School of Dentistry, Shiraz University of Medical Sciences, Shiraz, Iran

Mosharaf A and Naderi A
Department of Oral and Maxillofacial Surgery, school of dentistry, Shiraz University of Medical Sciences, Shiraz, Iran

Abedi H, Gholamrezaee Saravi M and Zarenejad N
Department of Restorative Dentistry, Faculty of Dentistry, Mazandaran University of Medical Sciences, Sari, Iran

Poureslami HR
Oral and Dental Diseases Research Center AND Kerman Social Determinants on Oral Health Research Center and Department of Pediatric Dentistry, School of Dentistry, Kerman University of Medical Sciences, Kerman, Iran

Hoseinifar Ra
Department of Operative Dentistry, School of Dentistry, Kerman University of Medical Science, Kerman, Iran

Hoseinifar Re
Department of Pediatric Dentistry, School of Dentistry, Kerman University of Medical Sciences, Kerman, Iran

Sharifi H
Regional Knowledge Hub, and WHO Collaborating Centre for HIV Surveillance, Kerman University of Medical Sciences, Kerman, Iran

Poureslami P
School of Dentistry, Mashhad University of Medical Sciences, Mashhad, Iran

Sharafeddin F
Department of Operative Dentistry and Biomaterial Research Center, School of Dentistry, Shiraz University of Medical Sciences, Shiraz, Iran

Farshad F
Student Research Committee and Department of Operative Dentistry, School of Dentistry, Shiraz University of Medical Sciences, Shiraz, Iran
Department of Operative Dentistry, School of Dentistry, Shahid Sadoughi University of Medical Sciences, Yazd, Iran

Azarian B
Tohid high school, Shiraz, Iran

Afshari A
Student Research Committee, School of Dentistry, Shiraz University of Medical Sciences, Shiraz, Iran

Karandish M
Health Policy Research Center, Shiraz University of Medical Sciences, Shiraz, Iran
Department of Orthodontics, Dental School, Shiraz University of Medical Sciences, Shiraz, Iran

Aalaei Sh
Dental Caries Prevention Research Center, Qazvin University of Medical Sciences, Qazvin, Iran

Nematollahi F
Department of Prosthodontics, Islamic Azad University, Dental Branch, Tehran, Iran

Vartanian M
General dentist, Qazvin, Iran

Beyabanaki E
Department of Prosthodontics, Faculty of Dentistry, Shahid Beheshti University of Medical Sciences, Tehran, Iran

Amiri M and Daneshkazemi A
Department of Operative Dentistry, Shahid Sadoughi University of Medical Sciences and Health Services, Yazd, Iran

Etemadifar Z
Department of Biology, University of Isfahan, Isfahan, Iran

Nateghi M
School of Dentistry, Shahid Sadoughi University of Medical Sciences and Health Services, Yazd, Iran

Daneshkazemi AR
Social Determinants on Oral Health Research Center and Department of Operative Dentistry, School of Dentistry, Shahid Sadoughi University of Medical Sciences, Yazd, Iran

Hajiahmadi Z
Yazd Dental School, Shahid Sadoughi University of Medical Sciences, Yazd, Iran

Moshkelgosha V
Orthodontic Research Center, Department of Orthodontics, School of Dentistry, Shiraz University of Medical Sciences, Shiraz, Iran

Mehrvarz Sh
Student Research Committee, School of Dentistry, Shiraz University of Medical Sciences, Shiraz, Iran

Saki M
Student Research Committee, Orthodontic Research Center and Department of Orthodontics, School of Dentistry, Shiraz University of Medical Sciences, Shiraz, Iran

Golkari A
Department of Dental Public Health , School of Dentistry, Shiraz University of Medical Sciences, Shiraz, Iran

Khaghani M and Alizadeh S
Young Researchers and Elite Club, Najafabad Branch, Islamic Azad University, Najafabad, Iran

Doostmohammadi A
Materials Department, Engineering faculty, Shahrekord University, Shahrekord, Iran

Salahi S and Moosaali F
Oral and Dental Diseases Research Center AND Kerman Social Determinants on Oral Health Research Center and Department of Periodontics, School of Dentistry, Kerman University of Medical Sciences, Kerman, Iran

Ghanbari M
General practitioner, Faculty of Dentistry, Kerman University of Medical Sciences, Kerman, Iran

Abrisham SM and Fallah Tafti A
Department of Prosthodontics, Yazd University of Medical Sciences, Yazd, Iran

Kheirkhah S
School of Dentistry, Shahid Sadoughi University of Medical Sciences, Yazd, Iran

Tavakkoli MA
Department of Orthodontics, School of Dentistry, Shiraz University of Medical Sciences, Shiraz, Iran

Nouzari A, Zohrei A and Mohammadi N
Department of Paediatrics, School of Dentistry, Shiraz University of Medical Sciences, Shiraz, Iran

Ferooz M
Melbourne Dental School, The University of Melbourne, Victoria, Australia

Sadeghi M and Deljoo Z
Undergraduate Student, Shiraz Dental School, Shiraz University of Medical Sciences, Shiraz, Iran

Bagheri R
Dental Materials Department and Biomaterials Research Centre, Shiraz Dental School, Shiraz University of Medical Sciences, Shiraz, Iran

Hajimaghsoodi S
Department of Oral Medicine, Shahid Sadoughi University of Medical Sciences, Yazd, Iran

Zandi H
Department of Microbiology, Shahid Sadoughi University of Medical Sciences, Yazd, Iran

Bahrami M
Shahid Sadoughi University of Medical Sciences, Yazd, Iran

Hakimian R
Department of Endodontics, School of Dentistry, Shahid Sadoughi University of Medical Sciences, Yazd, Iran

Farmani S and Sookhakiyan M
Student Research Committee, Shiraz Dental School, Shiraz University of Medical Sciences, Shiraz, Iran

Orandi S
Postgraduate Student , Department of Prosthodontics, School of Dentistry, Shiraz University of Medical Sciences, Shiraz, Iran

Mese A
Department of Prosthodontics, School of Dentistry, Dicle University, Diyarbakir, Turkey

Jafari AA
Department of Medical Parasitology and Mycology, School of Medicine, Shahid Sadoughi University of Yazd Medical Sciences, Yazd, Iran

Lotfi-Kamran MH
Department of Prosthodontics, School of Dentistry, Shahid Sadoughi University of Yazd Medical Sciences, Yazd, Iran

Ghafoorzadeh M
Paramedical School, Shahid Sadoughi University of Yazd Medical Sciences, Yazd, Iran

Shaddel SM
Department of Prosthodontics, ShahidSadoughi University of Yazd Medical Sciences, Yazd, Iran

Moosavi H and Moghaddas MJ
Associate Professor, Dental Materials Research Center, Department of Operative Dentistry, Mashhad Dental School, Mashhad University of Medical Sciences, Mashhad, Iran

Ghapanchi J
Associate Professor, Oral and Maxillofacial Medicine Department, School of Dentistry, Shiraz University of Medical Sciences, Shiraz, Iran

Kordnoshahri F
General Dentist, Mashhad Dental School, Mashhad University of Medical Sciences, Mashhad, Iran

Zanjani M
Department of Operative Dentistry, Mashhad Dental School, Mashhad University of Medical Sciences, Mashhad, Iran

Abdulrazzaq Naji S
Foundation of Technical Education, College of Health and Medical Technology, Baghdad, Iraq and Department of Dental Biomaterials, School of Dentistry, International Campus, Tehran University of Medical Sciences, Tehran, Iran

Jafarzadeh Kashi T
Associate professor, Iranian Tissue Bank and Research Center, Department of Dental Biomaterials, School of Dentistry, Tehran University of Medical Sciences, Tehran, Iran

Behroozibakhsh M
Assistant professor, Research Center for Science and Technology in Medicine, Department of Dental Biomaterials, School of Dentistry, Tehran University of Medical Sciences, Tehran, Iran

Hajizamani H
Research Center for Science and Technology in Medicine, Department of Dental Biomaterials, School of Dentistry, Tehran University of Medical Sciences, Tehran, Iran

Habibzadeh S
Assistant Professor, Department of Prosthodontics, Tehran University of Medical Sciences, International Campus, School of Dentistry, Tehran, Iran

Shafiei F
Assistant professor, Department of Dental Biomaterials, School of Dentistry, Tehran University of Medical Sciences, Tehran, Iran

Ashnagar A
Pharm-D, School of Pharmacy, Shahid Beheshti University of Medical Sciences, Tehran, Iran

Ghavami-Lahiji M
Research Center for Science and Technology in Medicine, Department of Dental Biomaterials, School of Dentistry, Tehran University of Medical Sciences, Tehran, Iran

Najafi F
Assistant professor, Department of Resin and Additives, Institute for Color Science and Technology, Tehran, Iran

Amin Marashi SM
Assistant professor, Department of Microbiology and Immunology, Alborz University of Medical Sciences, Karaj, Iran

Ghapanchi J
Associated Professor, Department of Oral and Maxillofacial Medicine, School of Dentistry, Shiraz University of Medical Sciences, Shiraz, Iran

Zangoei Boushehri M
Oral and Maxillofacial Radiologist, Shiraz, Iran

Haghnegahdar AA
Assistant Professor, Department of Oral and Maxillofacial Radiology, School of Dentistry, Shiraz University of Medical Sciences, Shiraz, Iran

Nayyrain SH
Under graduate Student, Shiraz University of Medical Sciences, International Branch, Shiraz, Iran

Shakibasefat H
Postgrduate student, Department of oral and maxillofacial medicine, School of Dentistry, Shiraz University of Medical Sciences, Iran

Paknahad M
Assistant Professor, Oral and Dental Disease Research Center, Department of Oral and Maxillofacial Radiology, School of Dentistry, Shiraz University of Medical Sciences, Shiraz, Iran

Tavangar MS
Department of Dental Materials, School of Dentistry, Shiraz University of Medical Sciences, Shiraz, Iran

Jafarpur D
Student Research Committee, School of Dentistry, Shiraz University of Medical Sciences, Shiraz, Iran

Bagheri R
Department of Dental Materials and Biomaterials Research Center, School of Dentistry, Shiraz University of Medical Sciences, Shiraz, Iran

Sharafeddin F
Professor, Department of Operative Dentistry, Biomaterials Research Center, School of Dentistry, Shiraz University of Medical Sciences, Shiraz, Iran

Azar MR
Associate Professor, Department of Endodontics, School of Dentistry, Shiraz University of Medical Sciences, Shiraz, Iran

Feizi N
Postgraduate Student, Department of Operative Dentistry, School of Dentistry, Shiraz University of Medical Sciences, Shiraz, Iran

Salehi R
Assistant Professor, Department of Operative Dentistry, School of Dentistry, Kashan University of Medical Sciences, Kashan, Iran

Motamedifar M
Department of Bacteriology, Shiraz Medical School & Shiraz HIV/AIDS Research Center, Institute of Health, Shiraz University of Medical Sciences, Shiraz, Iran

Nozari A
Department of Pediatric Dentistry, School of Dentistry, Shiraz University of Medical Sciences, Shiraz, Iran

Azhdari Ghasrodashti E
Student Research Committee, School of Dentistry, Shiraz University of Medical Sciences, Shiraz, Iran

Lavaee F
Assistant Professor, Oral and Dental Disease Research Center, School of Dentistry, Shiraz University of Medical Sciences, Shiraz, Iran

Motamedifar M
Professor, HIV/AIDS Research Center, Institute of Health, Shiraz University of Medical Sciences, Shiraz, Iran & Department of Bacteriology and Virology, School of Medicine, Shiraz University of Medical Sciences, Shiraz, Iran

Sorourian S
Student Research Committee, School of Dentistry, Shiraz University of Medical Sciences, Shiraz, Iran

Alaghemand H
Department of Restorative Dentistry, Head of the Dental Materials Research Center, Faculty of Dentistry, Babol University of Medical Sciences, Babol, Iran

Ramezani M
Department of Endodontics, Faculty of Dentistry, Mazandaran University of Medical Sciences, Sari, Iran

Sabokseir A
Oral and Dental Disease Research Center and Department of Dental Public Health, School of Dentistry, Shiraz University of Medical Sciences, Shiraz, Iran

Golkari A
Oral and Dental Disease Research Center and Department of Dental Public Health, School of Dentistry, Shiraz University of Medical Sciences, Shiraz, Iran Research Department of Epidemiology and Public Health, University College London, London, UK

Sheiham A and Watt RG
Research Department of Epidemiology and Public Health, University College London, London, UK

Blane D
Department of Social Science and Medicine, Imperial College London, London, UK

Sharifi M
Department of Paediatric Dentistry, School of Dentistry, Rafsanjan University of Medical Sciences, Rafsanjan, Iran

Khoramian Tusi S
Department of Paediatric Dentistry, School of Dentistry, Alborz University of Medical Sciences, Karaj, Iran

Index

S

Salmonella Typhimurium, 94

Scanning Electron Microscope, 135-136, 138, 172, 180

Scotch Bond, 144, 146-147

Sensikin Gel, 97, 100-102

Shear Bond Strength, 24, 54-55, 57-59, 150-168, 170-174

Sodium Fluoride Gel, 97

Sof-lex Disc, 135-137

Spearmint Extract, 92-95

Staining Solutions, 135, 139-140

Streptococcus Mutans, 9-10, 12-14, 17-18, 43, 52-53, 56-58, 129-133, 179-180

T

Tetric N Ceram Bulk Fill, 121, 123, 125

Thermocycled, 70, 144, 171

Titanium Dioxide, 52-55, 57, 60, 67

Tooth Bleaching, 150-151

V

Veneering Techniques, 160

Visual Analogue Scale, 98-99

Z

Zirconia Restorations, 164, 168

Zirconium-oxide, 164

www.ingramcontent.com/pod-product-compliance
Lightning Source LLC
Chambersburg PA
CBHW050436200326
41458CB00014B/4967